Advances in Laminitis, Part II

Guest Editor

CHRISTOPHER C. POLLITT, BVSc, PhD

VETERINARY CLINICS OF NORTH AMERICA: EQUINE PRACTICE

www.vetequine.theclinics.com

Consulting Editor
A. SIMON TURNER, BVSc, MS

August 2010 • Volume 26 • Number 2

SAUNDERS an imprint of ELSEVIER, Inc.

W.B. SAUNDERS COMPANY
A Division of Elsevier Inc.

1600 John F. Kennedy Boulevard • Suite 1800 • Philadelphia, Pennsylvania 19103

http://www.vetequine.theclinics.com

VETERINARY CLINICS OF NORTH AMERICA: EQUINE PRACTICE Volume 26, Number 2
August 2010 ISSN 0749-0739, ISBN-13: 978-1-4377-2501-8

Editor: John Vassallo; j.vassallo@elsevier.com

Veterinary Clinics of North America: Equine Practice (ISSN 0749-0739) is published in April, August, and December by Elsevier Inc., 360 Park Avenue South, New York, NY 10010-1710. Business and Editorial Offices: 1600 John F. Kennedy Blvd., Suite 1800, Philadelphia, PA 19103-2899. Subscription prices are $222.00 per year (domestic individuals), $339.00 per year (domestic institutions), $111.00 per year (domestic students/residents), $259.00 per year (Canadian individuals), $424.00 per year (Canadian institutions), $299.00 per year (international individuals), $424.00 per year (international institutions), and $151.00 per year (international and Canadian students/residents). To receive student/resident rate, orders must be accompanied by name of affiliated institution, date of term, and the signature of program/residency coordinator on institution letterhead. Orders will be billed at individual rate until proof of status is received. Foreign air speed delivery is included in all *Clinics* subscription prices. All prices are subject to change without notice. **POSTMASTER:** Send address changes to *Veterinary Clinics of North America: Equine Practice*, 3251 Riverport Lane, Maryland Heights, MO 63043. Customer Service (orders, claims, online, change of address): Elsevier Health Sciences Division, Subscription Customer Service, 3251 Riverport Lane, Maryland Heights, MO 63043. Tel: 1-800-654-2452 (U.S. and Canada); 314-447-8871 (outside U.S. and Canada). Fax: 314-447-8029. E-mail: journalscustomerservice-usa@elsevier.com (for print support); E-mail: journalsonlinesupport-usa@elsevier (for online support).

Reprints. For copies of 100 or more of articles in this publication, please contact the Commercial Reprints Department, Elsevier Inc., 360 Park Avenue South, New York, NY 10010-1710. Tel.: 212-633-3812; Fax: 212-462-1935; E-mail: reprints@elsevier.com.

Veterinary Clinics of North America: Equine Practice is covered in *MEDLINE/PubMed (Index Medicus)*, *Excerpta Medica, Current Contents/Agriculture, Biology and Environmental Sciences*, and *ISI*.

Printed and bound in the United Kingdom
Transferred to Digital Print 2011

Contributors

CONSULTING EDITOR

A. SIMON TURNER, BVSc, MS

Diplomate, American College of Veterinary Surgeons; Professor, Department of Clinical Sciences, College of Veterinary Medicine and Biomedical Sciences, Colorado State University, Fort Collins, Colorado

GUEST EDITOR

CHRISTOPHER C. POLLITT, BVSc, PhD

Professor, Australian Equine Laminitis Research Unit, School of Veterinary Science, The University of Queensland, Gatton, Queensland, Australia; The Laminitis Institute, University of Pennsylvania School of Veterinary Medicine, New Bolton Center, Kennett Square, Pennsylvania

AUTHORS

SIMON R. BAILEY, PhD, MRCVS

Senior Lecturer, School of Veterinary Science, University of Melbourne, Parkville, Victoria, Australia

SÉBASTIEN H. BAUQUIER, DMV

Lecturer in Anesthesia, Section of Critical Care, Department of Clinical Studies-Philadelphia, School of Veterinary Medicine, University of Pennsylvania, Philadelphia, Pennsylvania

DANIELE BERNARDINI, DVM, PhD

Professor of Internal Medicine, Department of Veterinary Clinical Sciences, University of Padua, Agripolis, Legnaro (Padova), Italy

SIMON N. COLLINS, PhD

School of Veterinary Science, The University of Queensland, Gatton, Queensland, Australia; Orthopaedic Research Group, Centre for Equine Studies, Animal Health Trust, Kentford, Newmarket, Suffolk, United Kingdom

LORENZO D'ARPE, DVM, PhD

Department of Veterinary Clinical Sciences, University of Padua, Agripolis, Legnaro (Padova), Italy

EMILY K. DEAN, DVM

C. B. Miller and Associates, North Salem, New York

MELODY A. DE LAAT, BVSc(Hons)

Australian Equine Laminitis Research Unit, School of Veterinary Science, The University of Queensland, Gatton, Queensland, Australia

BERND DRIESSEN, DVM, PhD
Diplomate, American College of Veterinary Anesthesiologists; Diplomate, European College of Veterinary Pharmacology and Toxicology; Professor of Anesthesiology, Section of Emergency/Critical Care and Anesthesia, Department of Clinical Studies-New Bolton Center, School of Veterinary Medicine, University of Pennsylvania, Kennett Square, Pennsylvania; Department of Anesthesiology, David Geffen School of Medicine, University of California Los Angeles, Los Angeles, California

ANDY DURHAM, BVSc, CertEP, DEIM, MRCVS
Diplomate, European College of Equine Internal Medicine; The Liphook Equine Hospital, Forest Mere, Liphook, Hampshire, United Kingdom

ROBERT A. EUSTACE, BVSc, CertEP, CertEO, FRCVS
The Laminitis Clinic, Mead House, Dauntsey, Chippenham, Wiltshire, United Kingdom

V.K. (SESHU) GANJAM, BVSc, MA (hc), PhD
Professor of Endocrinology, Department of Biomedical Science, College of Veterinary Medicine, University of Missouri, Columbia, Missouri

RAYMOND J. GEOR, BVSc, MVSc, PhD
Diplomate, American College of Veterinary Internal Medicine (Large Animal Internal Medicine); Professor and Chairperson, Department of Large Animal Clinical Sciences, Veterinary Medical Center, College of Veterinary Medicine, Michigan State University, Lansing, Michigan

PHILIP J. JOHNSON, BVSc(Hons), MS, MRCVS
Diplomate, American College of Veterinary Internal Medicine (Large Animal Internal Medicine); Diplomate, European College of Equine Internal Medicine; Professor of Equine Internal Medicine, Department of Veterinary Medicine and Surgery, College of Veterinary Medicine, University of Missouri, Columbia, Missouri

ALISON LACARRUBBA, DVM
Diplomate, American Board of Veterinary Practitioners; Clinical Instructor of Equine Clinical Practice, Department of Veterinary Medicine and Surgery, College of Veterinary Medicine, University of Missouri, Columbia, Missouri

CATHERINE M. MCGOWAN, BVSc, MACVSc, PhD, FHEA, MRCVS
Diplomate, European College of Equine Internal Medicine; Director of Equine Professional Studies, Faculty of Health and Life Sciences, School of Veterinary Science, University of Liverpool, Leahurst, United Kingdom

NICOLA J. MENZIES-GOW, MA, VetMB, PhD, CertEM(Int.med), MRCVS
Diplomate, European College of Equine Internal Medicine; Lecturer in Equine Medicine, Department of Veterinary Clinical Science, Royal Veterinary College, Hertfordshire, United Kingdom

NAT T. MESSER IV, DVM
Diplomate, American Board of Veterinary Practitioners; Professor of Equine Medicine, Department of Veterinary Medicine and Surgery, College of Veterinary Medicine, University of Missouri, Columbia, Missouri

SCOTT MORRISON, DVM
Rood & Riddle Equine Hospital, Lexington, Kentucky

STEPHEN E. O'GRADY, DVM, MRCVS
Veterinarian and Farrier, Northern Virginia Equine, Marshall, Virginia

JAMES A. ORSINI, DVM
Diplomate, American College of Veterinary Surgeons; University of Pennsylvania, School of Veterinary Medicine, Kennett Square, Pennsylvania

CHRISTOPHER C. POLLITT, BVSc, PhD
Professor, Australian Equine Laminitis Research Unit, School of Veterinary Science, The University of Queensland, Gatton, Queensland, Australia; The Laminitis Institute, University of Pennsylvania School of Veterinary Medicine, New Bolton Center, Kennett Square, Pennsylvania

PATRICK T. REILLY
Chief, Farrier Services, University of Pennsylvania, School of Veterinary Medicine, Kennett Square, Pennsylvania

MARTIN N. SILLENCE, PhD
Professor, Faculty of Science and Technology, Queensland University of Technology, Brisbane, Queensland, Australia

ANDREW VAN EPS, BVSc, PhD
Diplomate, American College of Veterinary Internal Medicine; School of Veterinary Science, The University of Queensland, Gatton, Queensland, Australia

DONALD M. WALSH, BS, DVM
Director of Clinical Research, Homestead Veterinary Hospital, Pacific, Missouri

KATHRYN WATTS, BS
Rocky Mountain Research & Consulting, Inc, Center, Colorado

CHARLES E. WIEDMEYER, DVM, PhD
Diplomate, American College of Veterinary Clinical Pathology; Assistant Professor of Veterinary Clinical Pathology, Department of Veterinary Pathobiology, College of Veterinary Medicine, University of Missouri, Columbia, Missouri

LAURA ZARUCCO, DMV, PhD
Assistant Professor in Large Animal Surgery, Dipartimento di Patologia Animale, Facoltà di Medicina Veterinaria, Università degli Studi di Torino, Via Leonardo da Vinci, Grugliasco, Turin, Italy

Contents

> In laminitis occurring in the field, as opposed to laminitis occurring during hospitalization or severe illness, endocrinopathic laminitis is the predominant form of laminitis. Prevalent causes of endocrinopathic laminitis are ECS and EMS. Exclusion of inflammatory or weight bearing causes of laminitis and focussing on the identification and treatment of underlying endocrine conditions will improve laminitis management strategies.

> Although much has been written about laminitis in the context of its association with inflammatory processes, recognition is growing that most cases of laminitis examined by veterinarians in private practice are those associated with pasture grazing, obesity, and insulin resistance (IR). The term endocrinopathic laminitis has been adopted to classify the instances of laminitis in which the origin seems to be more strongly associated with an underlying endocrinopathy, such as either IR or the influence of corticosteroids. Results of a recent study suggest that obesity and IR represent the most common metabolic and endocrinopathic predispositions for laminitis in horses. IR also plays an important role in the pathogenesis of laminitis that develops when some horses or ponies are allowed to graze pastures at certain times of the year. The term equine metabolic syndrome (EMS) has been proposed as a label for horses whose clinical examination results (including both physical examination and laboratory testing) suggest heightened risk for developing laminitis as a result of underlying IR.

> Laminitis occurring in association with hyperinsulinemia is frequently encountered in today's equine population. New evidence suggests that hyperinsulinemia is the direct cause of this form of laminitis, rather than insulin resistance per se. The mechanism by which elevated serum insulin concentrations result in lamellar dysfunction is currently under investigation by many researchers and the use of a new insulin infusion model for investigating the pathogenesis of insulin-associated laminitis will doubtless enhance progress in this field of research. By focusing on the metabolic and vascular actions of insulin in the lamellar microenvironment, our research group is trying to gain an insight into the pathophysiological

processes involved in this complex problem, in order to better understand the disease.

Epidemiologic studies indicate that most laminitis cases occur in horses and ponies kept at pasture, hence the term pasture-associated laminitis. Clinical cases of laminitis most often occur under conditions that favor accumulation of rapidly fermentable nonstructural carbohydrates (fructans, simple sugars, or starches) in pasture, and animals with an equine metabolic syndrome (EMS) phenotype (insulin resistance, abnormal insulin dynamics, +/– obesity) seem to be at highest risk for developing the condition. Although the mechanisms linking consumption of pasture forage with development of lamellar failure have not been fully elucidated, a systemic inflammatory response that accompanies hindgut carbohydrate overload likely initiates lamellar inflammatory events (including infiltration and activation of leukocytes) that contribute to destruction of lamellar epithelium and extracellular matrix. This article reviews current knowledge on the epidemiology and risk factors for pasture-associated laminitis, including the role of forage carbohydrates and metabolic/endocrine predispositions, and also discusses the pathophysiology of this condition.

A direct causal association between corticosteroid use and laminitis has yet to be proven scientifically, and there have been few studies specifically addressing this aspect. New evidence, however, is improving the understanding of the causes of laminitis, particularly related to endocrine factors. The focus of this article is discussing the circumstances under which steroids might cause this condition.

Supporting limb laminitis poses a threat to all horses suffering from severe unilateral lameness. Despite its devastating effects, relatively little is known about the precise pathologic processes that lead to its development. This article reviews the potential mechanisms of supporting limb laminitis, and the authors present some preliminary data based on advanced imaging and computer-based modeling techniques aimed at further elucidating the etiology of this unique form of laminitis. Gaining a better understanding of the pathologic processes that lead to supporting limb laminitis is essential to enable the development of appropriate countermeasures to safeguard horses at risk of the disease.

Although the treatment and management of laminitis in the horse requires a holistic and often multidisciplinary approach from the veterinarian, farrier, and nutritionist, this review focuses on pharmacologic interventions that might have prophylactic benefit, specifically in the horse with laminitis as a result of pituitary pars intermedia dysfunction and equine metabolic syndrome.

Managing pain in horses afflicted by chronic laminitis is one of the greatest challenges in equine clinical practice because it is the dreadful suffering of the animals that most often forces the veterinarian to end the battle with this disease. The purpose of this review is to summarize our current understanding of the complex mechanisms involved in generating and amplifying pain in animals with laminitis and, based on this information, to propose a modified approach to pain therapy. Furthermore, a recently developed pain scoring technique is presented that may help better quantify pain and the monitoring of responses to analgesic treatment in horses with laminitis.

Clinical diagnostic venography allows in vivo visualization of the digital venous system and the effects of venocompression related to foot load and laminitis pathology. Venography has predictive potential and helps the clinician anticipate and treat laminitis tissue damage before it is detectable by plain radiography. The authors describe the podiatry radiographic technique to correctly perform digital venography and the modifications they have developed. The authors provide guidelines for the interpretation of laminitis venograms in the context of laminitis chronology. Frequent venographic monitoring of laminitis helps clinicians understand the sometimes puzzling chronology of the disease process and improves therapeutic outcome.

The sugar, starch, and fructan content (collectively referred to as nonstructural carbohydrates [NSC]) of pasture plants is dependent on the environmental conditions under which they have grown. Pasture that is stressed by cold, drought, or lack of nutrients can be 2 to 3 times higher in NSC than pasture that grows quickly in warm weather and is adequately watered and fertilized. Horses at risk for laminitis should have access to pasture limited or be removed completely when environmental conditions are conducive to high levels of NSC accumulation.

Certain individual animals appear predisposed to recurrent pasture-associated laminitis, but the exact mechanisms underlying their predisposition remain a fundamental question in laminitis research. The risk of endocrinopathic laminitis can be reduced if steps are taken to improve insulin sensitivity and reduce inflammation using strategies based on exercise and diet. Exercise has been shown to reduce insulin resistance and suppress inflammation, and dietary manipulation can significantly affect insulin sensitivity.

rehabilitated back to athletic soundness, light use, breeding, or pasture soundness, whereas others suffer from permanent instability and never enjoy an acceptable level of comfort. To understand how to minimize damage in the acute laminitic foot or rehabilitate the chronic laminitic foot, the veterinarian should have an understanding of the normal supporting structures of the digit, the biomechanical forces acting on the foot, and the structural failure that results when these otherwise normal forces act on a diseased, damaged foot.

Maggot debridement therapy is a nontraumatic, minimally invasive method to treat infections in a foot compromised by chronic laminitis. A mechanical strategy must first be in place to address the instability of the distal phalanx and hoof capsule. Adverse reactions to maggot debridement therapy are uncommon and the only side effect observed has been irritation or hypersensitivity at the site. Chronic laminitic cases of sepsis/necrosis within the hoof benefit from this procedure due to the noninvasive, continuous debridement and healing properties provided by the larvae.

The goals of mechanical treatment during the acute phase of laminitis are to preserve the lamellar interface by reducing the forces that are compromising its integrity and to make the horse more comfortable. Early decision making is important in managing acute laminitis. This article helps the practitioner to identify some of the commonly used and accepted methods of protecting the laminitic foot. The materials available and the theories behind their use are also described. The laminitic foot needs to be understood before determining methods for its support. Most treatment options involve shifting the weight-bearing forces from compromised areas of the foot (ie, the lamellar interface) to areas more capable of supporting the patient's weight, remembering that the sum of the forces should remain the same. The many treatment options available allow for flexibility and effective management and permit each modality to be combined in infinite ways for hoof support. The goal of therapy is to support the foot and stop the progression of the disease to the chronic phase.

FORTHCOMING ISSUES

RECENT ISSUES

THE CLINICS ARE NOW AVAILABLE ONLINE!

Access your subscription at:
www.theclinics.com

Preface

Advances in Laminitis, Part II

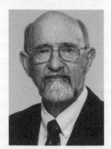

Christopher C. Pollitt, BVSc, PhD
Guest Editor

If knowledge can create problems, it is not through ignorance that we can solve them.

—Isaac Asimov (1920–1992)

The current importance of laminitis is reflected in the decision by the editors to dedicate not just one, but two editions to the topic of laminitis. The first edition dealt mainly with laminitis associated with septic/inflammatory conditions (*Veterinary Clinics of North America: Equine Practice. Advances in Laminitis, Part 1. Volume 26, Number 1, April 2010*) and this second edition concentrates on metabolic and endocrinopathic laminitis. Both have articles on treatment/preventive strategies and how to cope with chronic laminitis, the aftermath of the acute stage.

Over 10 years have passed since Dr. David Hood guest edited the landmark edition in the *Veterinary Clinics of North America: Equine Practice* series entitled Laminitis. Readers consulting the 1999 issue will find much that is current and not covered in either parts of the 2010 volume. However, in the 1999 volume, the word insulin was hardly mentioned and the term "equine metabolic syndrome" had yet to be coined.[1] Obesity was thought to influence laminitis outcome because of the weight factor, and the focus of endocrinology was corticosteroids and thyroid hormone. The systemic components of laminitis were consequential to laminitis, and pathology of the endocrine system was not perceived as a direct laminitis risk factor. Thus, in the intervening 10 years, there has been a veritable explosion of research into endocrinopathic laminitis, reflected in Part II by 9 of the 17 articles dedicated to this topic.

Laminitis associated with equine Cushing's syndrome, iatrogenic corticosteroid administration, pasture consumption, and equine metabolic syndrome are reviewed by various authors (McGowan, Johnson et al, Geor, Bailey, Durham, Menzies-Gow, and Walsh). Common to all these conditions is insulin resistance and hyperinsulinemia. Horses and ponies that have lost insulin sensitivity and have high serum insulin concentrations are more likely to develop laminitis and be euthanized soon thereafter. Insulin resistance and hyperinsulinemia, as genuine risk factors for laminitis, unify the pathophysiology of equine

Vet Clin Equine 26 (2010) xiii–xv
doi:10.1016/j.cveq.2010.06.008

Cushing's syndrome, iatrogenic corticosteroid administration, pasture-associated laminitis, and equine metabolic syndrome. Studies involving prolonged intravenous infusion of supraphysiologic insulin into first ponies[2] and then horses[3] provide experimental evidence in support of the laminitogenic potential of insulin and is reviewed here by de Laat et al. An article on pasture management and another on diet and exercise further acknowledge the link between glucose metabolism, insulin, and laminitis.

In Advances in Laminitis, Part I, the information generated by computed tomographic scanning was manipulated into a virtual 3-dimensional model to illustrate the lamellar wedge of chronic laminitis. In Part II, Mimics software is used again, this time in conjunction with an intravascular contrast agent, to illustrate the effect of weight-bearing on the arterial circulation of the foot. Supporting limb laminitis (SLL) has long been the bane of orthopedic surgeons performing complex restorative operations on fractures in the opposite limb in horses. The article by van Eps et al reviews what little information there is on SLL and posits that a highly evolved mechanism, normally of benefit in circulating blood through the horse's foot during locomotion, traps the horse in a unique pathologic process that results in SLL.

The pain of chronic laminitis often becomes refractory to conventional treatment regimens. A new concept for laminitis science is the article by Driessen, which suggests this may be due to neuropathic pain (ie, pain due to a lesion or dysfunction of the sensory transmission pathways in both the peripheral and the central nervous systems). Understanding that laminitis pain is being amplified and is the product of complex neuropathologic processes affecting both the peripheral and the central somatosensory nervous system should lead to rethinking of how analgesia is achieved for our equine patients. Many of the foot support techniques we employ are inherently painful and effective analgesia is needed to gain sufficient time to assess their effectiveness. Thus, effective multimodal combinations of agents, targeting different sites within the nociceptive system, coupled with effective monitoring, must now be embraced if we are to claim "best practice" for our equine patients. More than just "bute" (phenylbutazone) is required.

Progress in understanding laminitis has certainly been made. In 2007, laminitis was described as "idiopathic inflammation or ischemia of the submural structures of the foot."[4] In 2010, even the author of that statement agrees that, while idiopathic means of unknown cause, it is a bit of a stretch to use it in laminitis. No one ever refers to navicular disease/syndrome as idiopathic, but we know more about the pathogenesis of laminitis than navicular disease (Andrew Parks, personal communication, 2010).

The language surrounding laminitis will always be evolving and editors may not get to completely dictate the terminology used in their editions.[5] There are many ways to describe the pathologic anatomy of laminitis and some of the few "experts" in the field have developed personal nomenclatures and neologisms to describe what they see. There is little unity and considerable confusion. Most have resisted "the call for unified terminology" addressed by Parks and Mair in 2009,[5] and we still have "founder distance" instead of "vertical coronet extensor process distance." The former is jargon and in common use among the cognoscenti (including myself), but the latter, much longer term, has precise meaning and can be used for morphometric studies of normal equid feet. It would be curious to use "founder distance" to measure the vertical distance between coronet and extensor process in the feet of normal horses that have never been touched by laminitis. Admittedly, for the purposes of objective measurement, coronet needs a precise definition and that of Eustace[6], ie, "rim of palpable mature horn distal to the perioplic ring (coronary band)," is satisfactory.

There are many examples of nomenclature disunity in the articles that follow and no apologies are offered. Some of the authors are busy practitioners and were invited to recount their personal approaches to the laminitis problem. Thus we have divergent current opinion on laminitis diagnosis, prognosis, and therapy. Confused readers are advised to consult Parks and Mair,[5] Eustace,[6] or even the *Illustrated Veterinary Anatomical Nomenclature,*[7] particularly if they believe a new phenomenon or treatment has been discovered and novel terminology has to be coined—may it be brief, accurate, and descriptive.

There is a tendency in the laminitis literature toward ideology and dogma. Instead of going where the evidence leads, selected data are presented to reinforce strongly held concepts. Discussion and speculation becomes self-evident fact and research is directed to prove it. When reading this publication, much has to be filtered and considered. There are divergent points of view and the reader is advised to apply the rules of evidence, objectivity, and rationality and draw their own conclusions. There is much that can be learned and it is important to bear in mind that nobody is right: laminitis has yet to reveal the secrets of its molecular pathogenesis.

The final articles offer a range of advice on managing the chronically affected foot and how best to care for afflicted horses in the hospital or "home" environment. Similar articles appeared in Part I and now more experts have been recruited to advance laminitis understanding.

I am grateful to Dr. Simon Turner and John Vassallo for the opportunity to serve as Guest Editor and author of the *Veterinary Clinics of North America: Equine Practice*. The contributing authors are thanked for devoting the time to share their knowledge and experience with an audience that will learn much about laminitis within the pages of Part I and II of Advances in Laminitis.

Christopher C. Pollitt, BVSc, PhD
Australian Equine Laminitis Research Unit
School of Veterinary Science
The University of Queensland Gatton Campus
Gatton, QLD 4343, Australia

The Laminitis Institute
University of Pennsylvania School of Veterinary Medicine
New Bolton Center
Kennett Square, PA 19348, USA

E-mail address:
c.pollitt@uq.edu.au

REFERENCES

1. Johnson PJ. The equine metabolic syndrome peripheral Cushing's syndrome. Vet Clin North Am Equine Pract 2002;18:271–93.
2. Asplin KE, Sillence MN, Pollitt CC, et al. Induction of laminitis by prolonged hyperinsulinaemia in clinically normal ponies. Vet J 2007;174:530–5.
3. De Laat MA, McGowan CM, Sillence MN, et al. Equine laminitis: Induced by 48 h hyperinsulinaemia in standardbred horses. Equine Vet J 2010;42:129–35.
4. O'Grady SE, Parks AW, Redden RF, et al. Podiatry terminology. Equine Vet Educ 2007;19:263–71.
5. Parks AH, Mair TS. Laminitis: A call for unified terminology. Equine Vet Educ 2009; 21:102–6.
6. Eustace RA. Laminitis—What's in a name? Vet J 2010;183:245–6.
7. Sack WO. Integumentum commune. In: Schaller O, editor. Illustrated veterinary anatomical nomenclature. Stuttgart: Ferdinand Enke Verlag; 1992. p. 542–61.

Endocrinopathic Laminitis

Catherine M. McGowan, BVSc, MACVSc, PhD, FHEA, MRCVS

KEYWORDS

- Insulin • Cortisol • Glucocorticoids
- Insulin resistance • Equine

Endocrinopathic laminitis has been defined as laminitis developing from hormonal influences rather than in association with proinflammatory and intestinal conditions.[1] Conditions associated with endocrinopathic laminitis fall into 2 basic categories associated with either:

1. glucocorticoids, including Equine Cushing's Syndrome (ECS), also called pituitary pars intermedia dysfunction (PPID), and iatrogenic corticosteroid administration or
2. insulin resistance, including pasture-associated laminitis and Equine Metabolic Syndrome (EMS).

These conditions are described in more detail in the ensuing articles of this issue. Common to all these conditions appear to be disturbed glucose and insulin regulation and, most importantly, the development of insulin resistance and hyperinsulinemia.

GLUCOCORTICOID-ASSOCIATED LAMINITIS

Iatrogenic laminitis associated with glucocorticoid administration may be attributed to the ability of corticosteroids to induce insulin resistance.[2] Insulin and cortisol have opposing actions on glucose metabolism such that hyperinsulinemia and insulin resistance are potential consequences of corticosteroid treatment. A single dose of triamcinolone at 0.05 mg/kg intramuscularly (IM) induced marked hyperglycemia for a period of 3 days and a higher dose of 0.2 mg/kg IM induced marked hyperglycemia and hyperinsulinemia for more than 6 days.[3] Three weeks of dexamethasone treatment at 0.08 mg/kg every 48 hours resulted in a 10-fold increase in basal insulin and insulin resistance demonstrated by the euglycemic-hyperinsulinemic clamp technique.[4]

Similarly, laminitis associated with ECS may be attributed to the effects of hyperadrenocorticism and the development of insulin resistance. Use of a 3β-hydroxysteroid dehydrogenase inhibitor (Trilostane), inhibiting cortisol production from the adrenal

School of Veterinary Science, Faculty of Health and Life Sciences, University of Liverpool, Leahurst, CH64 7TE, UK
E-mail address: C.M.Mcgowan@liverpool.ac.uk

Vet Clin Equine 26 (2010) 233–237
doi:10.1016/j.cveq.2010.04.009
0749-0739/10/$ – see front matter © 2010 Elsevier Inc. All rights reserved.

gland, ameliorated laminitis in 13 of 16 horses with ECS and laminitis.[5] Supporting the importance of the development of insulin resistance in the pathogenesis of laminitis in horses with ECS is the importance of insulin as a prognostic indicator for survival. Horses with very high serum insulin concentration at presentation (>188 μIU/mL) were much more likely to develop laminitis and survive fewer than 2 years after diagnosis, than those with only moderate elevations or normal insulin concentrations (<62 μIU/mL).[6]

INSULIN-ASSOCIATED LAMINITIS

Laminitis associated with EMS has been linked to insulin resistance and hyperinsulinemia in both field studies[7–9] and in experimental studies.[10,11] Pasture-associated laminitis and other forms of insulin-resistance syndrome in horses have recently been grouped into the umbrella term of EMS, owing to the commonality of risk factors for laminitis.[12] EMS describes a syndrome of obesity, insulin resistance, and laminitis (or a predisposition to laminitis) and has been reviewed extensively in the literature.[1,2,12,13] More detail on the proposed pathogenesis of EMS, pasture-associated laminitis, and insulin-induced laminitis will be covered in subsequent articles of this issue.

From a clinical and epidemiologic perspective, the spectrum of EMS is an important point to consider. Pasture-associated laminitis or pre-laminitic metabolic syndrome (PLMS), the least severe end of the spectrum, is seasonal and tends to occur when horses become overly obese and/or insulin resistant during the summer months with an associated risk of summer pasture-associated laminitis.[14] Much of the research to date has been performed on horses at this end of the spectrum, with a naturally occurring predisposition to seasonal laminitis.[7,15–17] Interestingly, of the spontaneously occurring cases of seasonal laminitis recorded in the literature, there is a predominance of pony breeds.[7,15,17] Frank and colleagues[16] report obesity and insulin resistance in a variety of horse breeds, but only 4 of 9 had a history of laminitis and 3 of 9 tested positive to ECS on the combined dexamethasone suppression thyrotropin-releasing hormone releasing test.

The most severe end of the spectrum is where insulin resistance and hyperinsulinemia are present year round and not dependant on access to nonstructural carbohydrate-rich pastures. Furthermore, even obesity may be absent, and de novo or recrudescent laminitis can occur at any time of the year. A few cases at this end of the spectrum have been reported; the first known cases reported were by Reeves and colleagues,[18] where 7 of 8 chronically laminitic ponies with demonstrated insulin resistance on intravenous insulin challenge were shown to test negative for ECS using the combined thyrotropin stimulation test and dexamethasone suppression test. McGowan and Riley[19] presented 19 cases, all in British breed ponies, as a conference abstract. More recently, Walsh and colleagues[9] presented 10 cases in the first series from the United States: 4 were Tennessee Walking Horses, 1 Arabian, 1 Arabian cross, and 4 Connemaras. Again, most of these published cases have been pony breeds or crosses. The assumption has been that these cases have progressed from PLMS or early forms of the disease, but more research on the pathogenesis of the disease is required to support or refute such an assumption. What stimulates such profound persistent insulin resistance in the severe end of the EMS spectrum and what precipitates insulin-resistant horses to develop laminitis is currently unknown, but it is clear there may be breed differences and other genetic factors complicating the link between these 2 conditions, in particular the association with British breed ponies and naturally occurring EMS.

EPIDEMIOLOGY
Glucocorticoid-Associated Laminitis

There have been few studies on the prevalence of iatrogenic glucocorticoid-associated laminitis; however, reported cases are few and a case series looking at "potentially at risk horses" undergoing intra-articular corticosteroid medication found the occurrence of adverse events low at 0.15% to 0.50%.[20,21] Of the 4 cases that did occur, 3 had a previous history of laminitis; the fourth was an aged horse and underlying insulin resistance was possible.

ECS is a common disorder affecting 15% of horses aged 15 years and older. Age is a significant risk factor with the risk of ECS increasing by 20% for every year of age over 15.[22] Based on several published clinical case series, between 50% and 80% of horses with ECS will have clinical laminitis.[5,23,24] Donaldson and colleagues[25] reported 70% of 40 cases of laminitis seen in first opinion practice were associated with a high adrenocorticotropic hormone (ACTH) value indicative of ECS. Although seasonality was not taken into consideration, this represents a high proportion of laminitis cases seen in a first opinion practice. A further 18% of horses in that study that were negative for ECS had laminitis associated with grazing lush pasture.[25]

Insulin-Associated Laminitis

The prevalence of all forms of EMS is unknown but the prevalence of pasture-associated laminitis or the least severe end of the spectrum of EMS is high, associated with indicators of obesity and apparently higher in pony breeds than relatively more obese horses. In a large survey of horse operations across the United States, the causes of laminitis as reported by the property manager were recorded. It was found that approximately 50% of all laminitis cases were associated with grazing lush pasture, whereas a further 27% were associated with "other known" problems including feed problems, pregnancy, and obesity.[26] The cause was unknown in 15%.

The prevalence of basal hyperinsulinemia among obese populations of horses in the United States and in normal pony populations in Australia has recently been reported. Research from the United States showed a prevalence of hyperinsulinemia in a random sample of 300 horses of 10%, with a positive correlation with age, body condition score, and cresty neck score.[27] Another study, using a lower cutoff value, had a prevalence of 22% in obese horses in the Ohio region, again with age and body condition score as risk factors.[28] Research from Australia, in a random selection of pony herds, showed the prevalence of hyperinsulinemia to be as high as 28% in pony breeds, including the Welsh Mountain pony and cob, Shetland, and Connemara ponies. Risk factors for the condition included increasing age, supplementary feeding, body condition score, and a history of laminitis.[29]

In laminitis occurring in the field, as opposed to laminitis occurring during hospitalization or severe illness, endocrinopathic laminitis is the predominant form of laminitis. Prevalent causes of endocrinopathic laminitis are ECS and EMS. Exclusion of inflammatory or weight bearing causes of laminitis and focussing on the identification and treatment of underlying endocrines conditions will improve laminitis management strategies.

REFERENCES

1. Johnson PJ, Messer NT, Slight SH, et al. Endocrinopathic laminitis in the horse. Clin Tech Equine Pract 2004;3:45–56.
2. Johnson PJ, Messer NT, Ganjam VK. Cushing's syndromes, insulin resistance and endocrinopathic laminitis. Equine Vet J 2004;36(3):194–8.

3. French K, Pollitt CC, Pass MA. Pharmacokinetics and metabolic effects of triamcinolone acetonide and their possible relationships to glucocorticoid-induced laminitis in horses. J Vet Pharmacol Ther 2000;23(5):287–92.
4. Tiley HA, Geor RJ, McCutcheon LJ. Effects of dexamethasone administration on insulin resistance and components of insulin signaling and glucose metabolism in equine skeletal muscle. Am J Vet Res 2008;69(1):51–8.
5. McGowan CM, Neiger R. Efficacy of trilostane for the treatment of equine Cushing's syndrome. Equine Vet J 2003;35(4):414–8.
6. McGowan CM, Frost R, Pfeiffer DU, et al. Serum insulin concentrations in horses with equine Cushing's syndrome: response to a cortisol inhibitor and prognostic value. Equine Vet J 2004;36:295–8.
7. Treiber KH, Kronfeld DS, Hess TM, et al. Evaluation of genetic and metabolic predispositions and nutritional risk factors for pasture-associated laminitis in ponies. J Am Vet Med Assoc 2006;228(10):1538–45.
8. Carter RA, Treiber KH, Geor RJ, et al. Prediction of incipient pasture-associated laminitis from hyperinsulinaemia, hyperleptinaemia and generalised and localised obesity in a cohort of ponies. Equine vet J 2009;41(2):171–8.
9. Walsh DM, McGowan CM, McGowan T, et al. Correlation of plasma insulin concentration with laminitis score in a field study of equine Cushing's Disease and Equine Metabolic Syndrome. J Equine Vet Sci 2009;29:87–94.
10. Asplin KE, Sillence MN, Pollitt CC, et al. Induction of laminitis by prolonged hyperinsulinaemia in clinically normal ponies. Vet J 2007;174:530–5.
11. DeLaat MA, McGowan CM, Sillence MN, et al. Equine laminitis: induced by 48 hours of hyperinsulinaemia in Standardbred horses. Equine Vet J 2009;42(2): 129–35.
12. Geor R, Frank N. Metabolic syndrome—From human organ disease to laminar failure in equids. Vet Immunol Immunopathol 2009;129(3–4):151–4.
13. Johnson PJ. The equine metabolic syndrome (peripheral Cushing's syndrome). Vet Clin North Am Equine Pract 2002;18(2):271–93.
14. Geor RJ. Pasture-associated laminitis. Vet Clin North Am Equine Pract 2009; 25(1):39–50.
15. Coffman JR, Colles CM. Insulin tolerance in laminitic ponies. Can J Comp Med 1983;47(3):347–51.
16. Frank N, Elliott SB, Brandt LE, et al. Physical characteristics, blood hormone concentrations, and plasma lipid concentrations in obese horses with insulin resistance. J Am Vet Med Assoc 2006;228(9):1383–90.
17. Bailey SR, Habershon-Butcher JL, Ransom KJ, et al. Hypertension and insulin resistance in a mixed-breed population of ponies predisposed to laminitis. Am J Vet Res 2008;69(1):122–9.
18. Reeves HJ, Lees R, McGowan CM. Measurement of basal serum insulin concentration in the diagnosis of Cushing's disease in ponies. Vet Rec 2001;149(15):449–52.
19. McGowan CM, Riley G. Long-term trilostane treatment for metabolic syndrome [abstract]. In: Proceedings 43rd British Equine Veterinary Association Congress, 2004.
20. McCluskey MJ, Kavenagh PB. Clinical use of triamcinolone acetonide in the horse (205 cases) and the incidence of glucocorticoid-induced laminitis associated with its use. Equine Vet Educ 2004;16(2):86–9.
21. Bathe AP. The corticosteroid laminitis story: 3. The clinician's viewpoint. Equine Vet J 2007;39(1):12–3.

22. McGowan TW, Hodgson DR, McGowan CM. The prevalence of equine Cushing's syndrome in aged horses. The prevalence of equine Cushing's syndrome in aged horses [abstract:113]. J Vet Intern Med 2007;21(3):603.
23. Schott HC, Coursen CL, Eberhart SW, et al. The Michigan Cushing's project. In: Proceedings of the 47th Annual Convention of the American Association of Equine Practitioners. 2001. p. 22–4.
24. Donaldson MT, Lamonte BH, Morresey P, et al. Treatment with pergolide or cyproheptadine of pituitary pars intermedia dysfunction (equine Cushing's disease). J Vet Intern Med 2002;16(6):742–6.
25. Donaldson MT, Jorgensen AJ, Beech J. Evaluation of suspected pituitary pars intermedia dysfunction in horses with laminitis. J Am Vet Med Assoc 2004;224(7): 1123–7.
26. USDA. Lameness and laminitis in US horses. In: USDA: APHIS: VS, CEAH. Fort Collins (CO): 2000.
27. Geor RJ, Thatcher CD, Pleasant RS, et al. Prevalence of hyperinsulinemia in mature horses: relationship to adiposity [abstract]. J Vet Intern Med 2007;21(3): 601.
28. Muno J, Gallatin L, Geor RJ, et al. Prevalence and risk factors for hyperinsulinemia in clinically normal horses in central Ohio [abstract]. J Vet Intern Med 2009; 23(3):721.
29. McGowan CM, McGowan TW. Prevalence and risk factors for hyperinsulinemia in ponies [abstract]. J Vet Intern Med 2008;22(3):734.

Laminitis and the Equine Metabolic Syndrome

Philip J. Johnson, BVSc(Hons), MS, MRCVS[a],*,
Charles E. Wiedmeyer, DVM, PhD[b], Alison LaCarrubba, DVM[a],
V.K. (Seshu) Ganjam, BVSc, MA (hc), PhD[c], Nat T. Messer IV, DVM[a]

KEYWORDS

- Endocrinopathic laminitis • Insulin resistance
- Equine metabolic syndrome • Obesity

Although much has been written about laminitis in the context of its association with inflammatory processes, such as dietary carbohydrate overload and endotoxemia,[1–5] recognition is growing that most cases of laminitis examined by veterinarians in private practice are those associated with pasture grazing, obesity, and insulin resistance (IR).[6,7] The term *endocrinopathic laminitis* has been adopted to classify the instances of laminitis in which the origin seems to be more strongly associated with an underlying endocrinopathy, such as either IR or the influence of corticosteroids.[8–11] Results of a recent study suggest that obesity and IR represent the most common metabolic and endocrinopathic predispositions for laminitis in horses.[6,12] IR also plays an important role in the pathogenesis of laminitis that develops when some horses or ponies are allowed to graze pastures at certain times of the year (pasture-associated laminitis [PAL]).[12–15] Moreover, IR is provoked by and contributes to pathophysiologic processes associated with endotoxemia and systemic inflammation under the more classic circumstances associated with risk for acute laminitis, such as grain overload, retention of fetal membranes, and gastroenteritis.[16,17] However, a recent study using the oligofructose model showed that experimentally induced laminitis was not associated with a loss of insulin sensitivity.[18]

The term *equine metabolic syndrome* (EMS) has been proposed as a label for horses whose clinical examination results (including both physical examination and laboratory

[a] Department of Veterinary Medicine and Surgery, College of Veterinary Medicine, University of Missouri, 900 East Campus Drive, Columbia, MO 65211, USA
[b] Department of Veterinary Pathobiology, Room 201 Connaway Hall, College of Veterinary Medicine, University of Missouri, 1600 Rollins Avenue, Columbia, MO 65211, USA
[c] Department of Biomedical Science, E102 Veterinary Medicine Building, College of Veterinary Medicine, University of Missouri, 1600 Rollins Avenue, Columbia, MO 65211, USA
* Corresponding author. Clydesdale Hall Veterinary Medical Teaching Hospital, 900 East Campus Drive, Columbia, MO 65211.
E-mail address: JohnsonPJ@missouri.edu

Vet Clin Equine 26 (2010) 239–255
doi:10.1016/j.cveq.2010.04.004
0749-0739/10/$ – see front matter © 2010 Elsevier Inc. All rights reserved.

testing) suggest heightened risk for developing laminitis as a result of underlying IR.[19] EMS is not a disease per se, but rather is a clustering of clinical abnormalities that, when identified collectively in a given patient, indicates that the likelihood of developing laminitis is greater than in individuals lacking the EMS criteria. Use of the term EMS is especially practical for distinguishing affected horses from those affected with either Cushing's (pituitary pars intermedia dysfunction [PPID]) or hypothyroidism, with which EMS is often confused.[19]

The clinical importance of diagnosing EMS centers on the fact that recognized risk factors for laminitis can subsequently be avoided in the affected individual. Preventive measures aimed at reducing the risk for laminitis should be rigorously emphasized in EMS-affected horses and ponies.

Recently, the American College of Veterinary Internal Medicine (ACVIM) commissioned a panel of EMS-interested specialists to develop a consensus statement that would help define the syndrome based on current knowledge.[20] During development of the consensus statement, contents of the working draft were presented and discussed at the ACVIM Annual Forum in Montreal, Canada and some of the following comments will be based on those discussions.[20] Ongoing experimental and clinical studies will help better define EMS (which is distinctly different to the human metabolic syndrome[21]) in the next few years.

DEFINING THE EQUINE METABOLIC SYNDROME: A WORK IN PROGRESS

IR represents the centerpiece of the pathophysiologic mechanisms that are at play in the equine metabolic syndrome.[6,19,20,22,23] Most EMS-affected horses and ponies are characterized by the development of obesity (either generalized or regional obesity). Regional obesity includes thickening in the crest of the neck (referred to as a *cresty neck*) and a pattern of expanded subcutaneous adipose tissue at the base of the tail, in the prepuce (male horses), near the mammary gland (females), and near the shoulders. However, not all EMS-affected horses are obese and not all obese horses develop IR. Horse owners commonly refer to affected horses as *easy keepers* or *good doers* because they perceive that these horses tend to easily maintain their obese body condition when being fed minimal rations. IR represents a risk factor for laminitis, and consequently the development of laminitis is sometimes used to support a diagnosis of EMS.[23] Although the physical or radiographic appearance of the hoof may indicate that laminitis had occurred in some EMS-affected equids, the owner may report that lameness (pain) per se has not been evident. Therefore, structural changes in the hoof–lamellar interface (HLI) may occur in the absence of laminitic pain in EMS-affected individuals. Moreover, EMS-affected equids seem to be especially prone to development of hoof pain after being allowed to graze pastures at certain times of the year.[24,25]

Some have argued that the existence of laminitis should not contribute to the definition for EMS because diagnosis of EMS is intended to predict a risk for laminitis. As is the case for the definition of the human metabolic syndrome, evidence now exists that EMS-affected horses and ponies may be characterized by up-regulated markers of inflammation[26,27] and a propensity to develop arterial hypertension.[28,29] Other clinical and laboratory abnormalities that may be helpful for defining the syndrome include infertility in mares, hypertriglyceridemia, and hyperleptinemia.[13,19,20]

HERITABILITY OF EQUINE METABOLIC SYNDROME

Some breeds seem to be at greater risk for the development of EMS, especially pony breeds (compared with horse breeds); Welsh, Shetland, and Dartmoor ponies are especially considered in this respect. The fact that pony breeds tend to be relatively insulin resistant when compared with horses may help to explain why the incidence of laminitis is greater in ponies.[23,30–33] Other breed predispositions that have been suggested include the Morgan breed, Miniature horses, Spanish Mustang, Saddlebred, Warmblood, Haflinger, Norwegian Fjord, Peruvian Paso, and Paso Fino breeds. EMS has also been recognized in some Quarter Horses and Tennessee Walking horses. However, Thoroughbreds and Standardbreds may be at less risk. Familial patterns are also recognized for EMS, and therefore specific genetic lines within any given breed might be at greater risk.[23] With the exception of published data supporting a genetic predisposition in certain pony breeding lines, most information pertaining to the inheritability of EMS is anecdotal and will surely be supplemented by new genetic mapping studies in the near future.

RECOGNITION AND OBJECTIVE MEASUREMENT OF OBESITY IN HORSES

An ideal index of body weight, such as the body mass index (BMI) described for humans based on the individual's height and sex, does not exist for horses. In fact, such an ideal standard would surely differ between different breeds. The body condition score (BCS; on a scale of 1–9, with 1 being emaciated and 9 being profoundly obese) is a commonly used visual estimate that serves to provide a subjective index of obesity in horses and ponies and does not require scales.[34] The BCS is better suited for evaluating adiposity in horses than it is for ponies. More recently, experts have suggested that the circumference of the neck (compared with the horse's height or girth) might be a practical index for suspicion of IR (similar to the use of waist circumference as an indicator of high BMI and IR in obese human patients).[35] A cresty neck score (CNS) has been suggested as a method of assessing subcutaneous adipose tissue expansion in the neck region with scores between 0 and 5 (CNS >3 implies EMS).[35]

A CNS of 3 is specifically described as follows: "Crest is enlarged and thickened, so fat is deposited more heavily in middle of the neck than toward poll and withers, giving a mounded appearance. Crest fills cupped hand and begins losing side-to-side flexibility."[35]

To determine the neck circumference-to-height at withers ratio, the circumference of the neck should be measured at the mid-point between the poll and the withers with the neck in a normal elevated position. In one study, when the ratio (with respect to the patient's height) exceeded 0.71, the affected pony was more likely to develop PAL.[35]

PATHOPHYSIOLOGY

A satisfactory and unifying explanation for the development of laminitis as a result of potentially diverse endocrinologic and metabolic influences is still lacking. However, several plausible and, in some cases, supportable hypotheses have been proposed. Endocrinologic perturbations that have been linked to risk for laminitis include hypercortisolism (Cushing's disease), pregnancy, obesity, and IR.[33,36–38] Certainly, IR is a component of hypercortisolism, pregnancy, and obesity. For the purposes of this discussion, aspects of obesity and IR that might play a role in the pathogenesis of laminitis are reviewed (obesity and IR are recognized contributors in EMS). Because of the complexity and extent of the discussion pertaining to theories regarding the pathogenesis of laminitis in the context of EMS, readers are strongly encouraged to seek out excellent reviews of this topic elsewhere in the literature.[6]

Glucose dysregulation is frequently cited as an explanation of the risk for laminitis associated with IR. This theory is derived from the observation that, using an in vitro explant model, hoof lamellar keratinocytes were shown to have a critical glucose requirement and that keratinocyte separation from underlying basement membrane occurs when glucose is insufficient.[39] More recently, insulin has been shown to not affect glucose uptake through HLI explants and the insulin-dependent glucose transporter (GLUT-4) is not present in hoof keratinocytes.[40] Therefore, if glucose dysregulation is pivotal to the risk for laminitis associated with IR, it is not based on an insulin-dependent glucose uptake mechanism through hoof–lamellar keratinocytes. Glucose dysregulation may contribute to risk for laminitis in an insulin resistant state because hyperglycemia may directly influence vascular endothelial cells (glucotoxic endotheliopathy).[19,41] Mild elevations in the plasma glucose concentration over time are sufficient to affect endothelial regulation of vasomotor tone (vasoconstrictive influence) and promote a prothrombotic endothelial phenotype.[41]

Vascular endothelial cells are also directly influenced by insulin in such a manner that interference with the action of insulin (IR) would likely promote vasoconstriction and platelet/leukocyte adhesion to endothelial surfaces.[6,42] Therefore, perturbations in the regulation and action of insulin and glucose could theoretically lead to a microvascular dysregulation basis for the risk of laminitis that attends IR. These increased vasoconstrictive influences likely contribute to hypertension that has been observed in both the human[43] and equine[28,29] forms of metabolic syndrome. Moreover, the increased platelet/leukocyte microvascular adhesiveness that is reported in insulin-resistant individuals likely augments the participating role of neutrophils in the development of laminitis resulting from endotoxemia, carbohydrate overload, systemic inflammation, and severe gastrointestinal disturbances.[44]

Recent experimental work showed that acute laminitis could be directly induced by insulin through maintenance of a supraphysiologic plasma insulin concentration over the course of several days in a euglycemic clamp experiment.[45,46] However, in these experiments, the plasma insulin concentrations that were associated with the development of laminitis significantly exceeded those that are reported for horses and ponies affected with EMS.[45] The fact that insulin can act as an independent trigger factor is important because under certain conditions it might act alongside concurrent trigger factors to cause laminitis at lesser circulating concentrations. Several explanations for a mechanism through which insulin might directly cause laminitis have been suggested and include hoof–lamellar hypoxia associated with insulin-induced microcirculatory dysregulation and increased tissue protease activity (including matrix metalloproteinases), both of which could increase the likelihood of structural failure at the level of the HLI.[45]

Although obesity is widely recognized as a risk factor for laminitis, a satisfactory mechanistic explanation is still lacking.[37] Plausible theories include increased weight-bearing, obesity-dependent IR, and the secretion of proinflammatory cytokines by adipose tissue. Although small quantities of cytokines are normally produced by cells in adipose tissue to exert autocrine and paracrine functions, the presence of prodigious quantities of adipose tissue in obese states leads to the secretion of much higher levels of these same cytokines (adipokines) that circulate to exert pathologic influence beyond the tissue of origin (endocrine effect).[37,47]

Numerous different cytokines that are derived from adipose tissue have been identified.[48,49] The adipokine repertoire produced by any single adipose repository is probably different depending on the location and many other factors.[50] Certain repositories of adipose tissue (e.g., omental and mesenteric fat in obese human patients) are characterized by the acquisition of an activated macrophage population that secretes proinflammatory cytokines into the venous effluent.[51,52] In obese individuals, these leukocyte-derived cytokines are released in substantial quantities and exert a systemic (endocrine) action.[51,52] Elevated circulating levels of proinflammatory signaling molecules have been suggested to contribute to the development of IR and the risk for laminitis in obese horses. Specifically, the circulating (blood) mRNA expression of both tumor necrosis factor-α (TNF-α) and interleukin-1β (IL-1β) are increased in obese horses.[26] In another study, a group of laminitis-prone ponies were characterized by elevated plasma TNF-α levels.[53] Elevated circulating TNF-α and IL-1β expression was identified as an independent risk factor for IR in one study.[26]

Macrophages that are identified in mesenteric adipose tissue in human and laboratory animal species are also characterized by the presence of 11β-hydroxysteroid dehydrogenase-1, a steroid-converting enzyme that converts cortisone, the plentiful inactive metabolite of cortisol, to active cortisol.[54–57] Therefore, the enhanced conversion of cortisol from cortisone in mesenteric adipose tissue leads to increased corticosteroid action in both the adipose tissue (where it stimulates activation of preadipocytes to adipocytes and promotes expansion of the adipose repository at this location) and the liver (downstream target organ, where it causes hepatic IR).[54–57]

In addition to cortisol and adipokines, mesenteric adipose tissue also releases free fatty acids (FFAs) into the circulation, and these FFAs contribute to the development of hepatic IR.[58] Elevated FFAs also stimulate inflammatory processes through enhanced Toll-like receptor 4 expression in macrophages.[59] Not all adipose tissue repositories are characterized by a population of leukocytes, and the circulating concentrations of other adipokines, such as leptin, resistin, and adiponectin, may be perturbed and contribute independently to the development of IR.[47] Elevated levels of circulating adipokines, such as TNF-α, may contribute independently to the development of IR and microvascular dysregulation. For example, enhanced vasospasticity (stimulated endothelin-1 production and reduced nitric oxide production), up-regulated oxidative stress, increased vascular permeability, increased expression of endothelial adhesion molecules, and inhibition of insulin signaling may all be attributed to the action of TNF-α.[42,60]

Different aspects of the metabolic syndrome (especially IR and obesity) may contribute diverse risk factors for laminitis, including increased weight-bearing of obesity, microvascular dysregulation in the HLI, hepatocellular dysfunction, enhanced inflammation, prothrombotic endothelial phenotype, increased endothelial adhesiveness, oxidative stress, and increased corticosteroid activity.

DIETARY FACTORS PRECIPITATE AND AGGRAVATE LAMINITIS IN EQUINE METABOLIC SYNDROME

A diagnosis of EMS implies that the individual is inherently at risk for laminitis when subjected to various and potentially diverse trigger factors. Horses and ponies that are affected with EMS seem to be especially sensitive to ingested nonstructural carbohydrate (NSC). One of the most commonly recognized trigger factors for laminitis in EMS patients is the ingestion of a ration that is characterized by a high NSC content. For example, grazing grass pastures is the most common cause for laminitis recognized by practicing veterinarians (PAL).[12] The total carbohydrate content of pasture grass is characterized by the carbohydrates that constitute the cell wall structure of plant cells (structural carbohydrates or fiber, such as cellulose and hemicellulose) that are indigestible by mammalian enzymes, and by NSCs (starch, soluble sugar, and fructans).[25,61] Modern pasture grassland species have been genetically selected for high NSC content as befits the needs of the food animal industry. Horses evolved to be nutritionally efficient on native grassland species that tend to have a lower NSC content.

A single and simple explanation does exist for why EMS horses tend to develop activated laminitis after ingestion of high NSC pasture grass. Several explanations are plausible: ingested NSC (starch and soluble sugars) cause both glycemic and insulinemic spiking that seems to be associated with aggravated laminitis; or certain types of fructan (not digested by the small intestine) may cause cecal/colonic floral perturbations leading to colonic acidulation, increased epithelial permeability, and the absorption of other laminitis triggers (bacterially derived exotoxins, endotoxins, and vasoactive amines).[12]

Studies have shown that the NSC content of common pasture grasses tends to increase at certain times of the year (eg, spring, fall) and that development of laminitis is more likely in EMS ponies at these times.[24,62] IR and elevated systemic blood pressure (both components of EMS) are also more prominent when ponies graze high NSC-content pastures.[28] The development of laminitis in equids during pasture grazing should alert veterinarians to the possibility of underlying EMS.

Diagnosis of Equine Metabolic Syndrome

Clinical suspicion of EMS is based on assessment of the patient's medical history, results of the physical examination, evaluation of radiographs of the feet, and the results of laboratory tests. The best laboratory tests for IR include the frequently sampled intravenous glucose tolerance test (FSIGT) and the euglycemic hyperinsulinemic clamp technique.[63,64] Unfortunately, these gold standard tests are impractical for practicing veterinarians and less-specific, alternative diagnostic approaches are generally recommended.

The easiest diagnostic test for IR is to simply determine the plasma insulin concentration. Compensatory hyperinsulinemia is a common finding in IR-affected equids.[65] Nevertheless, veterinarians should be cautious when interpreting the results of single-sample insulin determinations without considering possible confounding factors. For example, serum insulin concentration can be influenced by many factors (in addition to the insulin sensitivity of the individual), including time since the animal was last fed; circulating cortisol concentration (diurnal variance, excitement, pain and stress, PPID); type of food on which the ration is based; reproductive status; and physiologic status (fitness/illness). However, fasting concentrations of both insulin and glucose tend to be relatively constant and may be used to provide insight into the patient's insulin sensitivity.

For purposes of measuring the circulating glucose and insulin concentrations, it is important to fast the patient for 8 to 10 hours and to obtain the samples between 8:00 and 10:00 AM (standardization).[20] It is also recommended that the patient should have been fed no more than one flake of low-NSC hay (per 500 kg horse) the previous evening (no later than 10:00 PM). Horses and ponies that are accommodated on pasture should be stalled or confined to a dry lot before the insulin and glucose concentrations are evaluated to determine insulin sensitivity.

Blood samples for insulin assay should be submitted to the same laboratory because different laboratories use different insulin assay procedures.[20] Therefore, for purposes of comparing data, serum insulin assays should be performed consistently using a method validated (by a specific laboratory) for horses (with an equine-specific reference range).

Horses and ponies affected with EMS tend to be characterized by a high normal or slightly elevated plasma glucose concentration (reference range, 80–115 mg/dL) and hyperinsulinemia (reference range, <20 μU/mL [<144 pmol/L]).[20] Because different laboratories use different assay methods, a universally accepted cutoff for significant hyperinsulinemia has not yet been determined. Furthermore, some EMS horses tend to develop reduced glycemic control (hyperglycemia, >150 mg/dL) and may be characterized with type 2 diabetes mellitus. The extent to which type 2 diabetes mellitus develops in mature IR-affected horses is currently unknown (it may be more common than generally believed).

Testing for IR in horses that are experiencing pain (or excitement) is not practical because any activation of the sympathetic nervous system will cause a reduction in insulin sensitivity. Therefore, testing patients that are presently affected with laminitic pain is not recommended. Moreover, determination of the serum insulin concentration may yield false-negative results in EMS-affected horses and ponies that have been fed a low-NSC ration. Therefore, dynamic endocrine testing is recommended for the potential EMS candidates in which the resting serum insulin and glucose concentrations are within reference intervals.[20]

Dynamic Testing for Insulin Resistance

A better diagnostic test for IR in clinical patients is the combined intravenous glucose–insulin test (CGIT).[66] Horses are tested through being administered both glucose and insulin (glucose, 150 mg/kg; insulin, 0.1 U/kg) and having the blood glucose concentration measured for 2 hours (12 blood glucose determinations at 0, +1, +5, +15, +25, +35, +45, +60, +75, +90, +105, and +120 minutes). Results of a CGIT are characterized by a two-phase curve with positive (hyperglycemic) and negative (hypoglycemic) portions. The test outcome is evaluated based on the time taken for the plasma glucose concentration to return to the (zero time) baseline level after administration of glucose and insulin. Normal insulin sensitivity is associated with a return to baseline within 45 minutes.[66] The testing conditions for a CGIT are the same as those for evaluating the patient's resting serum insulin and glucose concentrations.

Patients have a very small risk for development of signs of insulin-provoked hypoglycemia (weakness, trembling and sweating) during the test. If signs of hypoglycemia develop, patients should be treated using intravenous 50% glucose infusion.[66] False-positive results (suggesting IR in a normal horse) may arise if any stressful or exciting event precedes or occurs during the test. Therefore, the test should always be performed in a quiet environment in patients that have been allowed to consume a simple grass hay–based ration. Intravenous catheters should be placed the day before the test. The CGIT represents a potentially practical clinical measurement of insulin sensitivity because it provides integrated information and more information than either the singular glucose tolerance test or an insulin sensitivity test.

Use of Continuous Glucose Monitors

Disadvantages of measuring the blood glucose and insulin concentrations in either a single sample or during dynamic testing include the possibility of the patient becoming excited (subsequently depressing insulin sensitivity) and the fact that the period of evaluation is short. Continuous glucose monitoring represents a technological innovation has been marketed in the human medical field for better studying glucose regulation in individuals with diabetes.[67,68] Briefly, this method entails placing a tiny glucose sensor in a subcutaneous location to render a computerized digital recording (Fig. 1). Using this method, it is possible to unobtrusively record the concentration of glucose in the interstitial compartment (equivalent to the blood glucose concentration) every 5 minutes over the course of up to 7 days (288 data points per 24-hour period).[67,68] A potential advantage of this method for equine practitioners includes the ability to monitor changes in interstitial tissue glucose concentration over time with minimal need for handling. Using this technique, the authors observed that the interstitial glucose concentration of lean, insulin-sensitive adult horses tends

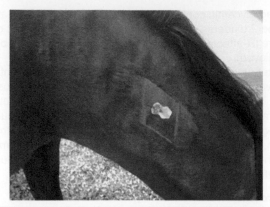

Fig. 1. A continuous glucose monitoring device secured to the neck of a horse.

to be maintained at the lower end of the reference range with minimal variance (horses being fed ad libitum low NSC grass hay) (**Fig. 2**A). In contrast, the interstitial glucose concentration of obese horses in which CGIT has shown IR tends to be more variable over time, runs relatively high within the reference range, and frequently exceeds the high end of the reference range (see **Fig. 2**B).

Diagnostic Controversy

Recently, it has become clear that PPID sometimes arises in teenage horses without the classic physical appearance (eg, inappropriate hirsutism, loss of musculature, polyuria/polydipsia).[69] In fact, the clinical presentation of PPID in young horses may be very similar to that of EMS. The extent to which EMS and PPID may be related is the subject of considerable controversy. Nevertheless, before EMS can be diagnosed, diagnostic tests such as the low-dose dexamethasone suppression test and measurement of the plasma adrenocorticotropic hormone concentration[70] may be undertaken to show that the patient's clinical signs are not resulting from PPID. In one study, the prognosis was reportedly worse for PPID-affected horses in which IR could easily be shown.[71]

PREVENTION, MANAGEMENT, AND TREATMENT RECOMMENDATIONS FOR EQUINE METABOLIC SYNDROME

The management and treatment options for EMS will be determined by a full evaluation of the individual patient's specific clinical circumstances. Ideally, however, veterinary clinical recognition of EMS will primarily prevent laminitis in EMS-affected horses and ponies.

If EMS is diagnosed before painful laminitis has occurred, the following preventive strategies should be used:

Reversal of obesity (when applicable), which entails both dietary change and physical activity.

Dietary changes aimed at reducing the energy and NSC components of the ration.

Increased level of physical activity.

Avoidance of pasture grazing for susceptible individuals, especially at certain times of the year and day.

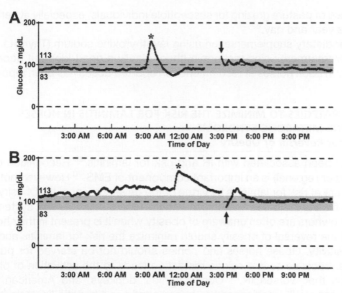

Fig. 2. (A) Graphic representation of interstitial glucose measurements obtained from a lean, healthy, 6-year-old physically active Arabian gelding fitted with a continuous glucose monitoring system (CGMS) for 24 hours of stall confinement. The arrow represents the beginning of the monitoring period and the asterisk indicates the point at which a combined intravenous glucose-insulin test (CGIT) was conducted. The gray zone represents the reference range for plasma glucose concentration in an adult horse (83–113 mg/dL). The interstitial glucose concentration tends to remain within the lower aspect of the reference range throughout the investigative period, and the outcome of the CGIT is consistent with normal insulin sensitivity (glucose concentration returns to baseline within 45 minutes). (B) Graphic representation of interstitial glucose measurements obtained from an obese, physically inactive, 14-year-old Quarter Horse gelding fitted with a CGMS for 24 hours of stall confinement. The arrow represents the beginning of the monitoring period and the asterisk indicates the point at which a CGIT was conducted. The gray zone represents the reference range for plasma glucose concentration in an adult horse (83–113 mg/dL). The interstitial glucose concentration tends to remain at the upper end of the reference range and drift into the hyperglycemic zone (poorly regulated glucose) throughout the investigative period, and the outcome of the CGIT is consistent with reduced insulin sensitivity (glucose concentration failed to return to baseline within 45 minutes).

Begin critical evaluations of the patient's hoof (based on appearance and radiographic characteristics) with a view to promoting hoof care practices (farriery) that should reduce the risk for laminitis (maintain photographic records).

If EMS is diagnosed after painful laminitis has occurred, the following management/ treatment strategies should be used:

Treatment of laminitis based on critical and objective evaluations of the patient's hoof (based on appearance and radiographic characteristics; this topic is reviewed elsewhere in this issue).

Reversal of obesity (when applicable), which must be based on dietary change because physical activity can exacerbate the HLI during painful laminitis.

Dietary changes aimed at reducing the energy and sugar/starch components of the ration.

Avoidance of pasture grazing for susceptible individuals, especially at certain times of the year and day.[62]

Consider dietary supplementation using levothyroxine sodium (Thyro-L).[72–74]

Consider treatment using metformin (theoretically a good idea but poor bioavailability in adult horses at recommended/reported doses has been reported).[75–77]

DIETARY STRATEGIES TO MINIMIZE THE RISK FOR LAMINITIS IN HORSES WITH EQUINE METABOLIC SYNDROME
Strategies for Reversal of Obesity

Obesity has been associated with IR and risk for laminitis.[20] Recognition of obesity (generalized or regional) is an important component of EMS.[20] However, not all obese individuals are at risk for laminitis by virtue of the development of IR. Obesity is clearly a common finding in horses and ponies under modern management systems. Moreover, horse owners are often unaware of obesity when it is present in their horses. It is logical that the reversal of obesity should minimize the risk for laminitis and promote insulin sensitivity. Obese horses and ponies should not be starved for purposes of weight loss, because severe calorie restriction leads to the activation of physiologic mechanisms that worsen IR.[78] Obese ponies, donkeys, and American Miniature Horses are especially predisposed to hyperlipemia and hepatic lipidosis (potentially fatal) when subjected to a calorie-restricted ration.[79] Strategies intended to reverse obesity should include increased physical activity and a reasonable restriction of dietary energy intake. Adjustments to the horse's ration should be instituted gradually, and progress with weight reduction should be evaluated objectively on a predetermined schedule.

Reduced dietary caloric intake coupled with increased physical activity represents the cornerstones of a successful weight-reduction program.[80] Unfortunately, the development of painful laminitis in some EMS-affected equids precludes the enhancement of exercise for purposes of promoting weight reduction. In those patients, dietary adjustments and the specific management of laminitis must be undertaken to better address obesity and IR.

The recommended dietary strategy for obesity reversal in patients with EMS is the provision of energy from structural carbohydrates (such as cellulose) rather than from NSCs (starch, soluble sugars, and fructans). Energy-dense food items such as sweet feed and grain should not be used. Because the NSC content of a batch of hay cannot be visually assessed, a forage analysis should be obtained for any hay that is intended for feeding of EMS-affected equids.[24,61,62] Ideally, the NSC content of hay used to both promote weight reduction and avoid glucose/insulin spiking should be less than 10% to 12%.[20] For more detailed information pertaining to the analysis of forage and the differences in how the analysis is performed and reported between forage analysis laboratories, the reader is directed elsewhere.[24,61,62] Weight reduction can generally be accomplished by providing 1.5% of the patient's targeted body weight as low-NSC hay, daily (feeding 2% of the patient's body weight failed to elicit weight reduction in one study). The daily forage intake should be provided as numerous small feedings throughout the day to minimize protracted periods of hunger and boredom. Recently, commercial horse feeding products (characterized by a certified low NSC content) have been marketed for EMS-affected equids and may be considered as a part of a weight-reduction program for obese or EMS-affected horses.

The nature of modern grassland species that are commonly found in horse pastures and paddocks have been genetically selected to support milk production and fattening of domesticated cattle, and are therefore characterized by a high NSC content in distinct contrast to the native grassland species on which horses evolved.[62] Therefore, discontinuation of pasture grazing should be emphasized for horses in which obesity reversal is important.[81,82] If completely eliminating pasture grazing is not practical, the practice of restricted pasture grazing may be adopted.[81,82] However, in one study, the authors showed that although time for grazing was reduced, significant weight loss did not occur because the consumption of grass increased in response to decreased time at pasture.[30] Other management strategies that might promote weight loss under a restricted pasture grazing program include the use of a grazing muzzle (ensuring that the patient can drink water), strategic mowing of the pasture, strip grazing, and depositing wood chips across an area of pasture.[81,82] That said, for purposes of weight reduction (and reduced NSC intake in general), strict avoidance of pasture grazing should be strongly recommended whenever possible for patients with EMS. Certainly, EMS-affected horses and ponies should never be grazed at the times of the year when pasture NSC levels are known to be elevated (spring bloom, early summer, and during the transition from fall to winter).

Strategies for Minimizing Dietary Nonstructural Carbohydrate Intake

In addition to addressing obesity, management of EMS-affected horses must also include a feeding regimen characterized by low NSC content and a low glycemic index.[61,81] Some patients with EMS are relatively refractory to dietary strategies aimed at reversing IR and remain susceptible to laminitis, even when fed relatively low NSC rations. It is important to be exceptionally diligent with respect to lowered NSC intake in these individuals and to monitor the patient's insulin sensitivity (serial serum insulin determinations on a regular basis) carefully over time. Other patients with EMS respond more favorably to less stringent dietary management strategies and may require a less rigorous and more practical approach. Practicing veterinarians should also consider consulting with specialist horse-oriented nutrition experts when formulating a suitable ration for EMS-affected horses and ponies.

For EMS-affected horses with relatively refractory IR, strict avoidance of pasture grazing must be considered and a forage-based diet characterized by a low (<10%–12%) NSC content should be provided. Limited (1–2 hours) pasture grazing may be allowed for horses with EMS and controlled IR at times of the day when the NSC content of grass is low (between 3:00 and 9:00 AM) but not at times of the year when seasonal and environmental conditions cause grass NSC to be relatively high (lush grass growth in spring and early summer; reactivated grass growth after rain in the summer; drought-affected pastures; and frost-affected pastures in the fall). The reader is directed to other literature sources for a more complete review of the seasonal and environmental factors that affect the NSC content of pasture grasses.[24,62,81,82]

The basic recommendation is to feed EMS-affected horses hay that is characterized by a low NSC and high fiber (structural carbohydrate) content. Affected horses should not be fed alfalfa, grain, or sweet feed. Selection of a suitable source of hay should be based on results of a forage analysis, because the NSC content of hay cannot be speculated. Soaking hay under a large volume of water for 60 minutes can sometimes reduce its NSC content.[62] Other potentially useful components of a suitable ration include (nonmolassed) sugar beet pulp and rice bran. If further dietary energy is required (for nonobese, athletic horses) at a level greater than that provided by forage, supplementing the ration with vegetable oil (typically corn or soy) should be considered.[81] Additionally, various commercial horse food products have been marketed with a certified low NSC content that will likely be helpful in some cases.

Providing low-NSC forage will likely not provide sufficient protein, vitamins, and minerals in the ration, and therefore a low-NSC, protein-enriched mineral and vitamin balancer should be considered as a part of the dietary plan (after evaluating forage analysis results with a nutritionist).[81] Although dietary supplementation using the

---

Box 1
Checklist for owners of horses with equine metabolic syndrome

- EMS identification. EMS is initially identified based on results of physical examination (body condition and signs of laminitis). Recognition of the phenotype may be an incidental finding during veterinary consultation for other unrelated problems. The development of obesity is common in contemporary horse management systems.

- Client education. Obesity and EMS represent important risk factors for laminitis. Discuss with client the health implications of obesity and feeding NSC-rich rations to physically inactive horses and ponies.

- Investigation. Review the patient's physical activity program and evaluate the feeding program based on the physical activity and nutritional requirements for the individual. Identify management and environmental factors that might increase risk for laminitis and counsel client regarding appropriate avoidance strategies.

- Promote a heightened level of physical activity for the patient (assuming laminitis is not present) and encourage maintenance of an exercise record.

- Help the owner obtain an accurate (calibrated scale at animal feed purveyor) or reasonably accurate (weight tape method) weight for the horse and determine an optimal weight to target after institution of both exercise and dietary strategies. Urge serial measurements of the patient's weight to evaluate progress.

- Record a primary evaluation of the patient's body condition and adiposity. Assess the patient's body condition score. Show the client how to measure the patient's neck circumference, height, and girth. Encourage the client to record these measurements on a regular basis.

- Undertake primary and follow-up endocrinologic evaluation of the patient to characterize insulin sensitivity (and to test for PPID, when appropriate). Serial endocrine testing might simply entail measurement of circulating insulin and glucose concentrations (using the same laboratory and ensuring that the samples are acquired as described earlier). Repeated testing will help to evaluate patient's responsiveness to instituted management strategies and owner's compliance.

- Obtain primary objective evaluation of the patient's feet (especially the forefeet). These objective evaluations may include photographs of the gross appearance of the hoof (including dorsal, lateral, and solar views) and radiographs (especially a carefully aligned lateromedial view).

- Provide specific guidance regarding the need for obesity reversal and minimizing NSC intake. Discuss the avoidance of grain, sweet feed, sugary treats, alfalfa, and pasture grazing. Consider obtaining specialist veterinary nutrition input. Obtain objective data for (especially) the nutritional quality of forage (NSC content in hay). Urge objective approach to feeding EMS-affected horses, including actually weighing the food to be provided. As a general rule, small quantities should be fed frequently, and providing infrequent large meals should be avoided. Sensitize the client to times of the year when environmental circumstances are such that the NSC content of pasture grass may be dangerously high.

- If avoiding pasture grazing is impossible, counsel the client regarding safer pasture management strategies that may help reduce the quantity of ingested grass or the NSC content of available grazing pastures (http://www.safergrass.com).

- Help the client develop a program of ongoing vigilance and monitoring of patients to prevent obesity and maintain good glycemic and insulinemic control.

micronutrients magnesium oxide and chromium picolinate has been recommended for promoting insulin sensitivity, evidence is not convincing that these products are helpful for managing EMS-affected equids.

Pharmacologic Strategies for the Management of Refractory Equine Metabolic Syndrome

Oral treatment using levothyroxine sodium seems to be helpful in managing refractory cases of obesity and EMS.[72–74] A favorable response to this treatment approach should not be used to justify a diagnosis of hypothyroidism, and the client and horse should not be subjected to life-long dependence on this medication. Recently, interest has been shown in the use of the biguanide, metformin, for treatment of EMS. Although some preliminary studies have reported a positive response after administration of metformin to EMS horses, much remains to be learned of the drug's pharmacokinetics and safety in the equine species.[75–77] EMS occurs in some older horses that are also affected with PPID.[70,71] If patients with EMS are concomitantly affected with PPID, treatment for PPID using low-dose pergolide (0.5–3.0 mg/d, orally, per 450 kg horse) should be instituted.[70]

WHAT CAN THE VETERINARIAN DO TO HELP OWNERS OF HORSES WITH EQUINE METABOLIC SYNDROME?

Specific aspects of the veterinarian's role in the management of EMS-affected horses and ponies are listed in **Box 1**.

REFERENCES

1. Belknap JK, Moore JN, Crouser EC. Sepsis-From human organ failure to laminar failure. Vet Immunol Immunopathol 2009;129(3–4):155–7.
2. Loftus JP, Johnson PJ, Belknap JK, et al. Leukocyte-derived and endogenous matrix metalloproteinases in the lamellae of horses with naturally acquired and experimentally induced laminitis. Vet Immunol Immunopathol 2009;129(3-4): 221–30.
3. Moore JN, Belknap JK. You say lamellae, I say laminae. Let's call. An overview of the Havemeyer workshop on laminitis pathophysiology. Vet Immunol Immunopathol 2009;129(3–4):149–50.
4. Bailey SR, Adair HS, Reinemeyer CR, et al. Plasma concentrations of endotoxin and platelet activation in the developmental stage of oligofructose-induced laminitis. Vet Immunol Immunopathol 2009;129(3–4):167–73.
5. Budak MT, Orsini JA, Pollitt CC, et al. Gene expression in the lamellar dermis-epidermis during the developmental phase of carbohydrate overload-induced laminitis in the horse. Vet Immunol Immunopathol 2009;131(1–2):86–96.
6. Geor R, Frank N. Metabolic syndrome-From human organ disease to laminar failure in equids. Vet Immunol Immunopathol 2009;129(3–4):151–4.
7. Pleasant RS, Thatcher C. Prevention of pasture-associated laminitis. In: Robinson NE, Sprayberry KA, editors. Current therapy in equine medicine. 6th edition. St Louis (MO): Saunders, Elsevier; 2009. p. 547–9.
8. Johnson PJ, Messer NT, Ganjam VK. Cushing's syndromes, insulin resistance and endocrinopathic laminitis. Equine Vet J 2004;36(3):194–8.
9. Johnson PJ, Messer NT, Slight SH, et al. Endocrinopathic laminitis in the horse. Clin Tech Equine Pract 2004;3(1):45–56.

10. Haffner JC, Eiler H, Hoffman RM, et al. Effect of a single dose of dexamethasone on glucose homeostasis in healthy horses by using the combined intravenous glucose and insulin test. J Anim Sci 2009;87(1):131–5.

11. Tiley HA, Geor RJ, McCutcheon LJ. Effects of dexamethasone on glucose dynamics and insulin sensitivity in healthy horses. Am J Vet Res 2007;68(7):753–9.

12. Geor RJ. Pasture-associated laminitis. Vet Clin North Am Equine Pract 2009; 25(1):39–50.

13. Carter RA, Treiber KH, Geor RJ, et al. Prediction of incipient pasture-associated laminitis from hyperinsulinaemia, hyperleptinaemia and generalised and localised obesity in a cohort of ponies. Equine Vet J 2009;41(2):171–8.

14. Usda-Nahms. Lameness and laminitis in US horses (monograph). In: United States Department of Agriculture National Animal Health Monitoring System. April 2000. #N318.0400.

15. Hinckley K, Henderson I. The epidemiology of equine laminitis in the UK. Warwick (UK): 35th Congress of the British Equine Veterinary Association; 1996. p. 62.

16. Tóth F, Frank N, Elliott SB, et al. Effects of an intravenous endotoxin challenge on glucose and insulin dynamics in horses. Am J Vet Res 2008;69(1):82–8.

17. Zhou MS, Schulman IH, Raij L. Vascular inflammation, insulin resistance, and endothelial dysfunction in salt-sensitive hypertension: role of nuclear factor kappa B activation. J Hypertens 2010;28(3):527–35.

18. Kalck KA, Frank N, Elliott SB, et al. Effects of low-dose oligofructose treatment administered via nasogastric intubation on induction of laminitis and associated alterations in glucose and insulin dynamics in horses. Am J Vet Res 2009; 70(5):624–32.

19. Johnson PJ. Equine metabolic syndrome ("Peripheral Cushing's Syndrome"). Vet Clin North Am Equine Pract 2002;18:271–93.

20. Frank N, Geor RJ, Bailey SR, et al. Equine Metabolic Syndrome. J Vet Intern Med 2010 Apr 2. [Epub ahead of print].

21. Robinson LE, Graham TE. Metabolic syndrome, a cardiovascular disease risk factor: role of adipocytokines and impact of diet and physical activity. Can J Appl Physiol 2004;29(6):808–29.

22. Kronfeld DS, Treiber KH, Hess TM, et al. Metabolic syndrome in healthy ponies facilitates nutritional countermeasures against pasture laminitis. J Nutr 2006; 136(Suppl 7):2090S–3S.

23. Treiber KH, Kronfeld DS, Hess TM, et al. Evaluation of genetic and metabolic predispositions and nutritional risk factors for pasture-associated laminitis in ponies. J Am Vet Med Assoc 2006;228(10):1538–45.

24. Longland AC, Byrd BM. Pasture nonstructural carbohydrates and equine laminitis. J Nutr 2006;136:2099S–102S.

25. Longland AC. Starch, sugar and fructans: what are they and how important are they in diets for horses? In: Harris PA, Hill SJ, Elliott J, et al, editors. The latest findings in laminitis research. The first WALTHAM-Royal Veterinary College Laminitis Conference. Suffolk (UK): Equine Veterinary Journal Limited; 2007. p. 7–14.

26. Vick MM, Adams AA, Murphy BA, et al. Relationships among inflammatory cytokines, obesity, and insulin sensitivity in the horse. J Anim Sci 2007;85(5):1144–55.

27. Vick MM, Murphy BA, Sessions DR, et al. Effects of systemic inflammation on insulin sensitivity in horses and inflammatory cytokine expression in adipose tissue. Am J Vet Res 2008;69(1):130–9.

28. Bailey SR, Habershon-Butcher JL, Ransom KJ, et al. Hypertension and insulin resistance in a mixed-breed population of ponies predisposed to laminitis. Am J Vet Res 2008;69(1):122–9.

29. Rugh KS, Garner HE, Sprouse RF, et al. Left ventricular hypertrophy in chronically hypertensive ponies. Lab Anim Sci 1987;37:335–8.
30. Buff PR, Johnson PJ, Wiedmeyer CE, et al. Modulation of leptin, insulin, and growth hormone in obese pony mares under chronic nutritional restriction and supplementation with ractopamine hydrochloride. Vet Ther 2006;7(1): 64–72.
31. Alford P, Geller S, Richrdson B, et al. A multicenter, matched case-control study of risk factors for equine laminitis. Prev Vet Med 2001;49(3–4):209–22.
32. Jeffcott LB, Field JR, McLean JG, et al. Glucose tolerance and insulin sensitivity in ponies and Standardbred horses. Equine Vet J 1986;18(2):97–101.
33. Field JR, Jeffcott LB. Equine laminitis—another hypothesis for pathogenesis. Med Hypotheses 1989;30(3):203–10.
34. Henneke DR, Potter GD, Kreider JL, et al. Relationship between condition score, physical measurements and body fat percentage in mares. Equine Vet J 1983; 15(4):371–2.
35. Carter RA, Geor RJ, Burton Staniar W, et al. Apparent adiposity assessed by standardized scoring systems and morphometric measurements in horses and ponies. Vet J 2009;179(2):204–10.
36. Johnson PJ, Messer NT, Ganjam VK, et al. Pregnancy-associated laminitis in mares. J Equine Vet Sci 2009;29(1):42–6.
37. Johnson PJ, Ganjam VK, Messer NT, et al. The obesity paradigm: an introduction to the emerging discipline of adipobiology. Presented at 52nd Annual Convention of the American Association of Equine Practitioners. San Antonio (TX), December 2–6, 2006.
38. Johnson PJ, Slight SH, Ganjam VK, et al. Glucocorticoids and laminitis in the horse. Vet Clin North Am Equine Pract 2002;18:219–36.
39. Pass MA, Pollitt S, Pollitt CC. Decreased glucose metabolism causes separation of hoof lamellae in vitro: a trigger for laminitis? Equine Vet J Suppl 1998;26:133–8.
40. Asplin KE, McGowan CM, Pollitt CC, et al. Role of insulin in glucose uptake in the equine hoof [abstract]. J Vet Intern Med 2007;21:668.
41. Poitout V, Robertson RP. Minireview: secondary beta-cell failure in type 2 diabetes—a convergence of glucotoxicity and lipotoxicity. Endocrinology 2002; 143:339–42.
42. Kim JK, Montagnani M, Koh KK, et al. Reciprocal relationships between insulin resistance and endothelial dysfunction: molecular and pathophysiological mechanisms. Circulation 2006;113:1888–904.
43. Spinler SA. Challenges associated with metabolic syndrome. Pharmacotherapy 2006;26(12 Pt 2):209S–17S.
44. Eades SC, Stokes AM, Johnson PJ, et al. Serial alterations in digital hemodynamics and endothelin-1 immunoreactivity, platelet-neutrophil aggregation, and concentrations of nitric oxide, insulin glucose obtained from horses following carbohydrate overload. Am J Vet Res 2007;68:87–94.
45. Asplin KE, Sillence MN, Pollitt CC, et al. Induction of laminitis by prolonged hyperinsulinaemia in clinically normal ponies. Vet J 2007;174(3):530–5.
46. Nourian AR, Asplin KE, McGowan CM, et al. Equine laminitis: ultrastructural lesions detected in ponies following hyperinsulinaemia. Equine Vet J 2009; 41(7):671–7.
47. Mora S, Pessin JE. An adipocentric view of signaling and intracellular trafficking. Diabetes Metab Res Rev 2002;18:345–56.
48. Trayhurn P, Beattie JH. Physiological role of adipose tissue: white adipose tissue as an endocrine and secretory organ. Proc Nutr Soc 2001;60:329–39.

49. Hotamisligal GS, Shargill NS, Spiegelman BM. Adipose expression of tumor necrosis factor-alpha: direct role in obesity-linked insulin resistance. Science 1993;259:87–91.

50. Matsuzawa Y. The role of fat topology in the risk of disease. Int J Obes (Lond) 2008;32(Suppl 7):S83–92.

51. Weisberg SP, McCann D, Desai M. Obesity is associated with macrophage accumulation in adipose tissue. J Clin Invest 2003;112:1796–808.

52. Xu H, Barnes GT, Yang Q, et al. Chronic inflammation in fat plays a crucial role in the development of obesity-related insulin resistance. J Clin Invest 2003;112:1821–30.

53. Treiber K, Carter R, Gay L, et al. Inflammatory and redox status of ponies with a history of pasture-associated laminitis. Vet Immunol Immunopathol 2009;129:216–20.

54. Masuzaki H, Paterson J, Shinyama H, et al. A transgenic model of visceral obesity and the metabolic syndrome. Science 2001;294:2166–70.

55. Seckl JR, Walker BR. Minireview: 11beta-hydroxysteroid dehydrogenase type 1—a tissue specific amplifier of glucocorticoid action. Endocrinol 2001;142:1371–6.

56. Rask E, Olsson T, Soderberg S, et al. Tissue specific dysregulation of cortisol metabolism in human obesity. J Clin Endocrinol Metab 2001;86:1418–21.

57. Kotelevtsev Y, Holmes MC, Burchell A, et al. 11beta-hydroxysteroid dehydrogenase type 1 knockout mice show attenuated glucocorticoid inducible responses and resist hyperglycemia on obesity or stress. Proc Natl Acad Sci U S A 1997;94:14924–9.

58. Boden G. Role of fatty acids in the pathogenesis of insulin resistance and NIDDM. Diabetes 1997;46:3–10.

59. Reyna SM, Ghosh S, Tantiwong P, et al. Elevated toll-like receptor 4 expression and signaling in muscle from insulin-resistant subjects. Diabetes 2008;57(10):2595–602.

60. Hotamisligil GS, Spiegelman BM. Tumor necrosis factor alpha: a key component in the obesity-diabetes link. Diabetes 1994;43:1271–8.

61. Harris P, Geor RJ. Primer on dietary carbohydrates and utility of the glycemic index in equine nutrition. Vet Clin North Am Equine Pract 2009;25(1):23–37.

62. Watts KA. Forage and pasture management for laminitic horses. Clin Tech Equine Pract 2004;3:88–95.

63. Treiber KH, Kronfeld DS, Hess TM, et al. Use of proxies and reference quintiles obtained from minimal model analysis for determination of insulin sensitivity and pancreatic beta-cell responsiveness in horses. Am J Vet Res 2005;66(12):2114–21.

64. Rijnen KE, van der Kolk JH. Determination of reference range values indicative of glucose metabolism and insulin resistance by use of glucose clamp techniques in horses and ponies. Am J Vet Res 2003;64(10):1260–4.

65. Firshman AM, Valberg SJ. Factors affecting clinical assessment of insulin sensitivity in horses. Equine Vet J 2007;39(6):567–75.

66. Eiler H, Frank N, Andrews FM, et al. Physiologic assessment of blood glucose homeostasis via combined intravenous glucose and insulin testing in horses. Am J Vet Res 2005;66(9):1598–604.

67. Wiedmeyer CE, Johnson PJ, Cohn LA, et al. Evaluation of a continuous glucose monitoring system for use in dogs, cats, and horses. J Am Vet Med Assoc 2003;223(7):987–92.

68. Wiedmeyer CE, Johnson PJ, Cohn LA, et al. Evaluation of a continuous glucose monitoring system for use in veterinary medicine. Diabetes Technol Ther 2005;7(6):885–95.

69. Donaldson MT, Jorgensen AJ, Beech J. Evaluation of suspected pituitary pars intermedia dysfunction in horses with laminitis. J Am Vet Med Assoc 2004; 224(7):1123–7.
70. Messer NT 4th, Johnson PJ. Evidence-based literature pertaining to thyroid dysfunction and Cushing's syndrome in the horse. Vet Clin North Am Equine Pract 2007;23(2):329–64.
71. McGowan CM, Frost R, Pfeiffer DU, et al. Serum insulin concentrations in horses with equine Cushing's syndrome: response to a cortisol inhibitor and prognostic value. Equine Vet J 2004;36(3):295–8.
72. Frank N, Sommardahl CS, Eiler H, et al. Effects of oral administration of levothyroxine sodium on concentrations of plasma lipids, concentration and composition of very-low-density lipoproteins, and glucose dynamics in healthy adult mares. Am J Vet Res 2005;66:1032–8.
73. Frank N, Elliott SB, Boston RC. Effects of long-term oral administration of levothyroxine sodium on glucose dynamics in healthy adult horses. Am J Vet Res 2008; 69:76–81.
74. Frank N, Buchanan BR, Elliott SB. Effects of long-term oral administration of levothyroxine sodium on serum thyroid hormone concentrations, clinicopathologic variables, and echocardiographic measurements in healthy adult horses. Am J Vet Res 2008;69:68–75.
75. Vick MM, Sessions DR, Murphy BA, et al. Obesity is associated with altered metabolic and reproductive activity in the mare: effects of metformin on insulin sensitivity and reproductive cyclicity. Reprod Fertil Dev 2006;18(6):609–17.
76. Durham AE, Rendle DI, Newton JE. The effect of metformin on measurements of insulin sensitivity and beta cell response in 18 horses and ponies with insulin resistance. Equine Vet J 2008;40(5):493–500.
77. Hustace JL, Firshman AM, Mata JE. Pharmacokinetics and bioavailability of metformin in horses. Am J Vet Res 2009;70(5):665–8.
78. Pajak B, Orzechowska S, Pijet B, et al. Crossroads of cytokine signaling—the chase to stop muscle cachexia. J Physiol Pharmacol 2008;59(Suppl 9):251–64.
79. Waitt LH, Cebra CK. Characterization of hypertriglyceridemia and response to treatment with insulin in horses, ponies, and donkeys: 44 cases (1995–2005). J Am Vet Med Assoc 2009;234(7):915–9.
80. Powell DM, Reedy SE, Sessions DR, et al. Effect of short-term exercise training on insulin sensitivity in obese and lean mares. Equine Vet J Suppl 2002;34:81–4.
81. Geor RJ, Harris P. Dietary management of obesity and insulin resistance: countering risk for laminitis. Vet Clin North Am Equine Pract 2009;25(1):51–65.
82. King C, Mansmann RA. Preventing laminitis in horses: dietary strategies for horse owners. Clin Tech Equine Pract 2004;3:96–102.

Hyperinsulinemic Laminitis

Melody A. de Laat, BVSc(Hons)[a],*,
Catherine M. McGowan, BVSc, MACVSc, PhD, FHEA, MRCVS[b],
Martin N. Sillence, PhD[c], Christopher C. Pollitt, BVSc, PhD[a,d]

KEYWORDS

• Hyperinsulinemia • Equine • Laminitis • Insulin resistance

An association between insulin resistance (IR) and the development of laminitis was first documented in the 1980s[1] and many subsequent studies have substantiated a link between hyperinsulinemia and laminitis.[2–4] Endocrine disorders such as equine Cushing's disease (ECD) and equine metabolic syndrome have been consistently implicated as risk factors for the development of IR, which is defined as a decline in the sensitivity of the tissues to the metabolic effects of insulin. The hyperinsulinemia in these conditions has been correlated with lamellar dysfunction.[4] Laminitis is commonly[5] associated with the ingestion of pastures with high starch, fructan, and sugar content with IR shown to play a role in this pasture-associated form of laminitis.[3,6] These nutritional risk factors promote obesity, and a reduction in insulin sensitivity has been shown to occur in obese horses when compared with those that are nonobese.[7] The term prelaminitic metabolic syndrome has been adopted to describe those equids with a phenotype of IR and obesity that are at an increased risk of developing laminitis.[8] Thus, dysregulated cortisol metabolism (secondary to ECD or iatrogenic corticosteroid administration), obesity, and a phenotypic or a genetic predisposition all appear to be significant predisposing factors for hyperinsulinemic laminitis, especially when combined with a significant glucose challenge. However, laminitis has also been induced experimentally in insulin-sensitive ponies[9] and horses[10] using prolonged insulin infusions to produce hyperinsulinemia, suggesting that insulin, as opposed to IR, may in fact be responsible for lamellar disease. The

---

This work was supported by The Rural Industries Research and Development Corporation, Australia.

[a] Australian Equine Laminitis Research Unit, School of Veterinary Science, The University of Queensland, Gatton, Queensland 4343, Australia
[b] Faculty of Health and Life Sciences, School of Veterinary Science, University of Liverpool, Leahurst CH64 7TE, UK
[c] Faculty of Science and Technology, Queensland University of Technology, Brisbane, Queensland 4001, Australia
[d] The Laminitis Institute, University of Pennsylvania School of Veterinary Medicine, New Bolton Center, Kennett Square, PA 19348, USA
* Corresponding author.
E-mail address: m.delaat@uq.edu.au

Vet Clin Equine 26 (2010) 257–264
doi:10.1016/j.cveq.2010.04.003
0749-0739/10/$ – see front matter © 2010 Elsevier Inc. All rights reserved.

mechanism by which hyperinsulinemia causes lamellar failure is not understood yet, and this is the current focus of the investigations in our laboratory.

NEW MODEL FOR STUDYING HYPERINSULINEMIC LAMINITIS

Restrospective analyses of cases of insulin-associated laminitis have advanced our understanding of the processes by which this disease occurs. Indeed, studies have successfully used serum and plasma insulin concentrations as predictive[11] and prognostic[2] indicators for ponies at risk of developing laminitis. The ability to accurately predict laminitis is essential for improving our capacity to prevent this debilitating disease and thus reduce its incidence. Although prevention is now feasible for many equids with known risk factors, an effective treatment for insulin-induced laminitis remains elusive. The development of such a treatment may be informed by a better understanding of the underlying pathophysiological processes that result in the final lesion. The inability to diagnose hyperinsulinemic laminitis until it is clinically overt has meant that early pathological change occurring in the prodromal stages of lamellar failure has not been described. Now, with the development of a model to reliably induce laminitis in ponies and horses,[10] researchers can focus on examining the pathophysiological events that occur throughout the disease process.

The model uses the euglycemic, hyperinsulinemic clamp (EHC) technique[12] to induce prolonged hyperinsulinemia with a constant rate, insulin infusion of 6 mIU/kgBW/min while maintaining blood glucose values at 5 ± 1 mM with a variable rate glucose infusion.[9] The clamp procedure produced mean serum insulin concentrations of more than 1000 µIU/mL in both ponies[9] and horses,[10] and although we have observed insulin concentrations in this range naturally in some ponies, they are substantially higher than those seen in most field cases of insulin-associated laminitis. However, Obel grade 2[13] laminitis developed after only 48 hours of this marked hyperinsulinemia in horses, which suggests that perhaps the model is an accelerated version of naturally occurring disease. The threshold for the onset of insulin-associated laminitis is unknown and most probably is quite variable among individuals and dependent on risk factors such as preexisting disease, obesity, and genetic predisposition. Development of the model to allow for manipulation of the mean serum insulin concentration reached during the clamp may improve our understanding of this complex issue and help in identifying a pathogenic threshold that significantly increases the risk for developing laminitis.

A significant feature of the model is its ability to induce laminitis in horses and ponies with normal insulin sensitivity; mean M-to-I ratio (ie, the amount of glucose metabolised per unit of insulin) (10^{-6}) is 3.07 ± 0.17 in horses and 3.5 ± 1.1 in ponies.[9,10] This is in direct contrast to our previous understanding that tissue resistance to insulin is *required* for horses to develop insulin-associated laminitis, or indeed our earlier hypothesis that laminitis was somehow caused by a failure of insulin action, for example a failure to stimulate glucose uptake in the hoof. Some degree of caution is required here, as insulin sensitivity was measured only at the beginning of the clamp procedure, and so in theory, some degree of tissue resistance to insulin could have developed during the infusion without being observed. However, given the rapid rate of induction of laminitis in our experiments, it is more likely that it is not the insensitivity of the tissues to insulin that causes laminitis, but rather a toxic effect of excessive insulin on lamellar tissues. In fact, lack of IR in these horses could have left them more susceptible to damage by the excessive circulating insulin concentrations. Interestingly, in the pony study, the most insulin-sensitive subject was the first to develop laminitis,[9] which may support this contention. Regardless of how closely the model mimics naturally occurring, insulin-associated laminitis, it does provide us with a clear link between hyperinsulinemia and laminitis and will be pivotal in augmenting our understanding of the pathophysiology.

INSULIN-MEDIATED LAMELLAR LESION

There are few detailed histopathological descriptions of cases of endocrinopathic laminitis. Hypercortisolemia has been reported to cause nonpainful lengthening of the primary and secondary epidermal lamellae (SEL) with a progressive separation of the lamellar basement membrane (BM) from the dermis of the pedal bone.[14] Basement membrane separation has also been documented 48 hours after induction of laminitis with carbohydrate,[15] oligofructose,[16] and hyperinsulinemia.[10] In addition to BM separation at the tips of the SEL, the hyperinsulinemic lamellar lesion is characterized by lengthening and attenuation of the SEL, rounding of the basal cell nuclei, and distortion of the normal architecture.[10] Interestingly, in experimentally induced hyperinsulinemic laminitis in ponies, BM degradation was mild[17]; and this may be attributable to their lower body weight when compared with horses.

PATHOPHYSIOLOGY OF HYPERINSULINEMIC LAMINITIS

Many theories on the pathogenesis of hyperinsulinemic laminitis have been proposed, including metabolic and vascular disturbances, inflammatory processes, and enzymatic degradation, and it is likely that more than one of these theories plays some role in the complicated disease process. Indeed, most of the individual theories can be interrelated to some degree, but the exact contribution and importance of these separate processes remains difficult to unravel. Insulin is an important metabolic and vascular hormone and as such, 2 major areas of focus for researching the pathogenesis of hyperinsulinemic laminitis include examining how hyperinsulinemia and IR affect glucose metabolism and vascular dynamics within the hoof.

Alterations in Glucose Metabolism

Studies in vitro have shown that the lamellae have a high requirement for glucose and that dermo-epidermal separation occurs when equine lamellar explants are incubated in the absence of glucose.[18,19] Furthermore, studies comparing the arterial and digital venous circulation have reported high levels of glucose uptake by hoof tissues.[20] This supports the suggestion that IR may interfere with GLUT-4–mediated glucose uptake in the hoof, thereby promoting lamellar separation and collapse. This idea can be further supported by a study that showed diminished immunolocalization of GLUT-4 receptors in lamellar tissue sections from laminitic horses.[21] However, this reliance on insulin-dependent glucose transport is not a feature of the integument in general[20] and raises the question of whether the lamellar tissue is a site for peripheral IR. The study by Mobasheri and colleagues[21] also found abundant expression of GLUT-1 receptors in the lamellae of normal horses and that GLUT-1 expression was substantially reduced in laminitic horses when compared with normal controls. Similarly, studies in vitro have shown that insulin does not affect glucose uptake by lamellar tissue.[22] These studies also confirmed the strong presence of GLUT-1 receptors in lamellar tissue,[22] suggesting that glucose uptake by the lamellae is likely to be largely insulin independent. Thus, a failure of glucose uptake by lamellar tissue during laminitis seems less feasible but remains a possibility if GLUT-1 transporters are reduced during laminitis. Further work on glucose utilization during laminitis is required.

Glucose uptake in vascular endothelial cells is also insulin independent, so local intracellular and extracellular glucose concentrations are similar.[20] This may predispose the tissue to glucose toxicity under circumstances of increased glucose delivery during hyperglycemia.[23] Microvascular studies in type 2 diabetic individuals have demonstrated that glucotoxicity increases vascular permeability, super oxide production, and adhesion molecule expression,[24] while glycosylation of normal cell proteins in vascular endothelial cells produces advanced glycation endproducts (AGEs).[25] The resultant cellular lipid peroxidation and release of reactive oxygen species (ROS)[26] may contribute to changes in vascular permeability and barrier dysfunction in diabetes, although the exact mechanism of glucotoxic endotheliopathy is poorly understood.[27] Although hyperglycemia is not often detected in insulin-resistant horses, and pancreatic shut down leading to diabetes is an uncommon equine disease, glucotoxicity could still play a part in lamellar failure. The onset of laminitis is often associated with a significant glucose challenge, for example following excessive sugar-rich pasture consumption, and this glucose load may be involved in the pathogenesis of hyperinsulinemic laminitis. The tight association between insulin and glucose, with hyperglycemia inevitably resulting in hyperinsulinemia, makes interpretation of existing data difficult and does not help to differentiate between an insulin or glucose cause.

Further work on the possibility of glucose overload and toxicity occurring in the lamellae of horses suffering from hyperinsulinemic laminitis is important. Glucose delivery to the lamellar region for uptake by the tissues may be affected by vascular dysfunction in the digital circulation and determining changes in blood flow to the lamellar tissue during hyperinsulinemic laminitis is another important step in understanding the pathogenesis.

Vascular Dysfunction

In addition to its metabolic actions, insulin is an important vasomediator. Overall, insulin's ability to influence blood flow relies on tight modulation of the release of nitric oxide (NO), a vasodilator, and endothelin-1 (ET-1), a vasoconstrictor, via the PI3-K and MAP-K insulin signaling pathways, respectively.[28] The principal vascular function of insulin is probably vasodilation, which it achieves by stimulating the production of NO by endothelial cells under physiological conditions. The consistently elevated hoof wall surface temperature (HWST) seen in insulin-sensitive, treated horses during the EHC[10] could be a result of insulin-mediated vasodilation via this NO pathway. The vascular actions of insulin are also thought to be coupled with insulin-mediated glucose disposal in skeletal muscle[29] with NO-mediated vasodilation promoting an increase in glucose delivery and hence an increase in glucose uptake. Potentially, vasodilation of digital vessels during hyperinsulinemic laminitis may increase the delivery of glucose and other potentially laminitogenic substances to the hoof. Data from naturally occurring cases of hyperinsulinemic laminitis, or pasture-associated cases is limited, although one study on a closed herd of ponies found that HWST was elevated in ponies that were prone to laminitis when compared with ponies that had never had laminitis.[11] However, these data were obtained using single measurements in an environment where ambient temperature was uncontrolled. Further studies on HWST or other indicators of digital vascular dynamics in field cases of insulin-associated laminitis are required.

Conversely, studies in lean, obese, and diabetic human patients have shown that the main metabolic pathway, the PI3-K signaling pathway, can become insulin resistant, while the MAP-K pathway controlling cell growth and gene expression functions normally.[30] This may suggest that in insulin-resistant horses, vasodilation in response to insulin action may be impaired and the balance pushed more toward vasoconstriction secondary to ET-1 release via the MAP-K pathway. In humans, an increase in the release of vasoconstrictors including ET-1 occurs secondary to endothelial dysfunction[31] and hyperinsulinemia,[32] with a resultant decrease in endothelial-dependent vasodilation.[33] A decline in NO concentration, either through reduced production or an increase in breakdown by ROS, can have severe consequences for endothelial health including impaired vasodilation, platelet and leucocyte aggregation, and vascular inflammation.[34] Digital vasoconstriction secondary to increased ET-1 release may occur in insulin-resistant horses, which in turn could lead to lamellar hypoxia, coagulopathies, endothelial dysfunction, and superoxide production secondary to ischemia and reperfusion. However, this theory is not supported by the elevated HWST that was seen during the induction of insulin-induced laminitis.[10] Findings from a recent EHC study on obese and lean human patients do not support the presumption that hyperinsulinemia associated with insulin resistance primarily augments ET-1–mediated vasoconstriction.[35] Instead, these authors postulated that insulin fails to activate the NO pathway during IR states, which results in reduced suppression and thus increased action of ET-1. Furthermore, human patients with insulinoma have been shown to have normal ET-1 levels.[36] The impedance of vascular and metabolic responses to insulin in insulin-resistant states is reported to be related to the degree of IR[37] and if true for horses these findings may mean that enhanced insulin-mediated glucose disposal secondary to increased perfusion is possible and may also explain why insulin-sensitive horses succumbed to laminitis after just 48 hours of hyperinsulinemia.[10] Perhaps the insulin-resistant state actually provides the lamellar structure with some protection against the effects of insulin in naturally occurring disease and may explain why many equids are able to be hyperinsulinemic and free from laminitis.

Hyperinsulinemia can also promote the development of a procoagulant state by interfering with the normally antithrombotic surface of endothelial cells and promoting platelet activation.[38] The synthesis of proinflammatory and prothrombotic molecules occurs via the MAP-K pathway,[39] which, as previously mentioned, appears to be unaffected during IR. Hyperinsulinemia also causes a reduction in the aggregating properties of platelets via an NO-mediated mechanism and a reduction in platelet function is evident in IR humans.[40] Increased platelet aggregation has been documented in the prodromal stages of alimentary laminitis, which may initiate clotting in the lamellar microcirculation and promote the diversion of blood away from the digital microcirculation through arteriovenous anastomoses shunts.[41] Similar events have not been documented to occur during hyperinsulinemic laminitis at this stage, but further investigation into vascular homeostasis in cases of insulin-induced laminitis in both insulin-resistant and insulin-sensitive individuals is necessary.

SUMMARY

Although significant advances in understanding the importance of IR and an appreciation of the direct correlation of hyperinsulinemia with laminitis have been made in recent years, our ability to fully describe the pathogenic processes involved and therefore provide adequate treatment, remains limited. However, with a new model available to actively examine the complex metabolic and vascular mechanisms underlying the disease process and the potential for more accurate quantification of the threshold for the onset of disease in insulin-sensitive and resistant individuals, significant progress in the near future is likely. At present, although much work in this area continues, preventive strategies to avoid the development of and careful management of existing cases of hyperinsulinemia remains our best approach to managing the unique problem of hyperinsulinemic laminitis.

REFERENCES

1. Coffman JR, Colles CM. Insulin tolerance in laminitis ponies. Can J Comp Med 1983;47:347–51.
2. McGowan CM, Frost R, Pfeiffer DU, et al. Serum insulin concentrations in horses with equine Cushing's syndrome: response to a cortisol inhibitor and prognostic value. Equine Vet J 2004;36:295–8.
3. Treiber KH, Kronfeld DS, Hess TM, et al. Evaluation of genetic and metabolic predispositions and nutritional risk factors for pasture-associated laminitis in ponies. J Am Vet Med Assoc 2006;228:1538–45.
4. Walsh DM, McGowan CM, McGowan T, et al. Correlation of plasma insulin concentration with laminitis score in a field study of equine Cushing's disease and equine metabolic syndrome. J Equine Vet Sci 2009;29:87–94.
5. USDA. In: System NAHM, editor. Lameness and laminitis in US horses. APHIS:VS, CEAH. Fort Collins (CO): USDA; 2000.
6. Bailey SR, Habershon-Butcher JL, Ransom KJ, et al. Hypertension and insulin resistance in a mixed-breed population of ponies predisposed to laminitis. Am J Vet Res 2008;69:122–9.
7. Hoffman RM, Boston RC, Stefanovski D, et al. Obesity and diet affect glucose dynamics and insulin sensitivity in thoroughbred geldings. J Anim Sci 2003;81: 2333–42.
8. Kronfeld DS, Treiber KH, Hess TM, et al. Metabolic syndrome in healthy ponies facilitates nutritional countermeasures against pasture laminitis. J Nutr 2006; 136:2090S–3S.
9. Asplin KE, Sillence MN, Pollitt CC, et al. Induction of laminitis by prolonged hyper-insulinaemia in clinically normal ponies. Vet J 2007;174:530–5.
10. de Laat MA, McGowan CM, Sillence MN, et al. Equine laminitis: induced by 48 h hyperinsulinaemia in standardbred horses. Equine Vet J 2010;42:129–35.
11. Carter RA, Treiber KH, Geor RJ, et al. Prediction of incipient pasture-associated laminitis from hyperinsulinaemia, hyperleptinaemia and generalised and local-ised obesity in a cohort of ponies. Equine Vet J 2009;41:171–8.
12. DeFronzo RA, Tobin JD, Andres R. Glucose clamp technique: a method for quantifying insulin secretion and resistance. Am J Physiol 1979;237: E214–23.
13. Obel N. Studies on the histopathology of acute laminitis. [Dissertation] Almqvist and Wiksells Boktryckeri AB, Uppsala, Sweden 1948.
14. Johnson PJ, Slight SH, Ganjam VK, et al. Glucocorticoids and laminitis in the horse. Vet Clin North Am Equine Pract 2002;18:219–36.
15. Pollitt CC. Basement membrane pathology: a feature of acute equine laminitis. Equine Vet J 1996;28:38–46.
16. van Eps AW, Pollitt CC. Equine laminitis induced with oligofructose. Equine Vet J 2006;38:203–8.
17. Nourian AR, Asplin KE, McGowan CM, et al. Equine laminitis: ultrastructural lesions detected in ponies following hyperinsulinaemia. Equine Vet J 2009. DOI: 10.2746/042516409X407648.
18. French KR, Pollitt CC. Equine laminitis: glucose deprivation and MMP activation induce dermo-epidermal separation in vitro. Equine Vet J 2004;36:261–6.

19. Pass MA, Pollitt S, Pollitt CC. Decreased glucose metabolism causes separation of hoof lamellae in vitro: a trigger for laminitis? Equine Vet J 1998;26: 133–8.
20. Wattle O, Pollitt CC. Lamellar metabolism. Clin Tech Equine Pract 2004;3:22–33.
21. Mobasheri A, Critchlow K, Clegg PD, et al. Chronic equine laminitis is characterised by loss of GLUT1, GLUT4 and ENaC positive laminar keratinocytes. Equine Vet J 2004;36:248–54.
22. Asplin KE. Investigating the role of impaired glucose uptake and hyperinsulinaemia in endocrinopathic laminitis. Brisbane (Australia): The University of Queensland; 2009. School of Veterinary Science.
23. Jansson PA. Endothelial dysfunction in insulin resistance and type 2 diabetes. J Intern Med 2007;262:173–83.
24. Singer G, Granger DN. Inflammatory responses underlying the microvascular dysfunction associated with obesity and insulin resistance. Microcirculation 2007;14:375–87.
25. Uemura S, Matsushita H, Li W, et al. Diabetes mellitus enhances vascular matrix metalloproteinase activity: role of oxidative stress. Circ Res 2001;88: 1291–8.
26. Giugliano D, Ceriello A, Paolisso G. Oxidative stress and diabetic vascular complications. Diabetes Care 1996;19:257–67.
27. Yuan SY, Breslin JW, Perrin R, et al. Microvascular permeability in diabetes and insulin resistance. Microcirculation 2007;14:363–73.
28. Muniyappa R, Montagnani M, Koh KK, et al. Cardiovascular actions of insulin. Endocr Rev 2007;28:463–91.
29. Clerk LH, Vincent MA, Lindner JR, et al. The vasodilatory actions of insulin on resistance and terminal arterioles and their impact on muscle glucose uptake. Diabetes Metab Res Rev 2004;20:3–12.
30. Cusi K, Maezono K, Osman A, et al. Insulin resistance differentially affects the PI3-kinase- and MAP kinase-mediated signalling in human muscle. J Clin Invest 2000;105:311–20.
31. Shankar P, Sundarka M. Metabolic syndrome: its pathogenesis and management. J Indian Acad Clin Med 2003;4:275–81.
32. Kim JA, Montagnani M, Koh KK, et al. Reciprocal relationships between insulin resistance and endothelial dysfunction—molecular and pathophysiological mechanisms. Circulation 2006;113:1888–904.
33. Reaven G. The metabolic syndrome or the insulin resistance syndrome? Different names, different concepts, and different goals. Endocrinol Metab Clin North Am 2004;33:283–303.
34. Imrie H, Abbas A, Kearney M. Insulin resistance, lipotoxicity and endothelial dysfunction. Biochim Biophys Acta 2010;1801:320–6.
35. Lteif AA, Fulford AD, Considine RV, et al. Hyperinsulinemia fails to augment ET-1 action in the skeletal muscle vascular bed in vivo in humans. Am J Physiol Endocrinol Metab 2008;295:E1510–7.
36. Piatti P, Monti LD, Conti M, et al. Hypertriglyceridemia and hyperinsulinemia are potent inducers of endothelin-1 release in humans. Diabetes 1996;45:316–21.
37. Mather K, Laakso M, Edelman S, et al. Evidence for physiological coupling of insulin-mediated glucose metabolism and limb blood flow. Am J Physiol Endocrinol Metab 2000;279:E1264–70.
38. Juhan-Vague I, Morange PE, Alessi MC. The insulin resistance syndrome: implications for thrombosis and cardiovascular disease. Pathophysiol Haemost Thromb 2002;32:269–73.

39. Anfossi G, Russo I, Doronzo G, et al. Contribution of insulin resistance to vascular dysfunction. Arch Physiol Biochem 2009;115:199–217.
40. Trovati M, Anfossi G. Influence of insulin and of insulin resistance on platelet and vascular smooth muscle cell function. J Diabetes Complications 2002;16:35–40.
41. Weiss DJ, Evanson OA, McClenahan D, et al. Evaluation of platelet activation and platelet-neutrophil aggregates in ponies with alimentary laminitis. Am J Vet Res 1997;58:1376–80.

Current Concepts on the Pathophysiology of Pasture-Associated Laminitis

Raymond J. Geor, BVSc, MVSc, PhD

KEYWORDS

• Laminitis • Nonstructural carbohydrates • Fructans
• Endotoxemia • Obesity • Insulin resistance • Hyperinsulinemia

Several disease conditions have been associated with laminitis, notably gastrointestinal disease (eg, surgical colic, colitis, duodenitis/proximal jejunitis), retained placenta or metritis, and severe infections (eg, pleuropneumonia).[1,2] However, survey studies have indicated that most laminitis cases occur in horses and ponies kept at pasture (hence the term *pasture-associated laminitis*).[3,4] In one survey in the United Kingdom, 61% of laminitis cases occurred in animals kept at pasture,[4] whereas the results of the 1998 National Animal Health Monitoring System (NAHMS) laminitis study showed that 46% of cases were associated with grazing on pasture.[3]

The mechanisms linking the consumption of pasture forage with development of lamellar failure have not been fully elucidated. Clinical cases of laminitis most often occur in conditions favoring accumulation of rapidly fermentable nonstructural carbohydrates (fructans, simple sugars, or starches) in grass and clover. Therefore, most believe that pasture laminitis is triggered by carbohydrate overload of the hindgut and the systemic absorption of substances that initiate lamellar failure.[1,2]

This hypothesis is supported by experimental studies in which laminitis is induced in healthy horses after the administration of large doses of oligofructose, a commercial fructan.[5] However, the extent to which this severe experimental model reflects events during development of naturally occurring laminitis is unknown, particularly considering the fact that only a very small proportion of any population develops pasture laminitis during periods of highest risk. Accordingly, recent research in this area has focused on reasons for the apparent increased susceptibility of certain horses and ponies, and evidence has emerged that animals with an insulin-resistant phenotype are at high risk for pasture-associated laminitis.[6–9] Moreover, the recent discovery that prolonged intravenous infusion of insulin induces laminitis in healthy animals

Department of Large Animal Clinical Sciences, D-202 Veterinary Medical Center, College of Veterinary Medicine, Michigan State University, East Lansing, MI 48824, USA
E-mail address: geor@cvm.msu.edu

Vet Clin Equine 26 (2010) 265–276
doi:10.1016/j.cveq.2010.06.001
0749-0739/10/$ – see front matter © 2010 Elsevier Inc. All rights reserved.

vetequine.theclinics.com

has widened the perspective on potential mechanisms that link ingestion of pasture forage to the development of laminitis.[10,11]

This article reviews current knowledge on the epidemiology and risk factors for pasture-associated laminitis, including the role of forage carbohydrates and meta-bolic/endocrine predispositions, and also discusses the pathophysiology of this condition.

EPIDEMIOLOGY AND RISK FACTORS

There have been few epidemiological studies and, as a consequence, knowledge of risk factors for pasture-associated laminitis is incomplete. Clinical observations indicate that pasture-induced laminitis often occurs at times of rapid grass growth and the accumulation of nonstructural carbohydrates in pasture forage, such as during the spring and early summer or after heavy rains. In support of these observations, the 1998 NAHMS survey of causes of lameness in horses reported that laminitis accounted for approximately 40% of foot problems in the spring and summer but only 20% of these problems in the winter.[3] Similarly, a 3-year retrospective study of pasture-kept horses and ponies in one region of the United Kingdom found the highest prevalence (2.39%) and incidence (16 cases/1000 animals) of laminitis in spring (May).[12] A statistically significant positive association between hours of sunshine and incident laminitis was also reported, but laminitis prevalence and incidence were not associated with regional rainfall or ambient temperature. The association between hours of sunshine and incident laminitis was presumed to reflect altered nutritional intake (ie, increased consumption of forage carbohydrates during periods of bright sunshine that promote plant photosynthesis and carbohydrate accumulation) rather than the direct effect of exposure of horses to sunlight.[12]

Another important aspect of pasture-associated laminitis is the clinical observation that certain horses or ponies tend to be affected more than others, with susceptible animals often prone to recurrent episodes.[6] This impression was supported by Katz and colleagues,[12] who reported that 35% of the animals diagnosed with laminitis had repeated episodes over the total study period, with many animals diagnosed multiple times within the same year. These observations suggest that phenotypic or genetic factors may confer susceptibility to laminitis. In this regard, experts now recognize that metabolic and endocrine factors, particularly obesity, insulin resistance, and hyperinsulinemia, are associated with increased risk of pasture laminitis.[7,8] Horses and ponies prone to pasture-associated laminitis, fitting the description of "easy keeper," are often overweight or obese (or have regional adiposity, such as a cresty neck), and may be persistently hyperinsulinemic.[7–9] The term *equine metabolic syndrome* (EMS) has been adopted to describe horses and ponies that exhibit generalized or regional adiposity, hyperinsulinemia, and subclinical (ie, hoof founder rings) or overt laminitis.[7–9,13–15]

Clinical observations linking insulin resistance and laminitis predisposition are supported by results of observational cohort studies in ponies. In an inbred herd of Welsh and Dartmoor ponies, the clustering of hyperinsulinemia, obesity, and hypertriglycer-idemia was associated with predisposition to pasture laminitis.[6] The term *prelaminitic metabolic syndrome* (PLMS) was used to describe the phenotype associated with laminitis risk. The PLMS criteria predicted 11 of 13 cases of clinical laminitis observed in May of the same year, with an odds ratio of 10.4 (ie, ponies with this insulin-resistant phenotype had an approximately 10-times higher risk for developing laminitis). A subsequent study of this population of ponies showed that the presence of general-ized or regional (cresty neck) obesity, hyperinsulinemia (insulin >32 mU/L when sampled on winter pasture), and hyperleptinemia (>7.3 ng/mL) were useful predictors of laminitis episodes when ponies were exposed to high-carbohydrate pasture.[13]

A study of outbred ponies in the United Kingdom confirmed the association between insulin resistance and predisposition to pasture laminitis, and provided evidence of hypertension in the high-risk ponies.[14] Signs of this metabolic syndrome (ie, insulin resistance and hypertension) were evident in summer but not winter, suggesting that environmental factors such as consumption of summer pasture forage affected expression of the phenotype.[14] In general, insulin sensitivity is markedly lower in ponies than in horse breeds,[6,16] potentially explaining the apparent higher susceptibility of pony breeds to pasture laminitis reported in some epidemiologic studies.[4,12]

Minimal published data are available on the possible association between insulin resistance and pasture-induced laminitis in horses. Nonetheless, the EMS phenotype has been described in many breeds, notably Morgans, Paso Finos, Arabians, and Norwegian Fjords,[7,9] and many of these horses are out on pasture when laminitis is first detected.[15] Insulin resistance may also contribute to laminitis predisposition in pituitary pars intermedia dysfunction (PPID),[17] also known as equine Cushing's disease, although no published studies have specifically evaluated PPID as a risk factor for pasture-associated laminitis.

Obesity and regional fat accumulation (eg, a cresty neck) may be independent risk factors for pasture-associated laminitis. Ponies at high risk for pasture laminitis had greater body condition scores (BCS >7) than animals without a history of laminitis, and a cresty neck was also common in these animals.[13] Pasture grazing may exacerbate obesity in easy keeper animals with high metabolic efficiency from the availability of abundant, nutrient-rich pasture. Mechanical trauma from increased load on the feet is one theory linking obesity with laminitis risk, but the increased risk of laminitis in obese equids is more likely related to other factors, such as insulin resistance and inflammation, which are consequences of obesity.[18–20] Not all obese horses are insulin-resistant and, conversely, insulin resistance can occur in nonobese animals. Therefore, clinical evaluation of adiposity alone is not sufficient to assess risk for pasture-associated laminitis.

One or more genetic polymorphisms may underlie the metabolic syndrome that heightens risk of pasture-associated laminitis.[6,14] In the study of Welsh and Dartmoor ponies, pedigree analysis suggested a dominant mode of inheritance for the metabolic syndrome phenotype, supporting the possibility of a genetic basis for the insulin resistance and laminitis predisposition in this population.[6] Further studies in more outbred populations are required to confirm these findings. Experts have proposed that these susceptible ponies have a "thrifty genotype," wherein insulin resistance is an adaptive strategy for survival in nutritionally sparse environments. However, this strategy may go awry when these animals are exposed to high-calorie diets, with development of obesity, exacerbation of insulin resistance and hyperinsulinemia, and increased risk of laminitis. A similar scenario may contribute to the suggested increased susceptibility of easy keeper horse breeds (eg, Morgan, Arabians, Paso Fino, Spanish Mustang) to EMS and pasture-associated laminitis.[7,9]

PATHOPHYSIOLOGY OF PASTURE LAMINITIS

Clinical observations and the results of epidemiologic studies have indicated that risk of laminitis is highest when horses or ponies are grazing "lush" (ie, green, actively photosynthetic) or "stressed" (ie, environmental conditions that restrict forage growth) pastures with high nonstructural carbohydrate content, such as fructans, simple sugars, or starch.[21] When pasture forage is abundant and rich in nonstructural carbohydrates, it is hypothesized that large quantities of carbohydrate are delivered to the hindgut. Rapid fermentation of these carbohydrates in the hindgut (cecum and large colon) may initiate intestinal disturbances that trigger a chain of events leading to development of laminitis.[1,2] Additionally, evidence shows that intake of feeds rich in these carbohydrate fractions may exacerbate hyperinsulinemia in predisposed animals, providing another potential mechanism for lamellar injury.[6]

Much of the current knowledge about the pathogenesis of pasture-associated laminitis has been extrapolated from experimental models of alimentary carbohydrate overload. A detailed discussion of these carbohydrate overload models is beyond the scope of this article, although several excellent, contemporary reviews of these models are available; these reviews include discussion on proposed mechanisms for lamellar failure after carbohydrate overload.[22,23]

In brief, alimentary carbohydrate overload is created by the bolus administration (through gastric gavage) of a mixture of cornstarch and wood flour (17 g/kg per body weight) or oligofructose (5.0–12 g/kg body weight).[5,22,23] In the oligofructose model, carbohydrate overload induces profound changes in the hindgut microbiome. These changes include disappearance of Escherichia coli and rapid proliferation of bacteria that preferentially ferment oligofructose and produce lactic acid as an end product of fermentation, particularly the equine hindgut streptococcal species (EHSS), Streptococcus bovis and S lutetiensis, formerly S equinus. Other events described include a sharp increase occurs in hindgut acidity, with pH values as low as 4; death and lysis of large numbers of bacteria and release of endotoxins, exotoxins, and other microbial components; and damage to hindgut epithelial cells with a resultant increase in intestinal permeability.[23,24] Evidence also shows an increase in the synthesis of vasoactive amines within the hindgut under conditions of carbohydrate overload.[25] The increase in intestinal permeability presumably favors absorption of exotoxins, endotoxins, other bacterial components, and vasoactive amines into the circulation.

In both models,[22,26] increased plasma endotoxin concentration has been detected 8 to 12 hours after carbohydrate overload and is associated with clinical signs of endotoxemia (eg, tachycardia, tachypnea, abdominal discomfort, fever) and evidence of a systemic inflammatory response (eg, increased inflammatory cytokine mRNA expression in blood, platelet activation, and activation of leukocytes) during the developmental phase of acute laminitis, but the precise role of endotoxemia in the pathogenesis of pasture-associated laminitis has not been determined. Intravenous infusion of endotoxin (lipopolysaccharide) does not induce development of laminitis in healthy horses.[27,28] However, a clinical study has identified endotoxemia as a risk factor for laminitis in hospitalized horses, although laminitis was associated with severe illness (gram-negative sepsis) rather than grazing on pasture.[29]

Endotoxin absorbed from the intestinal tract may play an important role during the developmental phase of pasture laminitis, perhaps by priming inflammatory and hemodynamic mechanisms involved in lamellar injury and failure. Tóth and colleagues[28] recently reported that pretreatment with lipopolysaccharide might increase the incidence and severity of laminitis induced by the administration of oligofructose (5 g/kg body weight). This novel finding merits further investigation.

The critical link between fermentation of carbohydrate in the intestine and development of acute laminitis remains to be identified. The systemic inflammation that occurs in response to carbohydrate overload likely initiates lamellar inflammatory events, including infiltration and activation of leukocytes, that contribute to destruction of lamellar epithelium and extracellular matrix.[1,2,22] Alterations in digital vascular hemodynamics associated with inflammation, platelet activation, and the action of vasoactive amines absorbed from the intestinal tract also may contribute to lamellar injury.[25,26,30]

Although the oligofructose model has gained favor over the starch model for the experimental induction of laminitis, its relevance to an understanding of naturally occurring pasture laminitis has been questioned. This limitation notwithstanding, under conditions that favor nonstructural carbohydrate storage in grasses, horses and ponies at pasture can clearly ingest substantial loads of nonstructural carbohy-drate–rich forage with consequent disturbances to the hindgut microbiome (and milieu) that may initiate events leading to development of laminitis. Accordingly, recent research has focused on the expansion of knowledge regarding the dynamics of carbohydrate storage in pasture grasses and how the interaction between animal pre-disposing factors (especially insulin resistance and hyperinsulinemia) and environ-mental conditions (especially the nutrient profile of pasture forage) alters risk for development of laminitis. These areas are discussed in the following sections.

Dynamics of Pasture Forage Nonstructural Carbohydrate Content

Forage in the form of pasture grasses or hay (or other preserved forage product) constitutes the major part of the diet for most horses.[21,31] Carbohydrates are the predominant component of forages, representing as much as 70% to 75% of dry matter (700–750 g/kg dry matter), and comprising both structural (cell wall constitu-ents, including cellulose, hemicellulose, lingo-cellulose, and lignin) and nonstructural forms.

The nonstructural carbohydrate fraction includes simple sugars (monosaccharides, disaccharides), starches, oligosaccharides (including fructans), and soluble fibers (gums, mucilages, and pectins). The structural carbohydrates are indigestible to mammals but provide nutritional value to the horse through microbial fermentation, primarily in the cecum and large colon. Similarly, mammals lack the enzymes needed for hydrolysis of fructans, and microbial fermentation is assumed to be the primary mechanism for the digestion of fructans in horses.

Starches and simple sugars are digested in the equine small intestine, but digestive capacity may be exceeded when large quantities are ingested, with undigested starch or sugar passing into the hindgut where it will undergo rapid fermentation. Much of the discussion on forage carbohydrates and laminitis risk has focused on fructans, but other components of nonstructural carbohydrates, especially the simple sugars and starches, also may be important.[6,21,31]

Pasture plants contain varying levels of simple sugars, fructans, and starch. The vegetative tissues of temperate (cool season or C3) pasture grasses, such as peren-nial ryegrass or fescue, accumulate fructan as the primary storage carbohydrate, with most fructan stored in the stem until required by the plant as an energy source.[21,31] In contrast, starch is the storage carbohydrate of the seed of temperate grasses and the seed and vegetative tissues of legumes (eg, clover) and warm season (C4) grasses such as Bermuda.[28]

Fructans are water-soluble polymers of fructose with either β-2,1 or β-2,6 linkages, all bonded to a terminal glucose moiety. The glycosidic bonds in fructan are not hydro-lyzed by host enzymes but may be susceptible to partial acid hydrolysis in the stomach, which could result in the release of fructose that is absorbed from the small intestine.[21] This process could contribute to risk of laminitis through exacerbation of hyperinsulinemia (discussed later). Some of the ingested fructan may be fermented in the foregut, but the bulk is thought to reach the hindgut where it is rapidly fermented.

In vitro studies have shown that inulin (a commercially available fructo-oligosaccharide derived from chicory) elicits a more rapid fall in cecal pH than an equal amount of corn starch.[32] The rate of fermentation is impacted by the biochemical structure of the fructan.[31] Inulin are linear molecules linked through β-2,1 bonds with low molecular weight and degree of polymerization (DP) less than 10, both of which favor rapid fermentation. The fructans in grasses (graminans) contain both β-2,1 and β-2,6 linkages, are highly branched, and have higher DP (40–100) compared with inulin; factors that contribute to a slower rate of fermentation.

The molecular size of fructans found in different species of grass varies considerably. Ryegrass fructans have DP of 30 to 40, whereas timothy or orchard grasses contain larger fructans with DP of 100 or more. Furthermore, in vitro studies have shown more rapid fermentation of the lower molecular weight fructans in ryegrass, suggesting that this species may pose a high risk for pasture-associated laminitis.[31]

Pasture forage nutrient composition (eg, protein, fiber, nonstructural carbohydrate) is highly dynamic and influenced by a large number of environmental factors, including the intensity and duration of sunlight, temperature (ambient and soil), soil fertility, water availability, and nitrogen status.[31,33] Studies in several Northern European countries have shown fructan content of perennial ryegrass to vary between less than 100 g and greater than 400 g/kg of dry matter depending on the season and growing conditions.[21,31]

In general, pasture nonstructural carbohydrate is highest in spring, lowest in mid-summer, and intermediate in fall. In northern Virginia pastures (tall fescue, Kentucky bluegrass mix), forage nonstructural carbohydrate content was highest in April and May (15%–20% dry matter; ie, 150–200 g/kg), intermediate in the fall, and lowest in mid-winter and summer (<5%–7% dry matter).[33,34] However, marked daily fluctuations can also coincide with patterns of energy storage (photosynthetic activity) and use. During periods of growth and intense photosynthetic activity, pasture nonstructural carbohydrate tends to rise during the morning, reaching maxima in the afternoon, and then declines overnight. In one study of spring pasture in northern Virginia, the nadir in forage nonstructural carbohydrate occurred between 0400 and 0500 hours (~15% nonstructural carbohydrate, dry matter basis), which peak values between 1600 and 1700 hours (~22%–24% nonstructural carbohydrate).[34] Under these conditions, therefore, horses may ingest a substantially greater quantity of NSC when grazing in the afternoon compared with nighttime or early morning. Stress conditions that restrict plant growth (and therefore energy demands) result in accumulation of nonstructural carbohydrate. These stress conditions include low temperatures, killing frosts, applications of nonlethal herbicides, and low soil fertility.[21,31]

At certain times of the year, the quantity of pasture nonstructural carbohydrate ingested by grazing equids may approach or exceed the amount of starch or fructan known to induce laminitis when administered as a single dose.[21,31] Although minimal data are available on rates of pasture forage intake by grazing equids, horses with 24-hour access to pasture may ingest between 2.5% and 3% of their body weight (as dry matter) per day, or 12.5 to 15 kg dry matter intake for a 500-kg horse.[21] Thus, nonstructural carbohydrate intake would range between approximately 1.25 and 1.5 kg dry matter per day and 3.75 and 4.5 kg dry matter per day for pastures with nonstructural carbohydrate content of 100 and 300 g/kg dry matter, respectively.

The higher end of forage nonstructural carbohydrate intake approaches the amount of fructan used for experimental induction of laminitis, albeit consumed over a 12- to 17-hour period rather than as a single bolus. However, the dosage of nonstructural carbohydrate (eg, as fructan) required to trigger digestive and metabolic disturbances in susceptible animals (ie, a horse or pony with an insulin-resistant phenotype) may be considerably lower than that needed to reliably induce disease in healthy experimental animals. Furthermore, subthreshold doses of nonstructural carbohydrate consumed over several days may induce multiple subclinical insults, with cumulative damage to the lamellae that ultimately manifests as clinical laminitis.

Role of Predisposing Factors in the Development of Laminitis

Recognition that certain horses and ponies are prone to repeated episodes of pasture-associated laminitis has stimulated research that seeks to elucidate mechanisms underlying this predisposition. Considerable evidence links an insulin-resistant phenotype (EMS) with susceptibility to laminitis, and current studies have begun to examine this link. Several questions arise concerning this association; for example, does insulin resistance per se play a direct role in the development of laminitis, or do factors associated with insulin resistance increase susceptibility to laminitis when the animal is exposed to conditions known to trigger development of the condition (eg, carbohydrate overload during grazing activity)?

The observation that laminitis can be elicited in healthy ponies and horses by maintaining prolonged hyperinsulinemia (serum insulin, ~1040 mU/L for 48 hours) has important implications for pasture-associated laminitis.[10,11] The mechanism through which hyperinsulinemia disrupts lamellar integrity has not been elucidated, although alterations in digital vascular hemodynamics leading to ischemic injury or direct toxic effects of insulin on lamellar epithelial cells have been proposed.[10] Regardless, these findings offer a potential explanation for episodes of laminitis in grazing horses and ponies.

Studies of grazing horses have shown a strong, positive relationship between pasture nonstructural carbohydrate content and circulating insulin concentrations,[34] and marked exacerbation of hyperinsulinemia has been observed in EMS ponies when grazing spring pasture (nonstructural carbohydrate, ~15%–18% dry matter).[6,35] In healthy, nonobese thoroughbred mares grazing spring (April) pasture in northern Virginia, serum insulin concentrations followed a circadian pattern that mirrored changes in forage nonstructural carbohydrate content, with peak insulin concentrations approaching 100 to 110 mU/L.[34] In a herd of Welsh and Dartmoor ponies kept at pasture, some of which were insulin-resistant and prone to recurrent pasture laminitis, serum insulin concentrations markedly increased during the months of April and May (values as high as 500–600 mU/L in some ponies), and this occurrence coincided with an increase in pasture grass nonstructural carbohydrate content.[35] Several ponies with the EMS phenotype developed laminitis 7 to 10 days after exacerbation of hyperinsulinemia was detected. Feeding inulin (to simulate intake of fructan from spring grass) to ponies elicits an exaggerated insulin response in animals predisposed to laminitis.[36]

Seasonal influences on insulin dynamics also may influence risk of pasture laminitis. A recent study showed exaggerated postdexamethasone insulin responses in previously laminitic ponies in April and July compared with responses in December. Additionally, the increase in serum insulin concentrations in response to dexamethasone administration was significantly higher in previously laminitic than in normal ponies.[37] Therefore episodes of laminitis in pasture-kept animals, especially those with an EMS phenotype, may be directly linked to increases in circulating insulin associated with season or the consumption of nonstructural carbohydrate–rich forage.

It can be argued that insulin does not play an essential role in the development of pasture-associated laminitis. Although insulin sensitivity has been shown to decrease after oligofructose administration,[28] hyperinsulinemia is not a feature of the laminitis that develops after experimental alimentary carbohydrate overload. However, this observation does not exclude the possibility that hyperinsulinemia contributes to lamellar injury in pasture-associated laminitis. In fact, it is tempting to speculate that the development of pasture-associated laminitis in susceptible animals (ie, equids with EMS) represents a "multi-hit" phenomenon, with lamellar injury occurring in response to inflammatory, oxidant, and vascular insults together with direct injury by insulin. Viewed another way, hyperinsulinemia may lower the threshold for laminitis in the face of other conditions that promote development of the condition, such as hindgut disturbances associated with rapid fermentation of fructan ingested in pasture forage that invoke a systemic inflammatory response and/or alter digital vascular hemodynamics.

Other components of the EMS phenotype may render the individual more susceptible to pasture-associated laminitis. Insulin resistance in humans and animal models of metabolic syndrome are characterized by vascular endothelial dysfunction that contributes to development of hypertension. Insulin is a vasoregulatory hormone, invoking vasodilatation through pathways similar to those of insulin-mediated glucose metabolism.[38,39] In insulin-resistant states, insulin's ability to counteract endothelin-1–associated vasoconstriction may be compromised because of decreased nitric oxide synthesis, whereas compensatory hyperinsulinemia might stimulate increased endothelin-1 production.[38] The resulting imbalance between the production of nitric oxide and secretion of endothelin-1 favors vasoconstriction and also contributes to platelet activation and leukocyte adhesion, all of which have been proposed as pathophysiologic mechanisms in the development of carbohydrate overload–induced laminitis.[1,2,25,30]

Bailey and colleagues[14] documented hypertension in insulin-resistant, laminitis prone ponies at summer pasture, suggesting that vascular endothelial dysfunction also is a component of the metabolic syndrome phenotype in equids. EMS animals may therefore be more susceptible to digital vasoconstriction, platelet aggregation, and neutrophil adherence and emigration into lamellar tissues under conditions of alimentary carbohydrate overload.[8]

The existence of a proinflammatory state in EMS also could enhance susceptibility to pasture-associated laminitis. In human obesity, progressive dysregulation of adipose tissue with recruitment of mononuclear cells, increased production and secretion of proinflammatory adipokines, and development of a chronic, low-grade inflammatory state occur.[18,19] In horses, blood tumor necrosis factor (TNF)-α and interleukin (IL)-1β mRNA expression were positively associated with body condition score (ie, adiposity), and increased expression of these cytokines was an independent risk for insulin resistance.[20] Additionally, increased serum TNF-α concentrations have been observed in a well-characterized population of laminitis-prone ponies that expressed the EMS phenotype.[8] Evidence from studies in humans patients and experimental animals suggests that the microvascular dysfunction (eg, platelet and leukocyte adhesion; leukocyte emigration) associated with sepsis or other inflammatory stimuli is exacerbated by obesity and insulin resistance.[40] Similarly, a proinflammatory state in EMS equids could amplify impairments to lamellar or digital vascular function associated with carbohydrate overload from pasture, thereby lowering the threshold for laminitis.

Another possibility is that susceptible horses and ponies have differences in their gut flora compared with animals less prone to laminitis, with heightened hindgut fermentative responses to a given load of nonstructural carbohydrate and increased production of substances that may be involved in the triggering of laminitis.[25] Studies by the laminitis research group at the Royal Veterinary College have focused on the potential for vasoconstrictor monoamines produced in the large intestine to contribute to the initiation of laminitis through hemodynamic disturbances in the digit (vasoconstriction and ischemic injury), and the possibility that equids with an EMS phenotype are more prone to digital vasoconstriction as a result of insulin resistance and associated vascular endothelial cell dysfunction.[25,41] They have shown that the cecal contents harvested from horses maintained on spring/summer pasture had two- to threefold higher concentrations of amines compared with cecal contents collected from horses fed hay or winter grass,[42] and that ponies who were sampled in winter had lower plasma concentrations of monoamines (tryptamine, tyramine, phenylethylamine, and isoamylamine) and semi–carbazide-sensitive amine oxidase, also known as *vascular adhesion protein-1*, than when they were sampled at summer pasture.[43]

In vitro and in vivo studies have documented marked increases in monoamine synthesis in cecal contents incubated with starch or inulin,[25,32] and increased fecal amine concentrations in ponies provided increased dietary inulin (3 g/kg body weight).[44] However, the decrease in fecal pH and increase in fecal amine concentrations associated with insulin feeding did not differ between normal ponies and those predisposed to laminitis.[44] Thus, circumstantial evidence implicates vasoactive amines in the pathogenesis of pasture-associated laminitis, but further research is needed to provide definitive proof and determine whether equids with the EMS phenotype are more susceptible to laminitis because of exaggerated amine-induced digital vasoconstriction.

SUMMARY

Epidemiologic studies indicate that most laminitis cases occur in horses and ponies kept at pasture, hence the term *pasture-associated laminitis*. Clinical cases of laminitis most often occur under conditions that favor accumulation of rapidly fermentable nonstructural carbohydrates (fructans, simple sugars, or starches) in pasture, and animals with an EMS phenotype (insulin resistance, abnormal insulin dynamics, +/– obesity) seem to be at highest risk for developing the condition. Although the mechanisms linking consumption of pasture forage with development of lamellar failure have not been fully elucidated, a systemic inflammatory response that accompanies hindgut carbohydrate overload likely initiates lamellar inflammatory events (including infiltration and activation of leukocytes) that contribute to destruction of lamellar epithelium and extracellular matrix. Alterations in digital vascular hemodynamics associated with inflammation, platelet activation, and the action of vasoactive amines absorbed from the intestinal tract also may contribute to lamellar injury. In horses and ponies with an EMS phenotype, increases in circulating insulin that are associated with season or the consumption of nonstructural carbohydrate–rich forage may contribute to development of laminitis. In addition, factors associated with the EMS phenotype, including hyperinsulinemia, vascular endothelial dysfunction, and a proinflammatory state, may act alone or in combination to lower the threshold for laminitis induction through carbohydrate overload–associated disturbances in the hindgut.

REFERENCES

1. Eades SC. Overview of current laminitis research. Vet Clin North Am Equine Pract 2010;26:51–63.
2. Bailey SR, Marr CM, Elliott J. Current research and theories on the pathogenesis of acute laminitis in the horse. Vet J 2004;167:129–42.
3. USDA-NAHMS. Lameness and laminitis in US horses. Fort Collins (CO): National Animal Health Monitoring System; 2000. p. 12.
4. Hinckley K, Henderson I. The epidemiology of equine laminitis in the UK. In: Proceedings of the 35th Congress of the British Equine Veterinary Association. Warwick (UK): 1996. p. 62.
5. van Eps AW, Pollitt CC. Equine laminitis induced with oligofructose. Equine Vet J 2006;38:203–8.

6. Treiber KH, Kronfeld DS, Hess TM, et al. Evaluation of genetic and metabolic predispositions and nutritional risk factors for pasture-associated laminitis in ponies. J Am Vet Med Assoc 2006;228:1538–45.
7. Johnson PJ. The equine metabolic syndrome: peripheral Cushing's syndrome. Vet Clin North Am Equine Pract 2002;18:271–93.
8. Geor R, Frank N. Metabolic syndrome – from human organ disease to laminar failure in equids. Vet Immunol Immunopathol 2009;129:151–4.
9. Frank N, Elliott SB, Brandt LE, et al. Physical characteristics, blood hormone concentrations, and plasma lipid concentrations in obese horses with insulin resistance. J Am Vet Med Assoc 2006;228:1383–90.
10. Asplin KE, Sillence MN, Pollitt CC, et al. Induction of laminitis by prolonged hyperinsulinaemia in clinically normal ponies. Vet J 2007;174:530–5.
11. De Laat MA, McGowan CM, Sillence MN, et al. Equine laminitis: induced by 48 h hyperinsulinaemia in Standardbred horses. Equine Vet J 2010;42:129–35.
12. Katz L, DeBrauwere N, Elliott J, et al. The prevalence of laminitis in one region of the UK. In: 40th British Equine Veterinary Association Congress. 2001. p. 199.
13. Carter RA, Treiber KH, Geor RJ, et al. Prediction of incipient pasture-associated laminitis from hyperinsulinemia, hyperleptinemia and generalized and localized obesity in a cohort of ponies. Equine Vet J 2009;40:171–8.
14. Bailey SR, Habershon-Butcher JL, Ransom KJ, et al. Hypertension and insulin resistance in a mixed-breed population of ponies predisposed to laminitis. Am J Vet Res 2008;69:122–9.
15. Frank N. Endocrinopathic laminitis, obesity-associated laminitis, and pasture-associated laminitis. In: Presented at the American Association of Equine Practitioners 54th Annual Convention. San Diego, December 6–10, 2008. p. 341–6.
16. Rijnen KE, van der Kolk JH. Determination of reference range values indicative of glucose metabolism and insulin resistance by use of glucose clamp techniques in horses and ponies. Am J Vet Res 2003;64:1260–4.
17. Donaldson MT, Jorgensen AJ, Beech J. Evaluation of suspected pituitary pars intermedia dysfunction in horses with laminitis. J Am Vet Med Assoc 2004;224: 1123–7.
18. Hutley L, Prins JB. Fat as an endocrine organ: relationship to the metabolic syndrome. Am J Med Sci 2005;330:280–9.
19. Wild SH, Byrne CD. ABC of obesity: risk factors for diabetes and coronary heart disease. Br Med J 2006;333:1009–11.
20. Vick MM, Adams AA, Murphy BA, et al. Relationships among inflammatory cytokines, obesity and insulin sensitivity in the horse. J Anim Sci 2007;85: 1144–55.
21. Longland AC, Byrd BM. Pasture nonstructural carbohydrates and equine laminitis. J Nutr 2006;136(Suppl 7):2099S–102S.
22. Pollitt CC, Visser MB. Carbohydrate alimentary overload laminitis. Vet Clin North Am Equine Pract 2010;26:65–78.
23. Milinovich GJ, Klieve AV, Pollitt CC, et al. Microbial events in the hindgut during carbohydrate-induced equine laminitis. Vet Clin North Am Equine Pract 2010; 26:79–94.
24. Milinovich GJ, Trott DJ, Burrell PC, et al. Changes in equine hindgut bacterial populations during oligofructose-induced laminitis. Environ Microbiol 2006;8: 885–98.
25. Elliott J, Bailey SR. Gastrointestinal derived factors are potential triggers for the development of acute equine laminitis. J Nutr 2006;136. 2103S–7S.

26. Bailey SR, Adair HS, Reinemeyer CR, et al. Plasma concentrations of endotoxin and platelet activation in the developmental stage of oligofructose-induced laminitis. Vet Immunol Immunopathol 2009;129:167–73.
27. Menzies-Gow NJ, Bailey SR, Katz LM, et al. Endotoxin-induced digital vasoconstriction in horses: associated changes in plasma concentrations of vasoconstrictor mediators. Equine Vet J 2004;36:273–8.
28. Toth F, Frank N, Chameroy KA, et al. Effects of endotoxaemia and carbohydrate overload on glucose and insulin dynamics and the development of laminitis in horses. Equine Vet J 2009;41:852–8.
29. Parsons CS, Orsini JA, Krafty R, et al. Risk factors for development of acute laminitis in horses during hospitalization: 73 cases (1997–2004). J Am Vet Med Assoc 2007;230:885–9.
30. Eades SC, Stokes AM, Johnson PJ, et al. Serial alterations in digital hemodynamics and endothelin-1 immunoreactivity, platelet-neutrophil aggregation, and concentrations of nitric oxide, insulin and glucose in blood obtained from horses following carbohydrate overload. Am J Vet Res 2007;68:87–94.
31. Longland AC. Starch, sugar and fructans: what are they and how important are they in diets for horses? In: Harris PA, Hill SJ, Elliott J, et al, editors. The latest findings in laminitis research. The 1st WALTHAM – Royal Veterinary College Laminitis Conference. London, Royal Veterinary College, March 24, 2007. p. 7–14.
32. Bailey SR, Rycroft A, Elliott J. Production of amines in equine cecal contents in an in vitro model of carbohydrate overload. J Anim Sci 2002;80:2656–62.
33. Cubitt TA, Staniar WB, Kronfeld DS, et al. Environmental effects on nutritive value of equine pastures in Northern Virginia. Pferdeheilkunde 2007;23:151–4.
34. Byrd BM, Treiber KH, Staniar WB, et al. Circadian and seasonal variation on pasture NSC and circulating insulin concentrations in grazing horses [abstract]. J Anim Sci 2006;84(Suppl 1):330–1.
35. Treiber KH, Carter RA, Harris PA, et al. Seasonal changes in energy metabolism of ponies coincides with changes in pasture carbohydrates: implications for laminitis [abstract]. J Vet Intern Med 2008;22:735–6.
36. Bailey SR, Menzies-Gow NJ, Harris PA, et al. Effect of dietary fructan and dexamethasone on the insulin response of ponies predisposed to laminitis. J Am Vet Med Assoc 2007;231:1365–73.
37. Borer KE, Menzies-Gow NJ, Berhane Y, et al. Seasonal influence on insulin and cortisol results from overnight dexamethasone suppression tests in normal and previously laminitic ponies. Presented at the 2nd AAEP Foundation Equine Laminitis Research Workshop. Palm Beach, November 4–5, 2009.
38. Kim JK, Montagnani M, Koh KK, et al. Reciprocal relationships between insulin resistance and endothelial dysfunction: molecular and pathophysiological mechanisms. Circulation 2006;113:1888–904.
39. Cosentino F, Luscher TF. Endothelial dysfunction in diabetes mellitus. J Cardiovasc Pharmacol 1998;32(3):S54–61.
40. Singer G, Granger DN. Inflammatory responses underlying the microvascular dysfunction associated with obesity and insulin resistance. Microcirculation 2007;14:375–87.
41. Bailey SR, Menzies-Gow NJ, Marr CM, et al. The effects of vasoactive amines found in the equine hindgut on digital blood flow in the normal horse. Equine Vet J 2004;36:267–72.
42. Bailey SR, Marr CM, Elliott J. Identification and quantification of amines in the equine caecum. Res Vet Sci 2003;74:113–8.

43. Bailey SR, Katz LM, Berhane Y, et al. Seasonal changes in plasma concentrations of cecum-derived amines in clinically normal ponies and ponies predisposed to laminitis. Am J Vet Res 2003;64:1132–8.

44. Crawford C, Sepulveda MF, Elliott J, et al. Dietary fructan carbohydrate increases amine production in the equine large intestine: implications for pasture-associated laminitis. J Anim Sci 2007;85:2949–58.

Corticosteroid-Associated Laminitis

Simon R. Bailey, PhD, MRCVS

KEYWORDS

• Laminitis • Corticosteroids • Glucocorticoids • Insulin

Corticosteroids are used widely in equine medicine, with glucocorticoids being the most effective, broad-acting, anti-inflammatory agents available. While several potential adverse effects may result from long-term use of corticosteroids, one of the most serious perceived risks associated with their use in horses is acute laminitis.[1–4]

The naturally occurring (endogenous) corticosteroids include the glucocorticoids, the mineralocorticoids (principally aldosterone), and the adrenal sex steroids. The glucocorticoids, including cortisol and synthetic derivatives with greater potency and specificity, are the most important in terms of clinical use[5] and in relation to the incidence of laminitis.[6] There is no evidence of mineralocorticoids causing laminitis, although there is a report in the literature of laminitis being induced experimentally following testosterone administration for 4 weeks, which suggested that the severity of laminitis was increased.[7] Nevertheless, this article will be concerned particularly with glucocorticoids and laminitis.

A direct causal association between corticosteroid use and laminitis has yet to be proven scientifically, and undoubtedly iatrogenic laminitis is a rare occurrence.[8] There is little case information and few experimental studies specifically addressing this aspect.[9] New evidence, however, is improving the understanding of the causes of laminitis, particularly related to endocrine factors, which is directing further understanding of the likely mechanisms and the circumstances under which steroids could cause this condition.

CLINICAL EVIDENCE: CIRCUMSTANCES WHERE GLUCOCORTICOIDS MIGHT CAUSE LAMINITIS
Exogenous Glucocorticoids

Reports first appeared in the 1980s to suggest that the administration of glucocorticoids may be a causative factor in laminitis.[1,3] Further reports followed; however, it was not clear in some cases whether other factors, such as gastrointestinal disease or metabolic dysfunctions, also may have played a role.[2,4]

School of Veterinary Science, University of Melbourne, Corner of Park Drive and Flemington Road, Parkville, Victoria 3052, Australia
E-mail address: bais@unimelb.edu.au

Vet Clin Equine 26 (2010) 277–285
doi:10.1016/j.cveq.2010.04.001
0749-0739/10/$ – see front matter © 2010 Elsevier Inc. All rights reserved.

Where large-scale studies have been conducted to determine links between particular risk factors and the incidence of laminitis, it becomes apparent that only a small percentage of cases have ever been associated with steroid administration; however, these cases have significant consequences for everyone involved. Hood and colleagues[10] identified 8 out of 525 cases that were considered to be drug-induced, but a further study by this group[11] observed that 3 out of 35 acute cases received glucocorticoids before the onset of laminitis. Four cases out of 211 referred animals in a UK study were attributed to the administration of corticosteroids.[12] Compared with the vast numbers of horses treated with standard therapeutic doses of corticosteroids each year, especially via the intra-articular route, the numbers of possible cases of laminitis subsequent to their use appears to be only a handful. Bathe [13] estimated that three cases of laminitis might have occurred subsequent to intra-articular steroid administration, out of 2000 horses receiving up to 20 to 45 mg of triamcinolone acetonide or 80 mg methylprednisolone acetate. Two of those cases occurred 2 to 3 months after treatment, long after the measurable systemic effects of these drugs would have been undetectable.[14] Therefore a causal link in those cases would be unlikely. In a study by McCluskey and Kavenagh,[15] out of 205 horses treated with up to 80 mg triamcinolone, one horse developed laminitis 7 days after receiving 40 mg triamcinolone, but this case had a prior history of laminitis.

There are numerous accounts of the administration of corticosteroids at moderately high doses to groups of experimental horses under controlled conditions, with no incidence of laminitis. These include dexamethasone at 1 mg/kg/d intravenously for 9 days, which did not cause signs of laminitis in mixed breed ponies,[16] and single doses of triamcinolone acetonide (0.2 mg/kg intramuscularly, equivalent to a total dose of approximately 80 mg).[17] The commonly recommended dose of triamcinolone is up to 20 mg.[18] It is unclear whether triamcinolone may be particularly associated with iatrogenic laminitis more than other steroidal compounds; this possibility[19] may be associated with the large numbers of cases treated with this compound. It was observed in one study, however, that the prior administration of triamcinolone (15 mg, 3 times a week for 4 weeks) markedly increased the severity of experimentally induced acute laminitis.[7]

Doses of triamcinolone far exceeding 80 mg appear to be linked with severe laminitis within a few days or weeks of administration. In one well publicized case in the United Kingdom in 2007, a French dressage horse was given 160 mg of triamcinolone (80 mg in each hock) plus 20 mg dexamethasone intramuscularly.[20] The horse developed severe laminitis shortly afterwards, necessitating euthanasia, and the veterinarians were found liable in court. In one report from Korea, a Thoroughbred filly received 20 mg of triamcinolone acetonide on each of 10 consecutive days (total dose 200 mg).[21] In this case, in addition to hepatopathy, laminitis became apparent 3 weeks later. Therefore extremely high doses of such compounds would appear to be required to elicit laminitis. The rare anecdotal reports of this condition resulting from recommended therapeutic doses of corticosteroids (Anon, personal communication) could be associated with the presence of other concurrent causative factors, whose effects were exacerbated by the drug.

Endogenous Glucocorticoids—PPID

Pituitary dysfunction has been associated with increased risk of laminitis.[22,23] Plasma cortisol levels, however, may not be consistently elevated in pituitary pars intermedia dysfunction (PPID),[24] but may be periodically increased.[25] The treatment of PPID cases with an inhibitor of 3-hydroxysteroid dehydrogenase (trilostane), a drug that reduces cortisol production, appeared to be successful in decreasing the incidence of chronic and recurrent laminitis in a large proportion of affected animals.[26]

The precise role of endogenous corticosteroids in the link between these conditions is unclear, and the relationship could be direct or indirect via other hormones, such as insulin. In addition to circulating cortisol levels, at the local tissue level, cortisone may be converted to cortisol by the enzyme 11β-hydroxysteroid dehydrogenase type 1 (11β-HSD-1), which is present in lamellar tissues.[27] The ketoreductase activity (cortisol-producing activity) of this enzyme was found to be increased fourfold in the acute phase of experimentally induced laminitis.[28]

POSSIBLE MECHANISMS INVOLVED IN GLUCOCORTICOID-ASSOCIATED LAMINITIS

To date, just as there is no scientific proof in the literature that steroids cause laminitis, no single mechanism has been proven to explain how glucocorticoids may cause the condition. Furthermore, there has been no detailed histopathological assessment of lamellar tissues from horses in the early stages of laminitis thought to be associated with corticosteroids. Despite this uncertainty, there are several plausible potential mechanisms that have been considered.

Interaction with Insulin

One of the more likely mechanisms by which glucocorticoids may cause laminitis is perhaps via an indirect effect on the lamellae, mediated by insulin, rather than a direct effect. This is informed by the remarkable findings at The University of Queensland that laminitis can be induced in normal ponies and horses by the administration of a prolonged infusion of insulin.[29,30] Insulin levels over approximately 1000 μIU/mL for 48 hours caused Obel grade 2 laminitis in normal, noninsulin-resistant Standardbred horses.[30] Although insulin-induced laminitis in smaller ponies produced relatively mild pathology and initially appeared to be a stretching rather than a complete detatchment of the basement membrane away from the epidermal lamellae,[29,31] the increased weight bearing in larger horses seemed to cause more dermo–epidermal detachment[30] similar to other models of laminitis.

Glucocorticoids may cause a relatively rapid increase in plasma insulin production, initially by stimulating hepatic gluconeogenesis and raising plasma glucose levels. This may occur after a single dose of long- or short-acting corticosteroids. Furthermore, prolonged administration of glucocorticoids may cause insulin resistance, by impairing glycogen synthase kinase 3 (GSK-3) phosphorylation in skeletal muscle, and resulting in decreased glycogen synthase activity in response to insulin.[32]

When 0.2 mg/kg triamcinolone acetonide (equivalent to a total dose of 80 mg for a 400 kg horse) was administered to five horses by the intramuscular route, there was a prolonged hyperglycemia and hyperinsulinemia, which lasted for more than 150 hours.[17] The peak insulin levels (approximately 150 μIU/mL) were nowhere near the levels used to induce acute laminitis in Standardbreds,[30] but did cause divergent growth rings to subsequently appear in the hooves of four out of the five horses. In laminitis-prone ponies that are insulin-resistant, the administration of a single, low dose of dexamethasone (0.04 mg/kg) may cause an exaggerated increase in plasma insulin measured 19 hours later.[33] In normal insulin-sensitive ponies, this dose did not increase serum insulin much outside of the normal laboratory reference range (up to 70 μIU/mL), but did increase insulin levels to between 100 and 400 μIU/mL in insulin-resistant ponies. Further studies with this dose of dexamethasone have shown that at certain times of year some ponies may respond with insulin values of 1000 μIU/mL or more.[34]

This author has not observed any cases of laminitis secondary to a standard dexamethasone suppression test, even in laminitis-prone ponies; this may be because very high levels of insulin first must be achieved and then sustained for several days, as in the experimental laminitis inductions.[30] To investigate further whether longer-acting compounds such as triamcinolone could increase insulin levels high enough and for long enough, sufficient to cause laminitis, insulin would need to be measured in normal horses or ponies after the administration of very large doses of triamcinolone, and also the approximate threshold level of insulin for causing laminitis would have to be determined.

There are other mechanisms involving glucose uptake and metabolism, by which corticosteroids might also have effects related to laminitis, although these may not directly be related to insulin. Lamellar epithelial cells are known to have a high requirement for glucose.[35–37] Steroids might impair lamellar glucose uptake by altering glucose transporter translocation, expression, or function.[37,38] This, however, is unlikely to be directly related to insulin resistance, since there is no evidence for the presence of insulin receptors on the epidermal basal epithelial cells that fail in laminitis. Whether vascular effects of insulin resistance may alter the delivery of glucose to these tissues remains to be determined.

Certainly insulin resistance may be an important mechanism related to laminitis risk,[39] and this metabolic state may be produced or exacerbated where glucocorticoids are administered over prolonged periods of time[32] or in the case of PPID.[40] Insulin resistance leads to a state of enhanced peripheral vasoconstriction,[41] due to a functional impairment of the vascular endothelium, and this may affect hemodynamic control within the lamellae and delivery of glucose to these tissues.

Apoptotic Effects

Apoptosis, (programmed cell death), occurs in the basal epidermal lamellar epithelial cells in both the black walnut and carbohydrate overload models of experimentally induced acute laminitis,[42] and also in the oligofructose model (Baily SR, PhD, MRCVS, unpublished observations, 2010). Apoptosis probably represents a response to cellular injury occurring in the developmental phase of laminitis, but it could be associated with loss of cell function and attachments to the basement membrane. Many different glucocorticoids may induce apoptosis in epithelial cells,[43,44] and this effect may be observed in cultured equine lamellar epithelial cells in vitro (Baily SR, PhD, MRCVS, unpublished observations, 2010). It is unclear, however, whether this mechanism may be relevant at therapeutic concentrations of corticosteroids.

Catabolic Effects

The catabolic effects of glucocorticoid steroids would be expected to become apparent quite slowly over weeks of therapy, which may not be consistent with a sudden widespread detachment of the lamellae, although corticosteroids could cause a weakness in these tissues. Thinning of the skin epidermis may be apparent after prolonged corticosteroid therapy[5] as well as poor healing.[45] Amino acids may be mobilized from many tissues, including the integument, and synthesis of collagen by fibroblasts also may be reduced.[46] Collagen IV and collagen VII are important components of the lamellar basement membrane,[47] and collagen I is present in the underlying dermal connective tissue.[48] These proteins have not been quantified in lamellar tissues from horses following prolonged corticosteroid treatment.

Production of keratin is also important for conferring mechanical strength to the hoof wall and laminar interface. Cortisol significantly decreased protein synthesis (including keratin) in bovine hoof explants cultured in vitro.[49] Therefore this would appear to be a direct effect of glucocorticoids, independent of effects on growth factor activity. Thus, long-term effects of glucocorticoid use may produce a weakening of the lamellar bonds or inhibit growth from the coronary band.

As well as decreasing tissue growth and protein use, corticosteroids may affect the integrity of the intestinal mucosa, impairing its barrier function. Intestinal damage or severe changes in the intestinal flora and contents may be an initiating cause of acute laminitis, and increased permeability of the large intestine is a feature of several experimental models of laminitis.[50-52] Loss of barrier function may allow potential toxins or laminitis trigger factors access from the intestinal contents into the circulation. This effect of corticosteroids has not been specifically demonstrated in horses, but is recognized in other species.[53]

Vascular Effects

Alterations in vascular function or blood flow may affect the lamellar tissues in a number of ways, and glucocorticoids may significantly increase blood vessel contractility in certain situations. Vasoconstriction, leading to ischemia or compartment syndrome, has been hypothesized as being involved in the early events occurring in the developmental phase of laminitis.[54-56]

Eyre and Elmes [57,58] showed that responses of isolated equine digital blood vessels and pump-perfused hooves to adrenaline and serotonin (5-HT) were enhanced by hydrocortisone. Additional studies ([59] and Baily SR, PhD, MRCVS, unpublished data, 2005) confirm that the vasoconstrictor response to 5-HT within the equine digit is markedly potentiated by corticosteroids (cortisol or dexamethasone), because they block the uptake (removal) of 5-HT or catecholamines from the circulation. Administration of dexamethasone to horses potentiated the effects of the α_1-adrenoceptor agonist, phenylephrine, in reducing skin blood flow.[60] Therefore, high plasma concentrations of corticosteroids could predispose horses to excessive peripheral vasoconstriction or digital vasospasm. This may reduce the delivery of glucose to the lamellar tissues (for which there is a high requirement)[37] or oxygen, or promote edema formation.

Immune Suppression

Although immune suppression is an important consequence of corticosteroid activity, it is unlikely that these actions would predispose to laminitis or worsen its severity. Recent research has shown that inflammation is a prominent feature in the pathology of laminitis, with influx of neutrophils[61] and increased expression of proinflammatory cytokines.[62] These changes have been described in the lamellar tissues during the developmental as well as the acute stage of the black walnut model of laminitis.[63-65] Comparing the black walnut model with the carbohydrate overload model, it appears that the inflammatory changes may only become evident in the acute phase of laminitis after carbohydrate overload.[66] Nevertheless, it has been suggested that some elements of the inflammatory tissue response in laminitis might be akin to the systemic inflammatory response syndrome (SIRS) seen in people with severe sepsis.[67]

The actions of glucocorticoids include inhibiting the expression of inflammatory mediators such as the interleukins, decreasing prostaglandin and leukotriene production, stabilizing neutrophil lysosomal membranes, and inhibiting leukocyte adhesion and migration.[5,68-70] They also may decrease matrix metalloproteinase enzyme expression.[71] These anti-inflammatory actions would not be consistent with glucocorticoids causing laminitis or worsening its outcome. In fact, these actions probably underlie the rationale for using steroids in the treatment of acute laminitis, as originally was advocated in the 1960s.[72]

SUMMARY

The evidence linking the administration of glucocorticoids directly with the induction of laminitis does not yet constitute absolute scientific proof, but circumstantial evidence points to very high doses (8 to 10 times the recommended therapeutic dose, for example 160 to 200 mg of triamcinolone acetonide) being associated with inducing laminitis. It remains a source of debate whether doses lower than this can precipitate the incidence of laminitis in previously normal animals, in the absence of other trigger factors. Anecdotal reports suggest that cases of laminitis may occasionally occur subsequent to the administration of lower doses of glucocorticoids, and therefore some individuals may be particularly susceptible. The reasons for this are not known. It has been shown, however, that corticosteroids such as triamcinolone may increase the severity of experimentally induced acute laminitis.

The exact mechanisms of cause and effect in the relationship between corticosteroids (both endogenous and exogenous) and laminitis remain unclear. There are, however, several possible ways in which glucocorticoids may weaken the lamellar tissues, or affect the activities of other hormones (such as insulin) that may themselves have detrimental effects on blood flow or tissue integrity. Further case data and prospective experimental studies are required to answer these questions.

REFERENCES

1. Lose MP. Drug-induced laminitis in a colt. Mod Vet Pract 1980;61:608–10.
2. Eustace RA, Redden RR. Iatrogenic laminitis. Vet Rec 1990;126(23):586.
3. Lawrence R, Fessler JF, Gall CM, et al. Clinical forum: questions and answers. Steroid-induced laminitis. Equine Pract 1985;7:31–2.
4. Frederick DM, Kehl M. Case report: back from the brink. Equus 2000;272:34–41.
5. Harkins JD, Carney JM, Tobin T. Clinical use and characteristics of the corticosteroids. Vet Clin North Am Equine Pract 1993;9(3):543–61.
6. Johnson PJ, Slight SH, Ganjam VK, et al. Glucocorticoids and laminitis in the horse. Vet Clin Equine 2002;18:219–36.
7. Hood DM, Stephens KA, Amoss MS. The effect of exogenous steroid on the carbohydrate overload model of equine laminitis: a preliminary report. Am Assoc Practic Newslett 1982;2:149–51.
8. US Food and Drug Administration. Cumulative Veterinary Adverse Drug Experience (ADE) Reports, 1987–2009.
9. Cornelisse CJ, Robinson NE. Glucocorticoid therapy and laminitis: fact or fiction? Equine Vet Educ 2004;16(2):90–3.
10. Hood DM, Grosenbaugh DA, Mostafa MB, et al. The role of vascular mechanisms in the development of acute equine laminitis. J Vet Intern Med 1993;7:228–33.
11. Slater MR, Hood DM, Carter GK. Descriptive epidemiological study of equine laminitis. Equine Vet J 1995;27:364–7.
12. Cripps PJ, Eustace RA. Factors involved in the prognosis of equine laminitis in the UK. Equine Vet J 1999;31(5):433–42.
13. Bathe AP. The corticosteroid laminitis story: 3. The clinician's viewpoint. Equine Vet J 2007;39(1):12–3.
14. Chen CL, Sailor JA, Collier J, et al. Synovial and serum levels of triamcinolone following intra-articular administration of triamcinolone acetonide in the horse. J Vet Pharmacol Ther 1992;15(3):240–6.
15. McCluskey MJ, Kavenagh PB. Clinical use of triamcinolone acetonide in the horse (205 cases) and the incidence of glucocorticoid-induced laminitis associated with its use. Equine Vet Edu 2004;16:86–9.

16. Tumas DB, Hines MT, Perryman LE, et al. Corticosteroid immunosuppression and monoclonal antibody-mediated CD5+ T lymphocyte depletion in normal and infectious anaemia virus-carrier horses. J Gen Virol 1994;75:959–68.
17. French K, Pollitt CC, Pass MA. Pharmacokinetics and metabolic effects of triamcinolone acetonide and their possible relationships to glucocorticoid-induced laminitis in horses. J Vet Pharmacol Ther 2000;23:287–92.
18. Bertone JJ, Horspool LJ. Drugs and dosages for use in equines. In: Bertone JJ, Horspool LJ, editors. Equine clinical pharmacology. 1st edition. Philadelphia: WB Saunders; 2004. p. 380.
19. McIlwraith CW. Diseases of joints, tendons, ligaments and related structures. In: Adams TS, editor. Adams' lameness in horses. Philadelphia: Lea and Febiger; 1987. p. 339–485.
20. Dutton H. The corticosteroid laminitis story: 1. Duty of care. Equine Vet J 2007; 39(1):12–3.
21. Ryu S, Kim B, Lee C, et al. Glucocorticoid-induced laminitis with hepatopathy in a Thoroughbred filly. J Vet Sci 2004;5(3):271–4.
22. Love S. Equine Cushing's disease. Br Vet J 1993;149:139–53.
23. McCue PM. Equine Cushing's disease. Vet Clin North Am Equine Pract 2002; 18(3):533–43.
24. van der Kolk JH, Wensing T, Kalsbeek HC, et al. Laboratory diagnosis of equine pituitary pars intermedia adenoma. Domest Anim Endocrinol 1995;12(1):35–9.
25. Haritou SJ, Zylstra R, Ralli C, et al. Seasonal changes in circadian peripheral plasma concentrations of melatonin, serotonin, dopamine and cortisol in aged horses with Cushing's disease under natural photoperiod. J Neuroendocrinol 2008;20:988–96.
26. McGowan CM, Neiger R. Efficacy of trilostane for the treatment of equine Cushing's syndrome. Equine Vet J 2003;35(4):414–8.
27. Johnson PJ. The equine metabolic syndrome peripheral Cushing's syndrome. Vet Clin North Am Equine Pract 2002;18(2):271–93.
28. Johnson PJ, Ganjam VK, Slight SH, et al. Tissue-specific dysregulation of cortisol metabolism in equine laminitis. Equine Vet J 2004;36(1):41–5.
29. Asplin KE, Sillence MN, Pollitt CC, et al. Induction of laminitis by prolonged hyperinsulinemia in clinically normal ponies. Vet J 2007;174:530–5.
30. DeLaat MA, McGowan CM, Sillence MN, et al. Equine laminitis: induced by 48 h hyperinsulinemia in Standardbred horses. Equine Vet J 2010;42(2):129–36.
31. Nourian AR, Asplin KE, McGowan CM, et al. Equine laminitis: ultrastructural lesions detected in ponies following hyperinsulinemia. Equine Vet J 2009;41(7): 671–7.
32. Tiley HA, Geor RJ, McCutcheon LJ. Effects of dexamethasone administration on insulin resistance and components of insulin signaling and glucose metabolism in equine skeletal muscle. Am J Vet Res 2008;69:51–8.
33. Bailey SR, Menzies-Gow NJ, Harris PA, et al. Effect of dietary fructans and dexamethasone administration on the insulin response of ponies predisposed to laminitis. J Am Vet Med Assoc 2007;231:1365–73.
34. Borer KE, Menzies-Gow NJ, Berhane Y, et al. Seasonal influence on insulin and cortisol results from overnight dexamethasone suppression tests (DST) in normal and previously laminitic ponies (abstract). J Equine Vet Sci 2010; 30(2):103.
35. Pass MA, Pollitt S, Pollitt CC. Decreased glucose metabolism causes separation of hoof lamellae in vitro: a trigger for laminitis? Equine Vet J Suppl 1998; 26:133–8.

36. French KR, Pollitt CC. Equine laminitis: glucose deprivation and MMP activation induce dermo-epidermal separation in vitro. Equine Vet J 2004;36(3):261–6.

37. Wattle O, Pollitt CC. Lamellar metabolism. Clin Tech Equine Pract 2004;3:22–33.

38. Sakoda H, Ogihara T, Anai M. Dexamethasone-induced insulin resistance in 3T3-L1 adipocytes is due to inhibition of glucose transport rather than insulin signal transduction. Diabetes 2000;49(10):1700–8.

39. Treiber KH, Kronfeld DS, Geor RJ. Insulin resistance in equids: possible role in laminitis. J Nutr 2006;136(Suppl 7):2094S–8S.

40. Johnson PJ, Messer NT, Ganjam VK. Cushing's syndromes, insulin resistance, and endocrinopathic laminitis. Equine Vet J 2004;36(3):194–8.

41. Caballero AE. Endothelial dysfunction in obesity and insulin resistance: a road to diabetes and heart disease. Obes Res 2003;11(11):1278–89.

42. Faleiros RR, Stokes AM, Eades SC, et al. Assessment of apoptosis in epidermal lamellar cells in clinically normal horses and those with laminitis. Am J Vet Res 2004;65(5):578–85.

43. Dorscheid DR, Wojcik KR, Sun S, et al. Apoptosis of airway epithelial cells induced by corticosteroids. Am J Respir Crit Care Med 2001;164:1939–47.

44. Tse R, Marroquin BA, Dorscheid DR, et al. Beta-adrenergic agonists inhibit corticosteroid-induced apoptosis of airway epithelial cells. Am J Physiol Lung Cell Mol Physiol 2003;285(2):L393–404.

45. Beer HD, Fassler R, Werner S. Glucocorticoid-related gene expression during cutaneous wound repair. Vitam Horm 2000;59:217–39.

46. McCoy BJ, Diegelmann RF, Cohen IK. In vitro inhibition of cell growth, collagen biosynthesis, and prolylhydroxylane activity by triamcinolone acetonide. Proc Soc Exp Biol Med 1980;153:216–22.

47. Pollitt CC, Daradka M. Equine laminitis basement membrane pathology: loss of type IV collagen, type VII collagen and laminin immunostaining. Equine Vet J Suppl 1998;26:139–44.

48. Pollitt CC. Anatomy and physiology of the inner hoof wall. Clin Tech Equine Pract 2004;3:3–21.

49. Hendry KA, MacCallum AJ, Knight CH, et al. Effect of endocrine and paracrine factors on protein synthesis and cell proliferation on bovine hoof tissue culture. J Dairy Res 1999;66:23–33.

50. Kreuger AS, Kinden DA, Garner HE, et al. Ultrastructural study of the equine caecum during onset of laminitis. Am J Vet Res 1996;47:1804–12.

51. Weiss DJ, Evanson OA, Macleay J, et al. Transient alteration in intestinal permeability to technetium Tc99m diethylenetriamino–pentaacetate during the prodromal phase of alimentary laminitis in ponies. Am J Vet Res 1998;59:1431–4.

52. McConnico RS, Holm AS, Eades SC, et al. The effect of Black Walnut extract on equine colonic histopathology and in vitro ion transport. In: Barton M, Love S, Merritt A, editors. Proceedings of the Sixth Colic Research Symposium. Manchester (England): Equine Veterinary Journal Ltd; 2002.

53. Kiziltas S, Imeryuz N, Gurcan T, et al. Corticosteroid therapy augments gastro-duodenal permeability to sucrose. Am J Gastroenterol 1998;93:2420–5.

54. Hunt RJ. The pathophysiology of acute laminitis. Compendium of Continuing Veterinary Education 1991;13(6):401–7.

55. Moore JN, Allen D. The pathophysiology of acute laminitis. Vet Med 1996;34:936–9.

56. Bailey SR, Marr CM, Elliott J. Current research and theories on the pathogenesis of acute laminitis in the horse. Vet J 2004;167(2):129–42.

57. Eyre P, Elmes PJ, Strickland S. Corticosteroid-potentiated vascular responses of the equine digit: a possible pharmacologic basis for laminitis. Am J Vet Res 1979; 40:135–8.
58. Eyre P, Elmes PJ. Corticosteroid-induced laminitis? Further investigations on the isolated, perfused hoof. Vet Res Commun 1980;4:139–43.
59. Bailey SR. A study of the vascular effects and factors regulating the concentration of 5-hydroxytryptamine in the equine digital circulation [PhD thesis]. London: University of London; 1998.
60. Cornelisse CJ, Robinson NE, Berney CA, et al. Thermographic study of in vivo modulation of vascular responses to phenylephrine and endothelin-1 by dexamethasone in the horse. Equine Vet J 2006;38(2):119–26.
61. Black SJ, Lunn DP, Yin C, et al. Leukocyte emigration in the early stages of laminitis. Vet Immunol Immunopathol 2006;109:161–6.
62. Belknap JK, Gigere S, Pettigrew A. Lamellar pro-inflammatory cytokine expression patterns in laminitis at the developmental stage and at the onset of lameness: innate vs. adaptive immune response. Equine vet J 2007;39(1):42–7.
63. Fontaine GL, Belknap JK, Allen D, et al. Expression of interleukin-1β in the digital laminae of horses in the prodromal stage of experimentally induced laminitis. Am J Vet Res 2001;62:714–20.
64. Waguespack RW, Kemppainen RJ, Cochran A, et al. Increased expression of MAIL, a cytokine-associated nuclear protein, in the prodromal stage of black walnut-induced laminitis. Equine Vet J 2004;36(3):285–91.
65. Waguespack RW, Cochran A, Belknap JK. Expression of the cyclooxygenase isoforms in the prodromal stage of black walnut-induced laminitis in horses. Am J Vet Res 2004;65(12):1724–9.
66. Leise BS, Johnson PJ, Faleiros RR, et al. Laminar inflammatory gene expression in the carbohydrate overload model of equine laminitis [abstract]. J Vet Int Med 2009;23(3):780.
67. Belknap JK, Moore JN, Crouser EC. Sepsis—from human organ failure to laminar failure. Vet Immunol Immunopathol 2009;129:155–7.
68. Lee SW, Tsou AP, Chan H, et al. Glucocorticoids selectively inhibit the transcription of the interleukin-1 beta gene and decrease the stability of interleukin-1 beta mRNA. Proc Natl Acad Sci U S A 1988;85(4):1204–8.
69. Shupnik MA, Chrousos GP, Siragy HM. Glucocorticoids and mineralocorticoids. In: Brody TM, Larner J, Minneman KP, editors. Human pharmacology: molecular to clinical. St. Louis (MO): Mosby, Incorporated; 1998. p. 485–97.
70. Liu L, Wang YX, Zhou J, et al. Rapid non-genomic inhibitory effects of glucocorticoids on human neutrophil degranulation. Inflamm Res 2005;54(1):37–41.
71. Richardson DW, Dodge GR. Dose-dependent effects of corticosteroids on expression of matrix-related genes in normal and cytokine-treated articular chondrocytes. Inflamm Res 2003;52(1):39–49.
72. Roberts D. Treatment of laminitis by intra-arterial infusion of adrenocorticoid steroids. Vet Med Small Anim Clin 1965;60(11):1109–13.

Supporting Limb Laminitis

Andrew van Eps, BVSc, PhD[a],*, Simon N. Collins, PhD[a,b],
Christopher C. Pollitt, BVSc, PhD[a,c]

KEYWORDS

• Laminitis • Horse • Supporting limb • Weight bearing

Laminitis in the unaffected supporting limb is a common and devastating secondary consequence of painful limb conditions in the horse (**Fig. 1**).[1–3]

Although there has been significant advancement in the techniques used for the treatment of painful limb conditions such as catastrophic fractures and orthopedic/synovial infections in horses, treatment success is still limited to those cases in which laminitis in the supporting limbs does not intervene. The actual incidence of supporting limb laminitis (SLL) in such cases has not been documented, although it is estimated to be at least greater than 10%.[4] Although the severity and duration of lameness are considered risk factors,[2,4] the development of SLL is still unpredictable, both in terms of timing and also with respect to which cases will succumb to it (and what degree of pain exhibited in the limb with the primary condition is necessary for SLL development).[5] The mortality on development of SLL is high (at least 50%),[2] and this type of laminitis tends to be commonly associated with rapid and severe failure of the suspensory apparatus of the distal phalanx (SADP), with subsequent distal displacement ("sinking") of the distal phalanx (DP) within the hoof capsule (**Figs. 2–4**).

There has been much research in recent years focusing on the pathogenesis of laminitis, particularly of the types that occur secondary to sepsis, or in association with insulin resistance. By contrast, there has been little or no primary research focused on the mechanisms that result in SLL. It is commonly believed that the pathogenesis of SLL has little in common with the other more comprehensively studied forms of the disease, at least until structural failure of the SADP begins to occur, at which time secondary inflammation, enzymatic activation, and vascular derangements are common sequelae. At present veterinary opinion is divided as to the precise causal mechanism resulting in SLL. On the one hand, it has been suggested that the gross

[a] School of Veterinary Science, The University of Queensland, Gatton Campus, Gatton, QLD 4343, Australia
[b] Orthopaedic Research Group, Centre for Equine Studies, Animal Health Trust, Lanwades Park, Kentford, Newmarket, Suffolk, UK
[c] The Laminitis Institute, University of Pennsylvania School of Veterinary Medicine, New Bolton Center, Kennett Square, PA 19348, USA
* Corresponding author.
E-mail address: a.vaneps@uq.edu.au

Vet Clin Equine 26 (2010) 287–302
doi:10.1016/j.cveq.2010.06.007
0749-0739/10/$ – see front matter © 2010 Elsevier Inc. All rights reserved.

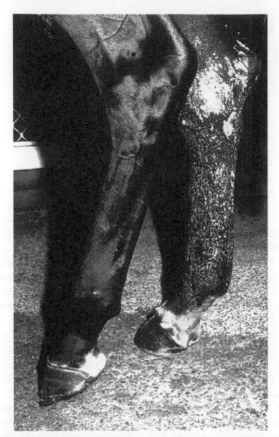

Fig. 1. A Standardbred horse with severe, septic arthritis of the right hock. For 12 days, after the initial injury, the painful right limb was non–weight bearing and the left hind limb supported most of the horse's hindquarter weight. Subsequently the left foot developed severe catastrophic laminitis, so painful that the horse transferred its weight to the injured right limb.

anatomic and histologic changes may be consistent with direct mechanical overload of the SADP.[6] Conversely, others suggest that inadequate perfusion of the lamellar tissue, due to reduced digital blood flow in the supporting limb associated with excessive and continuous compensatory weight-bearing loads is the most likely pathogenesis of SLL.[4,7–10] Although there is no direct experimental evidence to support this proposed vascular mechanism, it is accepted that the horse must unload the digit for a period of time to facilitate digital (and in particular dorsal lamellar) blood flow when at rest.[4] However, there is no evidence documenting the required duration or frequency of these periods of unloading, and furthermore no information regarding what amount of blood flow is adequate and how sensitive the lamellar tissues are to hypoperfusion.

This article discusses the pathophysiology of SLL, including the consequences of excessive and prolonged weight bearing on the digit. Other potential contributors to lamellar damage in horses with a painful primary unilateral limb lameness are also considered. For detailed discussion of treatment and preventative measures the reader is directed elsewhere.[4,7]

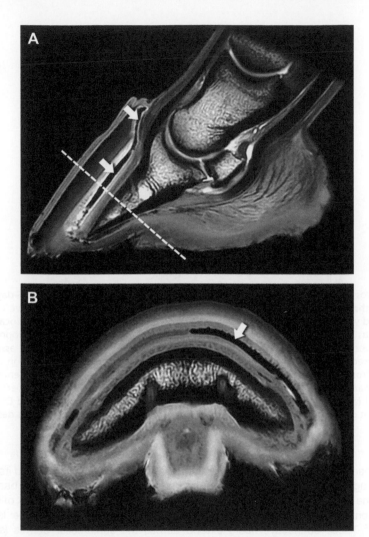

Fig. 2. High-resolution 3-dimensional T1 spoiled gradient echo magnetic resonance (MR) images in the sagittal (*A*) and transverse (*B*) planes (at the level indicated by the *dotted line* in *A*), of laminitis in a supporting foot 5 days after carpal arthrodesis in the opposite forelimb. The extensive separation between the dorsal hoof wall and the underlying dermis, in the coronary and lamellar regions (*arrow* in *A* and *B*), is diagnostic of severe and catastrophic failure of the suspensory apparatus of the distal phalanx (SADP), and was associated with extensive hemorrhage into the submural void.

LAMINITIS AS A CONSEQUENCE OF MECHANICAL OVERLOAD: MECHANISMS
Review of Normal Mechanics of the Digit

The horse foot displays a highly modified anatomic organization in which the appendicular skeleton is suspended within the hoof capsule via the SADP.[11–13] This anatomic structure (referred to elsewhere as the hoof-bone attachment apparatus) unites the DP and hoof wall via the lamellar dermis. The SADP is formed by the interdigitation of the dermal and epidermal lamellae (*stratum lamellatum*), and is facilitated

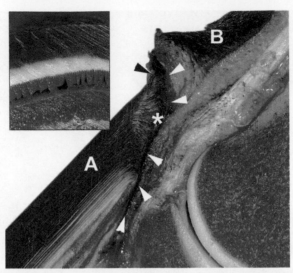

Fig. 3. Gross, midline anatomic section of the coronary region of foot with SLL 5 days after carpal arthrodesis (same horse as in **Fig. 2**) showing the extensive degenerative changes associated with distal dislocation of the DP (following failure of the SADP). Dislocation of the DP has resulted in distortion of the proximal hoof wall (A) and the development of a pronounced and palpable, supracoronary depression (B). This condition is associated with marked reorientation of the dermal papillae and complete physical separation of these papillae from the proximal hoof wall (*asterisk*). There is a shear lesion that extends along the coronary interface from the proximal lamellar region to the external aspect of the hoof wall (*arrowheads*). A transverse section through the dorsal hoof wall and DP (*inset*) shows that global lamellar separation has occurred and the case fits the laminitis descriptor "sinker."

by the basement membrane (which forms the dermoepidermal junction) and its structural linkage to the DP. The basal epidermal cells are attached to the basement membrane (BM) via hemidesmosomes, which in turn are linked to a network of collagenous connective fibers contained within the extracellular matrix of the lamellar dermis.[14] These connective fibers extend across the sublamellar dermis (*stratum reticulare*), and finally insert onto the periosteum of the DP via Sharpey's fibers. This complex anatomic association unites the hoof capsule with the DP,[13–15] and enables these structures to act as a single structural and functional entity.[16–19] This SADP is of major biomechanical importance in force transference between ground and skeleton.

This anatomic arrangement (the unguligrade stance/posture), is unique to the ungulate foot, and results in a unique mode of weight bearing. Indeed, in the horse it constitutes the principal mechanism by which weight-bearing forces are accommodated/resisted, and pain-free[14,20–22] force transfer is achieved between the ground and the appendicular skeleton.[13,15] Unlike the digitigrade and plantigrade foot, weight-bearing forces do not act through the digital cushion and the sole. Instead, they are redirected to the hoof wall via the SADP,[23,24] with the hoof wall acting as the major weight-bearing component. The biomechanical response of the horse foot to static weight bearing is summarized in **Fig. 5**.

It is widely accepted that the foot responds to loading in the manner described by the "depression theory,"[23,24] and in accordance with Newton's third law of motion, a vertically directed ground reaction force (G) is generated during weight bearing,

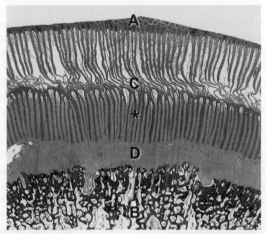

Fig. 4. Photograph of the transverse section of the hoof (A) and DP (B) from the horse in **Fig. 2.** There is marked, physical lamellar separation (C) with the original epidermal lamellae empty of dermal lamellar connective tissue. Dysplastic epidermal lamellae have reformed (*asterisk*) but, no longer attached to the hoof wall proper, they will contribute little to the now severely compromised SADP. D, sublamellar dermis (H&E stain).

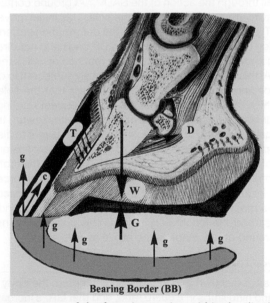

Bearing Border (BB)

Fig. 5. Diagrammatic summary of the force interaction within the distal limb during static weight bearing to illustrate the force interaction in the sagittal plane of the foot (Collins 2004,[20] after Müller 1936,[12] modified after Pellmann 1995,[13] Budras and Huskamp 1999[17]). c, resolved compressive component of g acting in a distoproximal direction within the hoof wall; D, action of deep digital flexor tendon; g, component of the ground reaction force acting on the bearing border; G, ground reaction force generated in response to W; T, tensile forces acting across the SADP; W, weight of horse acting through the center of the hoof.

which is directed through the center of the solear aspect of the hoof, to counter the weight of the horse (W) that acts through the DP. However, as the distal margin of the hoof wall (BB) represents the weight-bearing element of the hoof, components of the ground reaction force (g) act via the BB. A resolved compressive force vector (c) is directed in a distoproximal direction, from the BB to the coronary band. The action of the force vectors (c and W) result in the generation of tensile forces (T) within the SADP. As a consequence of this force interaction, and the geometric shape of the hoof, the hoof capsule deforms in a consistent manner[25,26] resulting in inward movement of the proximal margin of the hoof wall, a decrease in the proximodistal height of the capsule, dorso-concavity of the dorsal aspect of the hoof wall, mediolateral heel expansion, and flattening of the sole. This deformation reflects the complex interaction between the external forces that act against the ground during weight bearing, and also the force changes that occur internally within the foot.[27] In this regard, the DP is subjected to 4 additional loading forces: compressive forces at the distal interphalangeal joint (DIPJ) due to the body weight of the animal; tensile forces at the extensor process due to the insertion and action of the common extensor tendon; tensile forces on the palmar surface due to the insertion and action of the deep digital flexor tendon; and compressive forces generated against the sole.

The pliant nature of the dermis and the SADP allows semi-independent movement of the DP relative to the hoof wall and sole (dislocation) in response to these force interactions. The dislocation of the DP is therefore dependent on the complex interaction of force vectors and the material properties of the SADP. In addition, as the foot acts as a unified functional entity, the dislocation of the DP is both influenced by, and influences, the hoof wall through the action of the SADP.[9] At ground contact, the DP is dislocated vertically away from the wall toward the sole. This initial movement generates the tensile forces (T) within the SADP. Although the deformation pattern of the hoof is in part a direct function of its geometric shape, the DP begins to act directly on the hoof capsule as loading forces increase, and a point is reached at which the sole cannot be displaced further. At this stage the solear dermis is likely subjected to compressive and shear forces. As loading increases, it has been argued that the sole further acts as a fulcrum about which the DP rotates, with the palmar aspect rotating distally, further flattening the solear surface, while the apex of the DP rotates toward the dorsal aspect of the hoof wall. Finally, lowering of the middle phalanx is thought to displace the digital cushion and further contribute to the degree of lateral heel expansion.

The magnitude of the ground reaction force (GRF) acting on the foot (and, intuitively, the resultant deformations, anatomic displacement, and internal forces) is dependent on several factors including: the weight of the horse (bwt); the speed of locomotion; the loading rate (as most biologic tissues display strain rate dependant viscoelastic material properties); and the locomotory gait (as this governs the number of feet in contact with the ground at any stage in the stride cycle).

Excessive Mechanical Load on the Digit

Force plate studies have shown that in the standing horse, the body mass is divided between the fore and hind limbs in a 60:40 ratio, and that GRFs increase progressively with speed-related gait change, with the foot being subjected to peak forces equivalent to 0.25 × bwt at the walk, 0.5 × bwt at the trot, and up to 3 × bwt at the gallop. Subtle changes in the GRF pattern have also been reported in association with limb lameness,[28,29] with the lame limb exhibiting significantly lower peak vertical GRF, less flexion of the DIPJ, and less extension of the metacarpophalangeal joint as compared with compensating limbs.[29] In unilateral forelimb as well as hind limb lameness, reduced loading of the lame limb is compensated primarily by the contralateral limb and, to a lesser extent, by the concurrently loaded ipsilateral or diagonal limb.[30] The weight-shifting mechanism corresponds to changes in body center of mass movement. Intuitively the change in the GRF pattern results in greater deformation of the hoof capsule, greater displacement of the DP, and greater internal force generation within the compensatory limbs. Although postural changes can occur during locomotion that can effectively negate the equivalent compensatory overload situation in the other limbs, it is not known whether a similar mechanism occurs to equivalent effect in the stall-rested, standing horse experiencing restricted activity.

Historical reports indicate that excessive mechanical overload of the foot can directly lead to SADP failure and traumatic lamellar damage, as is the case with classic "road founder" and, in recent times, in the sports horse following high-intensity work. Indeed it can be argued that lamellar damage seen in the modern sports horse may be considered as a latter-day equivalent to "road founder," and represents an example of traumatic laminitis. However it seems unlikely, from a mechanical perspective, that the modest compensatory load redistributions associated with unilateral limb lameness can per se be sufficient to induce traumatic lamellar damage in cases of SLL. Indeed, it is difficult to envisage a situation whereby such compensatory load redistribution can, in the standing horse, exceed the mechanical "strength" of the SADP, given that it can normally withstand up to 3 times the weight of the horse without adverse mechanical effect. Linford[31] developed a model to study "traumatic" laminitis. A single hoof was excessively trimmed, and horses were housed and exercised on concrete surfaces over a 4-month period. Lameness in the overtrimmed digit was associated with solar bruising and changes in the DP, with minimal detectable laminitis pathology. Increased weight bearing in the contralateral (control) limb resulted in more notable laminitis pathology, though the changes were still very mild. There are currently no other published studies documenting experimental laminitis induced by excessive weight bearing.

It is worthwhile considering that SLL cases often show severe, extensive, and catastrophic lamellar separation, which extends circumferentially around the entire hoof capsule (see **Figs. 2–4**). This dermoepidermal separation often extends across the coronary dermis, resulting in a pronounced shear lesion seen at the height of the coronary band. It does not seem plausible that excessive mechanical load on the SADP alone could be responsible for such severe changes, given the inherent strength of the SADP in the normal hoof. It therefore seems more likely that SADP failure occurs as a consequence of changes or disturbances to normal foot function, which result as a secondary effect of these modest load redistributions. Lamellar damage is more likely to be the result of metabolic, vascular, and/or lymphatic compromise occurring secondary to prolonged and enforced changes in load distribution; decreased cyclical loading of the digit; and/or inflammatory responses to these events within the compensatory limb(s).

Vascular Supply to the Digit and Its Association with Weight-Bearing Load

Many have pondered the mechanics of the circulation of blood through the horse foot. Situated some distance from the heart and subjected to large fluctuations in hydraulic pressure and centrifugal force, especially during the stance phase of the high-speed gallop, several physical problems have to be overcome for blood and lymph to complete their mandated physiologic circuit. Bouley's insightful observations in 1851 described the horse's foot as an additional heart working as "a pushing and sucking pump".[32] The "pushing" phase (venous return) comes from descent of bones, tendons, and cartilage into the semirigid hoof capsule, compressing the corium and the blood vessels contained within. The low-resistance veins and lymphatic vessels are more affected by the pressure than the thick-walled arteries, and conduct blood and lymph away from the foot. The absence of valves in the majority of the extensive anastomosing network of digital veins ensures an unencumbered, rapid outflow of blood (and coincidentally facilitates retrograde venography). Valves are present mid-pastern (in the proper digital vein) and in the coronary, subcoronary, and caudal hoof veins.[33] For a pump to operate effectively, no back flow must occur. Bouley assumed that blood pressure in the completely valveless palmar arteries was the mechanism preventing retrograde arterial flow. However, it is important to appreciate that the horse foot experiences loading forces during the stance phase equivalent to 3 × bwt at the gallop, which intuitively induce internal forces that far exceed systolic pressure. Hence without the presence of other protective mechanisms to safeguard the digital circulation, turbulent arterial backflow would occur. When the loading (pressure) phase ends veins are refilled (the "sucking" phase) ready for the next cycle. This phase is easily demonstrated on cannulated, cadaver distal limb specimens that have the distal check ligament intact.[34]

A more complete understanding of foot circulation was derived in 1982 from the pioneering, angiographic studies of van Kraayenburg and colleagues,[35,36] using contrast agent injected into the palmar digital arteries of conscious, standing horses. With the foot relaxed and unloaded, contrast medium injected into digital arteries of horses of Arabian descent completely filled the terminal arch within the DP. From the terminal arch arterial branches exited via numerous foramina in the dorsal parietal surface of the DP to supply the dorsal, lamellar region. However, when one forelimb was lifted and then contrast was injected into the palmar artery of the now supporting limb, arterial constrictions were evident that prevented blood flow in the terminal arch and the dorsal lamellae. The arterial termination points were adjacent to the medial and lateral extremities of the distal sesamoid bone and within the terminal arch itself. Although technical difficulties prevented this being demonstrated in vivo in all the horses in the study, it was readily replicated in cadaver limbs subjected to calibrated loads in a hydraulic press. Each increment of load caused greater flexion of the DIPJ until flow in the palmar digital arteries was terminated. The load required was less than the forequarter mass of the horses; 262 ± 52 kg.[35,36]

Thus it was established that for each limb there was a mechanical load that could occlude arterial blood flow to the foot. Arterial closure was considered essential and physiologic in normal horses, and was the likely mechanism preventing arterial back flow during the compressive load phase of the stride. Thus, approximately 130 years after the Parisian veterinarian Bouley proposed that blood pressure prevented arterial back flow during the stance phase, it was the South African farrier van Kraayenburg that completed the explanation by discovering that, complementary to arterial blood pressure, there was a valve-like, closing mechanism in the digital arteries of the loaded distal limb.

van Kraayenburg's angiography of the cadaver distal limb under load has been replicated in the authors' laboratory; first using digital subtraction angiography in 1992,[34] and recently using computed tomography (CT) and Mimics modeling software (Materialise NV, Leuven, Belgium), with barium sulfate as a vascular contrast medium (Pollitt, van Eps, and Collins, unpublished data, 2010). Mimics models were created according to the method of Collins and colleagues.[37] Barium sulfate is a suspension of particles too large to enter capillaries, so either arteriograms or venograms can be obtained by infusing the appropriate vessels. Barium arteriograms of normal, non-loaded Standardbred feet showed the expected vascular pattern (see "The Anatomy and Physiology of the Suspensory Apparatus of the Distal Phalanx" by C.C. Pollitt in Advances in Laminitis, Part 1 of *Veterinary Clinics of North America: Equine Practice*,

2010). Contrast in the medial and lateral digital arteries, entering the solear canal on the palmar aspect of the DP, showed no evidence of constrictions (**Fig. 6**).

When the distal limb was moderately loaded (**Fig. 7**), Mimics models of the CT data showed occlusion of the medial and lateral digital arteries adjacent to the extremities of the navicular bone (see white arrows in **Fig. 7**A) thus confirming the results of van Kraayenburg and colleagues.[35] However, proximal to the navicular bone a large segment of both the medial and lateral digital arteries was also void of contrast (see blue arrows in **Fig. 7**A). There was reduced arterial contrast in the heels and quarters of the foot (see asterisk in **Fig. 7**A). Addition of the deep digital flexor tendon (DDFT) to the Mimics model (see **Fig. 7**B) showed that the medial and lateral margins of the insertion of the DDFT closely overlaid the points of arterial occlusion. During limb loading, tension in the DDFT may have compressed the arteries and thus participated in the closing mechanism.

A lateral view of the Mimics model (**Fig. 8**) shows the reduced perfusion of the heels and quarters (see asterisk in **Fig. 8**A) and the extent of occlusion in the medial and lateral digital arteries (distal to the blue arrow in **Fig. 8**A). Although the arteries entering the solear canal are occluded, the terminal arch (see white arrow in **Fig. 8**B) is nevertheless filled, apparently by anastomosing branches of the proximal and middle phalangeal arteries. The dorsal branches of the medial and lateral palmar arteries (see black arrow in **Fig. 8**A) have escaped occlusion and may have contributed to filling of the terminal arch via anastomoses from the circumflex and other arteries.

When the distal limb was heavily loaded (**Fig. 9**) and the common digital artery infused with barium sulfate, there was no filling of any artery below the coronary band. Increased tension within the flexor tendons and the digital annular ligaments, as well as global compression of the corium between bone and hoof, prevents arterial blood entering the foot. This degree of DIPJ flexion would be encountered during locomotion at even moderate speeds. Thus, the horse's foot appears to routinely experience a short period of total arterial occlusion during the limb cycle that coincides with venous and lymphatic outflow from the foot. During the nonloaded, swing phase of the stride, arterial flow to the foot is restored and veins and lymphatic vessels are refilled.

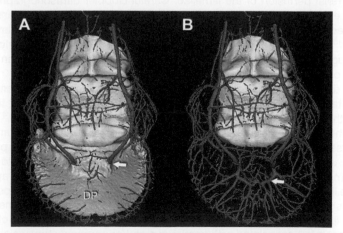

Fig. 6. Mimics models of computed tomography data of normal Standardbred cadaver foot with barium sulfate infused into the common digital artery. The medial and lateral branches of the artery enter the solear canal of the DP via foramina (*arrow* in *A*). Within the DP the arteries anastomose and form the terminal arch (*arrow* in *B*).

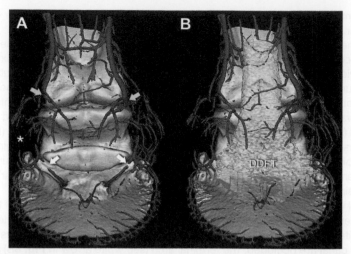

Fig. 7. Palmar views of Mimics models of a moderately loaded distal limb with the common digital artery infused with barium sulfate. There is occlusion of the medial and lateral digital arteries adjacent to the extremities of the navicular bone (*white arrows* in A). A large segment of both the medial and lateral digital arteries is also void of contrast (distal to the *blue arrows* in A). There is reduced perfusion of the heels and quarters of the foot (*asterisk* in A). The deep digital flexor tendon (DDFT) has been added to the Mimics model in B. The medial and lateral margins of the insertion of the DDFT closely overlay the points of arterial occlusion.

These filling and emptying events alternate in the heart-like manner proposed in 1851 by Bouley.[32]

This cyclically reduced/absent arterial blood flow to the foot is a possible explanation for the pathogenesis of SLL. A horse standing on either one fore or one hind foot, for long periods of time, may recruit the arterial closing mechanism and experience reduced arterial perfusion of the lamellae. Careful Doppler ultrasonography studies show that even moderately increased weight bearing increases resistance in the vascular bed of the foot and decreases blood velocity in the distal palmar digital arteries.[38–40] Thus, a highly evolved mechanism, normally of benefit in circulating blood through the horse's foot during locomotion, could trap the horse in a unique pathologic process.

To avoid digital ischemia, it appears that cyclic loading of the feet plays an essential role in digital homeostasis for the horse at rest. Reduced frequency of this cyclic loading is thought to be a major risk factor for the development of SLL,[4] and may represent the major pathophysiological mechanism. Indeed even while standing, the normal horse will shift weight in the forelimbs approximately 1 to 5 times per minute (Refs.[41,42]; van Eps and Pollitt, unpublished data, 2010), presumably to maintain hemodynamic balance within the foot. The average standardbred horse appears to tolerate the lifting of one forelimb for approximately 8 to 10 minutes (van Eps and Pollitt, unpublished data, 2010). It is unclear after this time why the horse begins to resent having the limb held off the ground; presumably it is either the restraint of the limb itself, or discomfort associated with continuous and/or compensatory weight bearing in the opposite limb. If the horse is then allowed to return the limb to the ground, even just momentarily, it will again tolerate another 8- to 10-minute period of weight bearing on the opposite limb. It is interesting to consider that a period of continuous weight

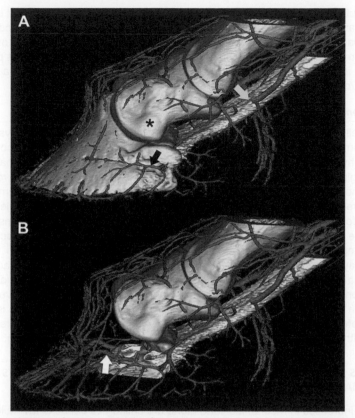

Fig. 8. Lateral views of Mimics models of a moderately loaded distal limb with the common digital artery infused with barium sulfate. There is reduced arterial contrast in the heels and quarters (*asterisk* in *A*) and extensive occlusion of the medial and lateral digital arteries (distal to the *blue arrow* in *A*). The terminal arch is filled (*white arrow* in *B*). The dorsal branches of the medial and lateral palmar arteries (*black arrow* in *A*) are not occluded and may have contributed to filling of the terminal arch via anastomoses from the circumflex and other arteries.

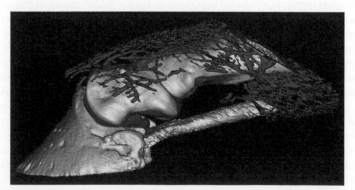

Fig. 9. Lateral view of a Mimics model of a heavily loaded distal limb with the common digital artery infused with barium sulfate. There is zero arterial contrast fill below the coronary band and the entire foot is devoid of arterial contrast.

bearing sufficient to cause ischemia of the lamellar/solear corium may result in a noci-ceptive/paresthetic stimulus that prompts the horse to unload the limb. It could then be speculated that in the horse with a severely painful limb condition there is overriding of this normal stimulus. It is also interesting to consider the possibility that profound analgesia in a horse at risk of SLL could also contribute to reducing such a stimulus to unload/cycle the supporting limb.

Consequences of Reduced Blood Supply to the Digit

Traditionally, lamellar ischemia had been implicated as the major pathophysiological mechanism in all forms of laminitis.[8] The role of ischemia in laminitis secondary to sepsis or hyperinsulinemia is now under question; however, ischemia, and particularly a lack of glucose delivery to the lamellar tissue, is likely to play a significant role in the development of SLL. The equine foot has been shown to consume large amounts of glucose relative to other tissues.[43] The foot contains no skeletal muscle and no capacity for the storage of glycogen, so it is reasonable to assume that consumption of glucose reflects the rate of glycolysis and oxidation through the citric acid cycle. Lamellar epidermal basal cells are rich in the glucose transporter GLUT1, and the lamellar layer seems to be able to rely on glycolysis for production of adenosine triphosphate.[43] The lamellar tissue has a high requirement for glucose,[43] and glucose deprivation results in a reduction in the mechanical force required to achieve lamellar separation in vitro.[44,45] Failure of glucose delivery to the lamellae (due to ischemia) may therefore be the primary means by which SADP failure ultimately occurs in asso-ciation with reduced perfusion during prolonged, increased weight bearing.

LAMINITIS AS A SYSTEMIC DISEASE: THE POSSIBLE CONTRIBUTIONS OF SYSTEMIC INFLAMMATION AND INSULIN-MEDIATED MECHANISMS TO SLL

Although increases in mechanical load alone are unlikely to cause SADP failure if the lamellar tissue itself is normal, it is reasonable to assume that a weakened lamellar interface could fail under conditions of even mildly increased load. Activation of lamellar matrix metalloproteinases decreases the force required to achieve lamellar separation in vitro.[44] Mild underlying systemic inflammation, or even hyperinsulinemia, could presumably lead to weakening of the lamellar interface as occurs in "general-ized" laminitis associated with these mechanisms. This weakening may be insufficient to result in failure of the SADP in the primarily injured/painful limb and the other more normally loaded limbs, but may be sufficient to cause SADP failure in the supporting limb. In general, investigators and clinicians have discounted the possibility that lami-nitis in the supporting limb is simply a severe manifestation of generalized laminitis (affecting all limbs). Although gross evidence of laminitis in limbs apart from the sup-porting limb is generally not reported in most clinical cases, there are no reports exam-ining for subtle evidence of laminitis in these limbs. It is the authors' experience that a small proportion of SLL cases do indeed develop clinical (and gross pathologic) evidence of laminitis in multiple limbs, particularly if the course has been more protracted.

The horse being treated for a painful limb injury or infection may also be suffering from elements of systemic inflammation and insulin resistance, known to be contrib-utors to "generalized" (multiple limb) laminitis. Stall confinement (hospitalization) alone can cause reduced insulin sensitivity.[46] Coupled with stress- or pain-related hypercor-tisolemia, this could lead to hyperinsulinemia that is severe enough to contribute to weakening of the lamellar interface via the same mechanisms that cause insulin-induced laminitis in multiple limbs.[47] Similarly, horses suffering from orthopedic and synovial infections may have low-grade systemic inflammation that is not severe enough to contribute to generalized laminitis, but is sufficient to weaken the lamellar interface in a limb subjected to increased load, thereby leading to acute failure of the SADP in that limb. After all, it has been suggested that it is the unique mechanical forces acting on the lamellar tissue that are the reason laminitis is the major manifestation of multiple organ dysfunction syndrome in the septic horse.[48] It should be noted that trauma alone (in the absence of septic inflammation), can cause systemic inflammatory response syndrome in human patients.[49] Similarly, a systemic inflammatory response may occur in equine patients with a severe traumatic limb injury, even in the absence of infection. The contribution of these "systemic" mechanisms to SLL may explain why some horses succumb to the condition whereas others do not, despite seemingly similar periods of prolonged compensatory limb loading.

SUMMARY

Although the pathophysiology remains unclear, SLL may occur as a consequence of reduced lamellar blood flow caused by a lack of normal cyclic loading. It is worthwhile considering the contributions of systemic inflammation and hyperinsulinemia to lamellar failure in the patient at risk of developing SLL. More research into the vascular and lamellar metabolic effects of prolonged and increased weight bearing on a single digit is necessary before specific recommendations for prevention and treatment can be made. Nevertheless, in the light of clear evidence that limb cycling is an essential component of the circulation, it would be prudent to heed the advice of Bramlage[3] and institute, whenever practicable, measures to improve foot circulation in horses at risk of SLL via either controlled exercise (walking) or physical therapy. Until further research is completed, the ideal frequency and duration of such preventive therapy remains unknown.

ACKNOWLEDGMENTS

The authors' specifically wish to thank Dr Davide Zani, University of Milan, Italy for his assistance in translating original manuscripts, Morag Wilson and Meg Day, University of Queensland, Australia for their expertise in CT image acquisition, and Ray Wright, Animal Health Trust, Newmarket, UK for histological preparations.

REFERENCES

1. Parsons CS, Orsini JA, Krafty R, et al. Risk factors for development of acute laminitis in horses during hospitalization: 73 cases (1997-2004). J Am Vet Med Assoc 2007;230:885–9.
2. Peloso JG, Cohen ND, Walker MA, et al. Case-control study of risk factors for the development of laminitis in the contralateral limb in equidae with unilateral lameness. J Am Vet Med Assoc 1996;209:1746–9.
3. Bramlage L. Research: goals and reality. J Equine Vet Sci 2003;23:77–8.
4. Redden RF. Preventing laminitis in the contralateral lib of horses with non-weightbearing lameness. Clin Tech Equine Pract 2004;3:57–63.
5. Richardson DW. Complications of orthopaedic surgery in horses. Vet Clin North Am Equine Pract 2008;24:591–610, viii.
6. Belknap JK. Pathogenesis of laminitis. In: Robinson NE, Sprayberry KA, editors. Current therapy in equine medicine. 6th edition. Philadelphia: Saunders; 2008. p. 541–3.

7. Baxter GM, Morrison S. Complications of unilateral weight bearing. Vet Clin North Am Equine Pract 2009;24:621–42.

8. Hood DM, Grosenbaugh DA, Mostafa MB, et al. The role of vascular mechanisms in the development of acute equine laminitis. J Vet Intern Med 1993;7:228–34.

9. Hood DM. The mechanisms and consequences of structural failure of the foot. Vet Clin North Am Equine Pract 1999;15:437–61.

10. Hood DM. The pathophysiology of developmental and acute laminitis. Vet Clin North Am Equine Pract 1999;15:321–43.

11. Budras KD, Hullinger RL, Sack WO. Light and electron microscopy of keratinization in the laminar epidermis of the equine hoof with reference to laminitis. Am J Vet Res 1989;50:1150–60.

12. Muller F. Der Pferdehuf im sagittalen Axialschnitt. Arch Wiss Prakt Tierheilk 1936; 70:296–301 [in German].

13. Pellmann R. Struktur und Funktion desHufbeinträgers beim Pferd [Structure and function of the suspensory apparatus of the distal phalanx in horses] [PhD thesis]. Diss Med Vet, Freie Univ Berlin, 1995 [in German].

14. Budras KD, Bragulla H, Pellmann R, et al. Das Hufbein mit Periost und Insertionszone des Hufbeinträgers. [The coffin bone with periosteum and insertion zone of the suspensory apparatus]. Wien Tierarztl Monatsschr 1996;84:241–7 [in German].

15. Pellmann R, Budras KD, Bragulla H. Structure and function of the suspensory apparatus of the coffin bone in the horse. Pferdeheilkunde 1997;13:53–64.

16. Hood DM. Laminitis in the horse. Vet Clin North Am Equine Pract 1999;15:287–94.

17. Budras KD, Huskamp B. Belastungshufrehe - Vergleichunde Betrachtungen zu anderen systemischen Hufreheerkrankungen. Pferdeheilkunde 1999;15:89–110 [in German].

18. Pollitt CC. Equine laminitis: a report for the Rural Industries Research and Development Corporation. RIRDC Publication 01/129. Kingston (Canada): RIRDC; 2001. p. 99.

19. Pollitt CC. Aetiology of fructan-induced laminitis; mechanism of fructan involvement, alteration of hindgut microflora and quantities required. In: Proceedings of the Dodson & Horrell Ltd. 4th International Conference on Feeding Horses, United Kingdom, 2002; p. 3–6.

20. Collins SN. A materials characterisation of laminitic donkey hoof horn [PhD thesis]. De Montfort University, Leicester; 2004.

21. Budras KD, Hinterhofer C, Hirschberg RM. [The suspensory apparatus of the coffin bone—part 1: the fan-shaped re-inforcement of the suspensory apparatus at the tip of the coffin bone in the horse]. Pferdeheilkunde 2009;25:96 [in German].

22. Collins SN, Van Eps AW, Pollitt CC, et al. The Lamellar Wedge. Vet Clin North Am Equine Pract 2010;26:179–95.

23. Peters F. Die Formveränderungen des Pferdeshufes bei der Einworkung der Last mit besonderrem Bezug auf die Ausdehungstheorie. Berlin: Verlag Paray; 1883.

24. Coleman E. Grundsätze des Hufbeschlages. Darmstadt (Germany): Georg Freidrich Heyer; 1805. Giessen.

25. Lungwitz A. The changes in the form of the horse's hoof under the action of the body-weight. J Comp Pathol Ther 1891;4:191–211.

26. Douglas JE. Morphological and material properties of the equine hoof wall and laminar junction [PhD thesis]. University of Guelph; 1998.

27. Leach DH. The structure and function of the equine hoof wall [PhD thesis]. University of Saskatchewan, Saskatoon; 1980.

28. Weishaupt MA. Compensatory load redistribution in forelimb and hindlimb lameness. Proceedings of the Annual Meeting American Association of Equine Practitioners 2005;51:126–9.
29. Clayton H. The science of lameness. USDF Connection September 29–32, 2001. Available at: http://cvm.msu.edu/research/research-centers/mcphail-equine-performance-center/publications/usdf-connection/USDF_Sept01.pdf. Accessed June 17, 2010.
30. Merkens HW. Evaluation of equine locomotion during different degrees of experimentally induced lameness. II: distribution of ground reaction force patterns of the concurrently loaded limbs. Equine Vet J Suppl 1988;6:107–12.
31. Linford RL. A radiographic, morphometric, histological and ultrastructural investigation of lamellar function, abnormality and the associated radiographic findings for sound and foot sore thoroughbreds and horses with experimentally induced traumatic and alimentary laminitis [PhD thesis]. University of California, Davis, USA; 1987.
32. Bouley MH. Treatise on the organisation of the foot of the horse, comprising the study of the structure, functions and diseases of that organ [book treatise]. Paris, 1851.
33. Mishra PC, Leach DH. Extrinsic and intrinsic veins of the equine hoof wall. J Anat 1983;136:543–60.
34. Pollitt CC. Equine foot studies. VideoVision, Information Technology Services. Brisbane: The University of Queensland, Queensland, Australia; 1992.
35. Van Kraayenburg FJ. A comparative study of haemodynamics in the equid digit [MSc thesis]. The University of Pretoria; 1982.
36. van Kraayenburg FJ, Fairall N, Littlejohn A. The effect of vertical force on blood flow in the palmar arteries of the horse. In: 1st International Congress on Equine Exercise Physiology, Cambridge; 1982. p. 144–54.
37. Collins SN, Murray RC, Kneissl S, et al. Thirty-two component finite element models of a horse and donkey digit. Equine Vet J 2009;41:219–24.
38. Hoffmann KL, Wood AKW, Griffiths KA, et al. Doppler sonographic measurements of arterial blood flow and their repeatability in the equine foot during weight bearing and non-weight bearing. Res Vet Sci 2001;70:199–204.
39. Pietra M, Guglielmini C, Nardi S, et al. Influence of weight bearing and hoof position on Doppler evaluation of lateral palmar digital arteries in healthy horses. Am J Vet Res 2004;65:1211–5.
40. Wongaumnuaykul S, Siedler C, Schobesberger H, et al. Doppler sonographic evaluation of the digital blood flow in horses with laminitis or septic pododermatitis. Vet Radiol Ultrasound 2006;47:199–205.
41. Hood DM, Wagner IP, Taylor DD, et al. Voluntary limb-load distribution in horses with acute and chronic laminitis. Am J Vet Res 2001;62:1393–8.
42. Hood DM, Hunter JF, Beltz WD. Digital loading patterns in the normal standing horse. In: Hood DM, Wagner IP, Jacobsen AC, editors. Proceedings of the hoof project. College Station (TX); Texas A&M University: 1997. p. 36–43.
43. Wattle O, Pollitt CC. Lamellar metabolism. Clinical Techniques in Equine Practice 2004;13:22–33.
44. French KR, Pollitt CC. Equine laminitis: glucose deprivation and MMP activation induce dermo-epidermal separation in vitro. Equine Vet J 2004;36:261–6.
45. Pass MA, Pollitt S, Pollitt CC. Decreased glucose metabolism causes separation of hoof lamellae in vitro: a trigger for laminitis? Equine Vet J Suppl 1998;(26): 133–8.

46. Toth F, Frank N, Geor RJ, et al. Effects of pretreatment with dexamethasone or levothyroxine sodium on endotoxin-induced alterations in glucose and insulin dynamics in horses. Am J Vet Res 2010;71:60–8.
47. Asplin KE, Sillence MN, Pollitt CC, et al. Induction of laminitis by prolonged hyperinsulinaemia in clinically normal ponies. Vet J 2007;174:530–5.
48. Belknap JK, Moore JN, Crouser EC. Sepsis—from human organ failure to laminar failure. Vet Immunol Immunopathol 2009;129:155–7.
49. Brun-Buisson C. The epidemiology of the systemic inflammatory response. Intensive Care Med 2000;26(Suppl 1):S64–74.

The Pharmacologic Basis for the Treatment of Endocrinopathic Laminitis

Andy Durham, BVSc, CertEP, DEIM, MRCVS

KEYWORDS

- Laminitis • Endocrine • Cushing's disease • PPID
- Metabolic syndrome • Treatment

The causal factors and pathophysiology of equine laminitis have been the subject of much research in the last 40 years. Evidence of possible endocrine involvement in the development of laminitis was first raised by an in vitro study by Eyre and colleagues[1] in 1979 who found that digital vasoconstriction induced by epinephrine, norepinephrine, and serotonin was potentiated in the presence of glucocorticoids. Subsequently, a few anecdotal reports describing laminitis following glucocorticoid therapy were published creating a contentious debate regarding the perceived risks of glucocorticoid use in equine practice.[2] During the 1980s, an association between laminitis and insulin resistance (IR) was first demonstrated[3–5] and this association has enjoyed a recent surge in interest following the review by Johnson[6] in 2002 in which the equine metabolic syndrome (EMS) was first proposed to explain the clustering of obesity, IR, and laminitis in certain individuals. In the meantime the complex age-related endocrinopathy associated with pituitary pars intermedia dysfunction (PPID, equine Cushing's disease) has become increasingly recognized by equine practitioners presented with ageing horses suffering from laminitis.[7] Other endocrine disturbances have been described in horses with laminitis including low concentrations of thyroid hormones and increased concentrations of testosterone, catecholamines, rennin, and aldosterone although any causal association between these findings and laminitis is considered unlikely.[8,9] Thus endocrinopathic laminitis, whereby endocrine disturbances cause or predispose to the development of laminitis, is regarded as comprising iatrogenic glucocorticoid-induced laminitis, PPID, and EMS.

Although the treatment and management of laminitis in the horse requires a holistic and often multidisciplinary approach from the veterinarian, farrier, and nutritionist, this

The Liphook Equine Hospital, Forest Mere, Liphook, Hampshire GU30 7JG, UK
E-mail address: andy@TheLEH.co.uk

Vet Clin Equine 26 (2010) 303–314
doi:10.1016/j.cveq.2010.04.006
0749-0739/10/$ – see front matter © 2010 Elsevier Inc. All rights reserved.

vetequine.theclinics.com

review focuses on pharmacologic interventions that might have prophylactic benefit, specifically in the horse with laminitis as a result of PPID and EMS.

PHARMACOLOGIC TREATMENT OF PPID

Laminitis is a prominent clinical feature of PPID with a combined prevalence of 56% of 223 PPID cases described in 7 recent studies.[7,10–15] Despite this, the pathophysiology of laminitis in PPID is not well understood and might involve endogenous glucocorticoid effects, IR, hyperinsulinemia, and/or other mechanisms. However, hypercortisolemia is not a consistent finding in PPID cases[16,17] and not all horses with PPID have IR or hyperinsulinemia.[18]

Dopamine Agonists

The fundamental pathophysiologic process that leads to development of PPID is believed to be oxidative damage to hypothalamic dopaminergic neurones that normally exert a tonic inhibitory influence on the melanotrophs of the pars intermedia of the anterior pituitary gland.[19] Reimposition of dopaminergic inhibition via exogenously administered dopamine agonists is a logical and attractive pharmacologic strategy, and has been shown experimentally to reduce secretion from the pars intermedia in the horse.[20] Pergolide mesylate, a combined D1/D2 dopamine receptor agonist, has become the first-line treatment of PPID in horses.[21–23] However, no pharmacokinetic data for pergolide in the horse have been published. In humans the drug is absorbed rapidly and has a long half-life leading to a relatively stable and physiologic plasma concentration profile.[24] Evidence of a rapid onset of effect has also been demonstrated in horses[25,26] and single daily dosing seems clinically efficacious.[21–23] In the past, pergolide was often administered to horses at doses as high as 0.010 mg/kg by mouth once a day[27] although following a 1995 report describing good efficacy of lower doses,[28] it is now widely accepted that between 0.001 and 0.003 mg/kg by mouth once a day is more appropriate.[22,23] The commonest adverse effect of pergolide therapy in horses is anorexia typically affecting 5% to 10% of treated cases, although colic and diarrhea are also reported rarely.[22,23] The problem of inappetance can usually be overcome by stopping treatment for a few days and then recommencing at a lower dose.[23] Although once prescribed for the treatment of Parkinson disease and Cushing's disease in humans, pergolide was withdrawn in the United States as a human medicine in 2007 because of concerns of increased risk of pulmonary and cardiac valvular fibrosis.[29] Compounding pharmacies continue to supply pergolide for veterinary species within the United States although, in Europe, any future withdrawal of pergolide as a human-licensed medicine could create problems for its continued equine use. Bromocryptine mesylate, another dopamine agonist, has also been reported as an effective treatment of PPID in horses at a dose of 0.005 to 0.03 mg/kg intramuscularly twice a day or 0.03 to 0.09 mg/kg by mouth twice a day[30] although this drug has not proved to be popular in equine practice. There are many other dopamine agonists used in human medicine that might be investigated in horses should the need arise.[31,32]

Cyproheptadine

Cyproheptadine hydrochloride, a serotonin, acetylcholine, and histamine antagonist has also been advocated for treatment of PPID in horses. The drug has been found to reduce corticotrophin secretion from corticotrophs in the pars distalis of humans via direct and antiserotonergic mechanisms and to have clinical benefits in some cases of human Cushing's disease.[33,34] However, the same effects have not been investigated in dysfunctional melanotrophs of the pars intermedia in horses with PPID. Nevertheless clinical and endocrine benefits of cyproheptadine therapy are described in horses receiving doses of 0.25 mg/kg by mouth once or twice a day.[35]

Inhibitors of Cortisol Synthesis

Despite the popularity and efficacy of pergolide and cyproheptadine in equine medicine, a similar pharmacologic strategy in human cases of Cushing's disease is generally of limited benefit.[36] Attempts to moderate adrenal biosynthesis of glucocorticoids is the favored medical approach in humans using the enzyme inhibitors ketoconazole, aminoglutethimide, metyrapone, and the enzyme inhibitor/adrenolytic agent mitotane (**Fig. 1**, **Table 1**).[36] The use of these agents in the horse has not been properly studied although mitotane is described as ineffective in a few anecdotal reports.[22] This author has used aminoglutethimide and metyrapone, at a dose of 2 to 4 mg/kg by mouth once a day, in several cases in the last 15 years with a generally favorable clinical impression and evidence of improvement in clinicopathologic tests in some cases. Trilostane, a 3β-hydroxysteroid dehydrogenase inhibitor, is not favored in human patients[37] but has been used successfully in pituitary-dependent hyperadrenocorticism in dogs[38] and is the only drug in this class subject to published investigation in horses. Trilostane was shown to inhibit the conversion of pregnenolone to progesterone after intravenous infusion in horses[39] and was subsequently investigated in PPID cases. A good clinical response was observed after 30 days of treatment with trilostane at 0.5 to 1.5 mg/kg by mouth once a day along with some improvement in endocrine tests in a study of 20 PPID cases although a control group was not compared.[40,41]

Drug Selection in PPID

A few comparative studies of the relative benefits of treatments for equine PPID cases have been published. These have generally found pergolide to be more efficacious

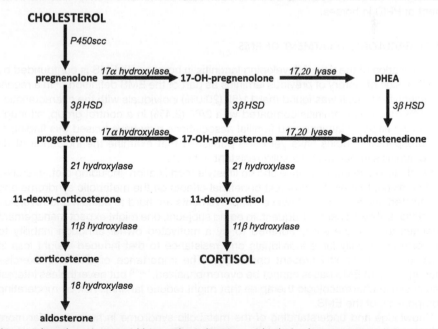

Fig. 1. Adrenal corticosteroid biosynthesis (P450scc, side chain cleavage enzyme; 3βHSD, 3β-hydroxysteroid dehydrogenase). See **Table 1** for enzymes targeted by therapeutic products.

Table 1
Enzyme targets of adrenal corticosteroid biosynthesis inhibitors (only trilostane has been the subject of a published study in the horse). See Fig. 1 for enzymatic actions (P450scc, side chain cleavage enzyme; 3βHSD, 3β-hydroxysteroid dehydrogenase)

	P450scc	17α-Hydroxylase	3βHSD	17,20-Lyase	11β-Hydroxylase
Aminoglutethimide	×				
Ketoconazole	×	×		×	
Metyrapone					×
Mitotane	×				×
Trilostane			×		

than cyproheptadine[12,13,27] although similar efficacy of the 2 drugs was shown by 1 study.[14] Comparison of the benefits of the herbal remedy *Vitex agnus castus* versus pergolide in 12 horses found no benefit of the former product but a good response to pergolide therapy in most cases.[42] Given the differing modes of action of many of the drugs used for PPID, there may be justification to consider drug combinations in poorly responsive cases and anecdotal reports exist describing the benefits of this approach.[22]

Cost of treatment is an important consideration in drug selection. Comparison of current costs in the United Kingdom reveal a standard dose of cyproheptadine (0.25 mg/kg twice a day) to be approximately 6 times the cost of pergolide (0.002 mg/kg once a day); and a standard dose of trilostane (1 mg/kg once a day) to be almost 20 times the cost of pergolide. The relative cost of these 3 drugs is similar in the United States depending on the source of pergolide (branded vs compounded). When this is considered alongside an appraisal of the published evidence outlined earlier then pergolide seems to be the unequivocal recommendation for first-line treatment of PPID in horses.

PHARMACOLOGIC TREATMENT OF EMS

Quantification of the risk of developing laminitis in horses with EMS is confounded by the inclusion of history of previous laminitis as part of the EMS definition.[43] In a recent prospective study, it was found that 11/55 (20.0%) individuals with the characteristics of EMS developed laminitis compared with 2/82 (2.4%) in a control group, although previous history of laminitis and familial associations may have biased this finding.[44] No prospective studies have yet been published that examine the incidence of de novo laminitis in obese and insulin-resistant subjects.

Most studies in humans have shown lifestyle modification, including diet, exercise, and smoking, to have the greatest beneficial effects on the metabolic syndrome and associated disease risk.[45] However, improvements are hard to sustain and reversion to previous lifestyle risks is frequent. In equid subjects, one might expect management changes to be more easily adhered to by a motivated owner although inability to exercise chronically lame individuals and resistance to diet-induced weight loss in easy-keeper types still present challenges. The importance of diet and exercise management of EMS cases cannot be overemphasized,[43,46] but nevertheless interest has arisen in pharmacologic therapies that might reduce laminitis risk by moderating components of the EMS.

Knowledge and understanding of the metabolic syndrome in humans is far more advanced than the analogous equine condition. There are multiple potential therapeutic aims for pharmacologic interventions in humans including management of obesity, IR, hyperinsulinemia, hyperglycemia, dyslipidemia, systemic inflammation, hypertension, and procoagulant status. Not all of these factors have been shown to be present and/or pathophysiologically relevant in EMS cases and therefore therapeutic ambitions of equine clinicians are currently unlikely to extend beyond the possible moderation of obesity, IR, hyperinsulinemia, and hyperglycemia (if present). Evidence supporting the pathophysiologic importance of obesity, IR, and hyperinsulinemia in laminitis risk has been published previously.[44,47,48] Hyperglycemia is an uncommon finding in EMS cases although statistical comparison with blood glucose in normal individuals has not been fully investigated. Even mild increases in blood glucose have been shown to promote endothelial dysfunction, inflammation, and coagulation in humans,[49] and therefore antihyperglycemic therapy might still be beneficial even in equine subjects with blood glucose within (upper) reference intervals.

L-Thyroxine

Currently the only pharmacologic treatment of horses with EMS that has a good evidence basis is L-thyroxine (eg, Thyro L, Lloyd Inc, Shenandoah, IA; Soloxine, Virbac Ltd, Bury St Edmunds, Suffolk, UK). In one study, daily administration of 0.1 mg/kg L-thyroxine was found to double the baseline insulin sensitivity of euthyroid horses following 16, 32, and 48 weeks of treatment.[50] The mechanism underlying the beneficial effect of L-thyroxine on insulin sensitivity is currently unclear and might involve direct effects on insulin-glucose metabolism and/or an indirect effect via induced weight loss.[50] L-Thyroxine treatment as described earlier has not been associated with significant adverse effects[51] although its use in nonobese insulin-resistant horses is questionable without further study. Current recommendations are to treat obese EMS cases with L-thyroxine at a dose of 0.1 mg/kg by mouth once a day for between 3 and 6 months during which time strict dietary control is essential. When satisfactory bodily condition has been achieved then L-thyroxine should be gradually withdrawn by administering a half dose for 2 weeks followed by a quarter dose for a further 2 weeks (Nicholas Frank DVM, PhD, DACVIM, Knoxville, TN, personal communication, November 2009).

Lessons from Human Metabolic Syndrome?

Based on efficacy, cost, and availability, the mainstays for medical management of the metabolic syndrome in humans are the biguanide metformin and the sulfonylurea glyburide (glibenclamide).[52,53] The other main therapeutic choices are listed in **Table 2**.[52–55] More than 50 natural products have also been suggested as having beneficial actions in insulin-resistant humans and horses but currently lack any strong evidence basis.[54,56,57] However, considerable caution should be exercised in the extrapolation of findings from human to equine studies as it is apparent that many significant differences exist between the 2 species in terms of pharmacokinetics and the pathophysiology of the metabolic syndrome in humans versus horses. Appetite suppressants have proved useful in the management of the metabolic syndrome in human patients but could well be hazardous in EMS because of the significant risks of inducing hyperlipemia in hypophagic insulin-resistant subjects. Inhibitors of carbohydrate digestion have been used to good effect in humans although the likely increased cecal carbohydrate delivery may actually increase laminitis risk in horses. Insulin secretagogues are commonly used in people who have lost effective compensatory pancreatic insulin secretion in response to chronic IR. Such cases would seem to be relatively uncommon in horses although glyburide (glibenclamide), the most commonly prescribed secretagogue in human subjects, has been administered to horses with type 2 diabetes mellitus.[25,58] Further concerns with the use of insulin

Table 2
Brief summary of the most commonly used pharmacologic agents for control of IR, hyperinsulinemia and/or hyperglycemia in human medicine[52-55]

Drug Class	Examples	Main Mode of Action
Biguanides	Metformin	Insulin-sensitization (hepatic)
Thiazolidinediones	Pioglitazone, Rosiglitazone	Insulin-sensitization
Sulfonylureas	Glyburide/Glibenclamide	Increased insulin secretion
Glinides	Repaglinide, nateglinide	Increased insulin secretion
Insulin and analogues	Insulin, insulin detemir	Compensation for reduced insulin secretion
α-Glucosidase inhibitors	Acarbose	Inhibition of carbohydrate digestion
Amylin analogues	Pramlintide	Glucagon suppression, appetite suppression
Incretin mimetics	Exenatide	Increased insulin secretion, β-cell regeneration, glucagon suppression, appetite suppression
Dipeptidyl peptidase IV antagonists	Sidagliptin, vildagliptin	Prolongation of glucagonlike peptide-1 (incretin) activity (see row above)

secretagogues and exogenous insulin therapy include the potential for inducing hypoglycemia and weight gain as well as the potentially adverse consequences of stimulating higher circulating insulin concentrations that could increase laminitis risk.[47,48,52,53,59,60]

Consideration of the pharmacologic properties of the various drugs used in the treatment of the metabolic syndrome in human patients has stimulated particular interest amongst equine clinicians in the insulin-sensitizing drugs, metformin and the thiazolidinediones. Although these drugs might seem logical choices for the treatment of IR in humans and horses, it is evident that they have multiple actions, not all of which are beneficial, and that adverse reactions are a serious consideration with novel deployment of any therapeutic product.

Metformin

Metformin, a biguanide, is a synthetic analogue of guanidine found naturally in the plant *Galega officinalis*. Metformin has been used for almost 50 years in Europe in human patients but was only made available in the United States in 1995. The mechanism(s) of action of metformin is not fully understood but it is suggested that it potentiates AMP-dependent protein-kinase (AMPK), a family of enzymes involved in intracellular energy homeostasis, carbohydrate and lipid metabolism, insulin secretion, and appetite.[61,62] Metformin's primary effect is widely quoted as antihyperglycemic as a result of suppression of hepatic gluconeogenesis,[63] although the potential beneficial effects of metformin are far wider than suppression of hyperglycemia. Other insulin-mediated effects of metformin include increased glucose uptake in peripheral tissues and reduction of plasma triglyceride concentrations suggesting a widespread insulin-sensitizing effect.[64-66] Furthermore, in the UK Prospective Diabetes Study, metformin was found to have a superior protective effect on the cardiovascular complications of IR in human subjects despite a similar degree of glycemic control compared with other drugs.[67] Moderation of endothelial hemostatic factors has been attributed to an endothelioprotective effect of metformin.[68] In contrast to other pharmacologic therapies for human IR, modest weight loss is a further unique benefit of metformin therapy in humans.[67]

The optimal dose of metformin in humans is approximately 25 mg/kg/d in 2 or 3 divided doses.[69] A study in obese mares found no convincing effect of metformin on insulin sensitivity when administered in doses up to 8.4 mg/kg by mouth twice a day.[70] A more recent study of 18 recurrently laminitic horses and ponies found a more favorable effect of metformin on estimates of IR and clinical signs of laminitis when administered at a dose of 15 mg/kg by mouth twice a day.[71] Fasting insulin and glucose and derived proxies were significantly improved in 10/11 subjects within 2 weeks of commencing therapy although this effect was not sustained in several of these. Studies conducted in human patients treated with metformin have generally reported significant decreases in circulating concentrations of glucose and insulin[72,73] although, as mentioned earlier, the potential benefits of metformin extend beyond insulin-glucose metabolism. Despite frequent gastrointestinal symptoms in human patients treated with metformin, no adverse effects of oral therapy have been reported in horses.[70,71,74,75] However, recent pharmacokinetic studies in horses have revealed poor bioavailability of metformin indicating the necessity for further evaluation of dosages and pharmacologic effects.[74,75]

Thiazolodinediones

The thiazolidinediones (TZDs) pioglitazone and rosiglitazone are 2 further insulin-sensitizing drugs commonly prescribed for humans.[66] TZDs are also suspected to promote AMPK although their major mode of action is more likely via stimulation of peroxisome proliferator-activated receptor gamma, a nuclear transcription factor that promotes genes involved in regulating glucose and lipid metabolism.[66] The main effect of TZDs seems to be increased glucose uptake by skeletal muscle cells and decreased lipolysis, typically increasing insulin sensitivity by 25% to 68%.[76,77] TZDs also lead to increased adiponectin synthesis (an insulin-sensitizing hormone), antiinflammatory effects, and improved endothelial function and fibrinolytic activity.[78–81] Comparative studies indicate a greater peripheral insulin-sensitizing effect and better control of hyperinsulinemia with TZDs compared with metformin in human subjects.[72,73] However, in contrast to metformin, treatment with TZDs is expensive, and associated with undesirable weight gain. Health concerns regarding hepatotoxicity and cardiovascular risk have also been published.[82–85]

SUMMARY

The treatment of endocrinopathic laminitis entails general therapeutic and management protocols applicable to other forms of laminitis. Targeting the underlying endocrinopathy is a further prophylactic aim of therapy and can be effectively accomplished in PPID cases with pergolide and, should this prove to be unsuccessful, alternative agents such as bromocryptine, cyproheptadine, and trilostane can be used. The preferred pharmacologic approach in obese EMS cases is L-thyroxine supplementation although further investigation of insulin-sensitizing agents such as metformin might bring about additional therapeutic options.

REFERENCES

1. Eyre P, Elmes PJ, Strickland S. Corticosteroid-potentiated vascular responses of the equine digit: a possible pharmacologic basis for laminitis. Am J Vet Res 1979; 40(1):135–8.

2. Bailey SR, Elliott J. The corticosteroid laminitis story: 2. Science of if, when and how. Equine Vet J 2007;39(1):7–11.
3. Coffman JR, Colles CM. Insulin tolerance in laminitic ponies. Can J Comp Med 1983;47(3):347–51.
4. Jeffcott LB, Field JR, McLean JG, et al. Glucose tolerance and insulin sensitivity in ponies and standardbred horses. Equine Vet J 1986;18(2):97–101.
5. Field JR, Jeffcott LB. Equine laminitis-another hypothesis for pathogenesis. Med Hypotheses 1989;30(3):203–10.
6. Johnson PJ. The equine metabolic syndrome: peripheral Cushing's syndrome. Vet Clin North Am Equine Pract 2002;18(2):271–93.
7. Hillyer MH, Taylor FGR, Mair TS, et al. Diagnosis of hyperadrenocorticism in the horse. Equine Vet Educ 1992;4(3):131–4.
8. Hood DM. Laminitis as a systemic disease. Vet Clin North Am Equine Pract 1999; 15(2):481–94.
9. Graves EA, Schott HC, Johnson PJ, et al. Thyroid function in horses with peripheral Cushing's syndrome. In: Proceedings of the 48th American Association of Equine Practitioners Annual Convention, Orlando (FL); 2002. p. 178–80.
10. van der Kolk JH, Kalsbeek HC, van Garderen E, et al. Equine pituitary neoplasia: a clinical report of 21 cases (1990–1992). Vet Rec 1993;133(24):594–7.
11. Couëtil L, Paradis MR, Knoll J. Plasma adrenocorticotropin concentration in healthy horses and in horses with clinical signs of hyperadrenocorticism. J Vet Intern Med 1996;10(1):1–6.
12. Schott HC, Coursen CL, Eberhart SW, et al. The Michigan Cushing's project. Proc AAEP 2001;47:22–4.
13. Donaldson MT, LaMonte BH, Morresey P, et al. Treatment with pergolide or cyproheptadine of pituitary pars intermedia dysfunction (equine Cushing's disease). J Vet Intern Med 2002;16(6):742–6.
14. Perkins GA, Lamb S, Erb HN, et al. Plasma adrenocorticotropin (ACTH) concentrations and clinical response in horses treated for equine Cushing's disease with cyproheptadine or pergolide. Equine Vet J 2002;34(7):679–85.
15. Frank N, Andrews FM, Sommardahl CS, et al. Evaluation of the combined dexamethasone/thyrotropin-releasing hormone stimulation test for detection of pars intermedia pituitary adenomas in horses. J Vet Intern Med 2006;20(4): 987–93.
16. van der Kolk JH, Wensing T, Kalsbeek HC, et al. Laboratory diagnosis of equine pituitary pars intermedia adenoma. Domest Anim Endocrinol 1995;12(1):35–9.
17. Haritou SJ, Zylstra R, Ralli C, et al. Seasonal changes in circadian peripheral plasma concentrations of melatonin, serotonin, dopamine and cortisol in aged horses with Cushing's disease under natural photoperiod. J Neuroendocrinol 2008;20(8):988–96.
18. Reeves HJ, Lees R, McGowan CM. Measurement of basal serum insulin concentration in the diagnosis of Cushing's disease in ponies. Vet Rec 2001;149(15): 449–52.
19. McFarlane D, Dybdal N, Donaldson MT, et al. Nitration and increased alpha-synuclein expression associated with dopaminergic neurodegeneration in equine pituitary pars intermedia dysfunction. J Neuroendocrinol 2005;17(2):73–80.
20. Orth DN, Holscher MA, Wilson MG, et al. Equine Cushing's disease: plasma immunoreactive proopiolipomelanocortin peptide and cortisol levels basally and in response to diagnostic tests. Endocrinology 1982;110(4):1430–41.
21. Muñoz MC, Doreste F, Ferrer O, et al. Pergolide treatment for Cushing's syndrome in a horse. Vet Rec 1996;139(2):41–3.

22. Schott HC. Pituitary pars intermedia dysfunction: equine Cushing's disease. Vet Clin North Am Equine Pract 2002;18(2):237–70.
23. Schott HC. Pituitary pars intermedia dysfunction: challenges of diagnosis and treatment. In: Proceedings of the 52nd American Association of Equine Practitioners Annual Convention, San Antonio (TX); 2006. p. 60–73.
24. Blin O. The pharmacokinetics of pergolide in Parkinson's disease. Curr Opin Neurol 2003;16(Suppl 1):S9–12.
25. Durham AE, Hughes KJ, Cottle HJ, et al. Type 2 diabetes mellitus with pancreatic β-cell dysfunction in 3 horses confirmed with minimal model analysis. Equine Vet J 2009;41(9):924–9.
26. Walsh DM, McGowan CM, McGowan T, et al. Correlation of plasma insulin concentration with laminitis score in a field study of equine Cushing's disease and equine metabolic syndrome. J Equine Vet Sci 2009;29(2):87–94.
27. Beech J. Treatment of hypophysial adenomas. Comp Cont Educ Pract Vet 1994; 16:921–3.
28. Peters DF, Erfle JB, Slobojan GT. Low-dose pergolide mesylate treatment for equine hypophyseal adenomas (Cushing's syndrome). In: Proceedings of the 41st American Association of Equine Practitioners Annual Convention, Lexington (MA); 1995. p. 154–5.
29. Antonini A, Poewe W. Fibrotic heart-valve reactions to dopamine-agonist treatment in Parkinson's disease. Lancet Neurol 2007;6(9):826–9.
30. Beck DJ. Effective long-term treatment of a suspected pituitary adenoma with bromocryptine mesylate in a pony. Equine Vet Educ 1992;4(3):119–22.
31. Stowe RL, Ives NJ, Clarke C, et al. Dopamine agonist therapy in early Parkinson's disease. Cochrane Database Syst Rev 2008;(2):CD006564.
32. Alexandraki KI, Grossman AB. Pituitary-targeted medical therapy of Cushing's disease. Expert Opin Investig Drugs 2008;17(5):669–77.
33. Ishibashi M, Yamaji T. Direct effects of thyrotropin-releasing hormone, cyproheptadine, and dopamine on adrenocorticotropin secretion from human corticotroph adenoma cells in vitro. J Clin Invest 1981;68(4):1018–27.
34. Tanakol R, Alagöl F, Azizlerli H, et al. Cyproheptadine treatment in Cushing's disease. J Endocrinol Invest 1996;19(4):242–7.
35. Couetil LL. Equine Cushing's disease: diagnosis and treatment. In: Proceedings of the 9th International Congress of the World Equine Veterinary Association, Marrakech (Morocco); 2006. p. 402–6.
36. Gross BA, Mindea SA, Pick AJ, et al. Medical management of Cushing disease. Neurosurg Focus 2007;23(3):E10.
37. Engelhardt D, Weber MM. Therapy of Cushing's syndrome with steroid biosynthesis inhibitors. J Steroid Biochem Mol Biol 1994;49(4–6):261–7.
38. Sieber-Ruckstuhl NS, Boretti FS, Wenger M, et al. Serum concentrations of cortisol and cortisone in healthy dogs and dogs with pituitary-dependent hyperadrenocorticism treated with trilostane. Vet Rec 2008;163(16):477–81.
39. Schutzer WE, Kerby JL, Holtan DW. Differential effect of trilostane on the progestin milieu in the pregnant mare. J Reprod Fertil 1996;107(2):241–8.
40. McGowan CM, Neiger R. Efficacy of trilostane for the treatment of equine Cushing's syndrome. Equine Vet J 2003;35(4):414–8.
41. McGowan CM, Frost R, Pfeiffer DU, et al. Serum insulin concentrations in horses with equine Cushing's syndrome: response to a cortisol inhibitor and prognostic value. Equine Vet J 2004;36(3):295–8.
42. Beech J, Donaldson MT, Lindborg S. Comparison of *Vitex agnus castus* extract and pergolide in treatment of equine Cushing's syndrome. In: Proceedings of

the 48th American Association of Equine Practitioners Annual Convention, Orlando (FL); 2002. p. 175–7.

43. Frank N, Geor RJ, Bailey SR, et al. Equine metabolic syndrome consensus statement. J Vet Intern Med 2010;24(3):467–75.

44. Treiber KH, Kronfeld DS, Hess TM, et al. Evaluation of genetic and metabolic predispositions and nutritional risk factors for pasture-associated laminitis in ponies. J Am Vet Med Assoc 2006;228(10):1538–45.

45. Knowler WC, Barrett-Connor E, Fowler SE, et al. Reduction in the incidence of type 2 diabetes with lifestyle intervention or metformin. N Engl J Med 2002; 346(6):393–403.

46. Geor RJ, Harris P. Dietary management of obesity and IR: countering risk for laminitis. Vet Clin North Am Equine Pract 2009;25(1):51–65.

47. Asplin KE, Sillence MN, Pollitt CC, et al. Induction of laminitis by prolonged hyperinsulinaemia in clinically normal ponies. Vet J 2007;174(3):530–5.

48. de Laat MA, McGowan CM, Sillence MN, et al. Equine laminitis: induced by 48 h hyperinsulinaemia in Standardbred horses. Equine Vet J 2010;42(2):129–35.

49. Shaw JE, Zimmet PZ, Alberti KG. Point: impaired fasting glucose: the case for the new American Diabetes Association criterion. Diabetes Care 2006;29(5):1170–2.

50. Frank N, Elliott SB, Boston RC. Effects of long-term oral administration of levothyroxine sodium on glucose dynamics in healthy adult horses. Am J Vet Res 2008; 69(1):76–81.

51. Frank N, Buchanan BR, Elliott SB. Effects of long-term oral administration of levothyroxine sodium on serum thyroid hormone concentrations, clinicopathologic variables, and echocardiographic measurements in healthy adult horses. Am J Vet Res 2008;69(1):68–75.

52. Inzucchi SE. Oral antihyperglycemic therapy for type 2 diabetes: scientific review. JAMA 2002;287(3):360–72.

53. Philippe J, Raccah D. Treating type 2 diabetes: how safe are current therapeutic agents? Int J Clin Pract 2009;63(2):321–32.

54. Hays NP, Galassetti PR, Coker RH. Prevention and treatment of type 2 diabetes: current role of lifestyle, natural product, and pharmacological interventions. Pharmacol Ther 2008;118(2):181–91.

55. Mohler ML, He Y, Wu Z, et al. Recent and emerging anti-diabetes targets. Med Res Rev 2009;29(1):125–95.

56. Althuis MD, Jordan NE, Ludington EA, et al. Glucose and insulin responses to dietary chromium supplements: a meta-analysis. Am J Clin Nutr 2002;76(1): 148–55.

57. Tinworth KD, Harris PA, Sillence MN, et al. Potential treatments for IR in the horse: a comparative multi-species review. Vet J, in press.

58. Johnson PJ, Scotty NC, Wiedmeyer C, et al. Diabetes mellitus in a domesticated Spanish mustang. J Am Vet Med Assoc 2005;226(4):584–8.

59. Garratt KN, Brady PA, Hassinger NL, et al. Sulfonylurea drugs increase early mortality in patients with diabetes mellitus after direct angioplasty for acute myocardial infarction. J Am Coll Cardiol 1999;33(1):119–24.

60. Marbury T, Huang WC, Strange P, et al. Repaglinide versus glyburide: a one-year comparison trial. Diabetes Res Clin Pract 1999;43(3):155–66.

61. Zhou G, Myers R, Li Y, et al. Role of AMP-activated protein kinase in mechanism of metformin action. J Clin Invest 2001;108(8):1167–74.

62. Musi N, Hirshman MF, Nygren J, et al. Metformin increases AMP-activated protein kinase activity in skeletal muscle of subjects with type 2 diabetes. Diabetes 2002;51(7):2074–81.

63. Hundal RS, Krssak M, Dufour S, et al. Mechanism by which metformin reduces glucose production in type 2 diabetes. Diabetes 2000;49(12):2063–9.
64. Sarabia V, Lam L, Burdett E, et al. Glucose transport in human skeletal muscle cells in culture. Stimulation by insulin and metformin. J Clin Invest 1992;90(4): 1386–95.
65. Kirpichnikov D, McFarlane SI, Sowers JR. Metformin: an update. Ann Intern Med 2002;137(1):25–33.
66. Bailey CJ. Treating insulin resistance in type 2 diabetes with metformin and thiazolidinediones. Diabetes Obes Metab 2005;7(6):675–91.
67. Turner RC. The U.K. prospective diabetes study. A review. Diabetes Care 1998; 21(Suppl 3):C35–8.
68. Charles MA, Morange P, Eschwège E, et al. Effect of weight change and metformin on fibrinolysis and the von Willebrand factor in obese nondiabetic subjects: the BIGPRO1 Study. Biguanides and the prevention of the risk of obesity. Diabetes Care 1998;21(11):1967–72.
69. Garber AJ, Duncan TG, Goodman AM, et al. Efficacy of metformin in type II diabetes: results of a double-blind, placebo-controlled, dose-response trial. Am J Med 1997;103(6):491–7.
70. Vick MM, Sessions DR, Murphy BA, et al. Obesity is associated with altered metabolic and reproductive activity in the mare: effects of metformin on insulin sensitivity and reproductive cyclicity. Reprod Fertil Dev 2006;18(6):609–17.
71. Durham AE, Rendle DI, Newton JE. The effect of metformin on measurements of insulin sensitivity and beta cell response in 18 horses and ponies with IR. Equine Vet J 2008;40(5):493–500.
72. Inzucchi SE, Maggs DG, Spollett GR, et al. Efficacy and metabolic effects of metformin and troglitazone in type II diabetes mellitus. N Engl J Med 1998;338(13): 867–72.
73. Yu JG, Kruszynska YT, Mulford MI, et al. A comparison of troglitazone and metformin on insulin requirements in euglycemic intensively insulin-treated type 2 diabetic patients. Diabetes 1999;48(12):2414–21.
74. Hustace JL, Firshman AM, Mata JE. Pharmacokinetics and bioavailability of metformin in horses. Am J Vet Res 2009;70(5):665–8.
75. Tinworth KD, Edwards S, Harris PA, et al. Pharmacokinetics of metformin in insulin-resistant ponies. Am J Vet Res, in press.
76. Miyazaki Y, Glass L, Triplitt C, et al. Effect of rosiglitazone on glucose and nonesterified fatty acid metabolism in type II diabetic patients. Diabetologia 2001; 44(12):2210–9.
77. Lebovitz HE, Banerji MA. Treatment of IR in diabetes mellitus. Eur J Pharmacol 2004;490(1–3):135–46.
78. Kruszynska YT, Yu JG, Olefsky JM, et al. Effects of troglitazone on blood concentrations of plasminogen activator inhibitor 1 in patients with type 2 diabetes and in lean and obese normal subjects. Diabetes 2000;49(4):633–9.
79. Yang WS, Jeng CY, Wu TJ, et al. Synthetic peroxisome proliferator-activated receptor-gamma agonist, rosiglitazone, increases plasma levels of adiponectin in type 2 diabetic patients. Diabetes Care 2002;25(2):376–80.
80. Paradisi G, Steinberg HO, Shepard MK, et al. Troglitazone therapy improves endothelial function to near normal levels in women with polycystic ovary syndrome. J Clin Endocrinol Metab 2003;88(2):576–80.
81. Libby P, Plutzky J. Inflammation in diabetes mellitus: role of peroxisome proliferator-activated receptor-alpha and peroxisome proliferator-activated receptor-gamma agonists. Am J Cardiol 2007;99(4A):27B–40B.

82. Diamant M, Heine RJ. Thiazolidinediones in type 2 diabetes mellitus: current clinical evidence. Drugs 2003;63(13):1373–405.
83. Rasouli N, Raue U, Miles LM, et al. Pioglitazone improves insulin sensitivity through reduction in muscle lipid and redistribution of lipid into adipose tissue. Am J Physiol Endocrinol Metab 2005;288(5):E930–4.
84. Isley WL. Hepatotoxicity of thiazolidinediones. Expert Opin Drug Saf 2003;2(6): 581–6.
85. Nissen SE, Wolski K. Effect of rosiglitazone on the risk of myocardial infarction and death from cardiovascular causes. N Engl J Med 2007;356(24):2457–71.

Neuropathic Pain Management in Chronic Laminitis

Bernd Driessen, DVM, PhD[a,b,*],
Sébastien H. Bauquier, DMV[c], Laura Zarucco, DMV, PhD[d]

KEYWORDS

- Horse • Laminitis • Neuropathic pain
- Nonsteroidal antiinflammatory drugs
- Analgesics • Gabapentin

Managing pain in horses afflicted by chronic laminitis is one of the greatest challenges in equine clinical practice because it is the dreadful suffering of the animals that most often forces the veterinarian to end the battle with this disease. The purpose of this review is to summarize our current understanding of the complex mechanisms involved in generating and amplifying pain in animals with laminitis and, based on this information, to propose a modified approach to pain therapy. Furthermore, a recently developed pain scoring technique is presented that may help better quantify pain and the monitoring of responses to analgesic treatment in horses with laminitis.

MECHANISMS OF PAIN IN LAMINITIS

Understanding the neuroanatomy of the equine foot and pathophysiological processes involved in triggering and modifying nociception during the course of laminitis, though incompletely understood, is essential when searching for effective pain-management strategies in affected animals. This point applies even more if one considers that up to 75% of horses affected by this disease eventually develop severe

[a] Section of Emergency/Critical Care and Anesthesia, Department of Clinical Studies, New Bolton Center, School of Veterinary Medicine, University of Pennsylvania, 382 West Street Road, Kennett Square, Philadelphia, PA 19348, USA
[b] Department of Anesthesiology, David-Geffen School of Medicine, University of California-Los Angeles, Los Angeles, CA, USA
[c] Section of Critical Care, Department of Clinical Studies-Philadelphia, School of Veterinary Medicine, University of Pennsylvania, 3850 Spruce Street, Philadelphia, PA 19104, USA
[d] Dipartimento di Patologia Animale, Facoltà di Medicina Veterinaria, Università degli Studi di Torino, Via Leonardo da Vinci 44, 10095 Grugliasco (TO), Italy
* Corresponding author. Section of Emergency/Critical Care and Anesthesia, Department of Clinical Studies, New Bolton Center, School of Veterinary Medicine, University of Pennsylvania, 382 West Street Road, Kennett Square, PA 19348.
E-mail address: Driessen@vet.upenn.edu

Vet Clin Equine 26 (2010) 315–337
doi:10.1016/j.cveq.2010.04.002
0749-0739/10/$ – see front matter © 2010 Elsevier Inc. All rights reserved.

or chronic lameness and debilitation.[1] As emphasized by Orsini and colleagues,[2] inflammation emerges as the common pathologic denominator in all cases of laminitis and disease-related pain. It is intimately associated with the cascade of events that may eventually lead to the complete failure of the lamellar dermal-epidermal bond. Inflammation and vascular dysfunction are evident in the early developmental phase of laminitis, when pain or other clinical symptoms are still absent.[3–5] During this prodromal phase, leucocyte extravasation and development of platelet microthrombi are accompanied by upregulated gene expression for key inflammatory cytokines (eg, interleukin [IL]-1β, IL-6), cyclooxygenase (COX)-2, and matrix metalloproteinases (MMPs) in the digital laminae.[5–9] Locally released and activated MMPs mediate degradation of the collagen components of the basement membrane (BM) that is interposed between the secondary dermal (SDL) and epidermal lamellae (SEL) and cause a separation of the SEL from the BM.[4,10–14]

Sensory innervation of the foot consists of thick myelinated A-fibers (largely A_β) transmitting low-threshold mechanical information and small, thin myelinated (A_δ-fibers) and unmyelinated afferents (C fibers), which express a variety of peptides and transmit high-threshold nociceptive information.[15–19] The A_β fibers innervate lamellated corpuscles (comparable with pacinian corpuscles) clustered below the digital cushion in the heel segment of the hoof that function as proprioceptors and provide a secure gait.[17,19] Both nociceptive A_δ- and C fibers that stain immunohistochemically positive for calcitonin gene-related peptide (CGRP) and substance P (SP) and are widely distributed throughout the base of the dermal layer (especially dermal papillae in the solar and bulbar segment and dermal lamellae in the parietal segment) and run parallel to blood vessels without innervating them.[17–19] In addition, slow-conducting unmyelinated nerve fibers of the autonomic (exclusively sympathetic) nervous system accompany the dense network of blood vessels and arteriovenous anastomoses within the hoof capsule.[19,20] As in visceral organs, these sympathetic nerves not only carry efferent fibers that regulate vasomotor tone, sweat glands, and pilo-erector muscles in the skin but also afferent viscerosensory fibers that signal information about vascular lumen, wall stress, and noxious stimulation or hypoxic/ischemic tissue conditions to the central nervous system (CNS).[19] Hence, they may contribute to sympathetically maintained nociceptive stimulation typically unresponsive to conventional analgesics.

The inflammatory and disadhesion processes that occur during the developmental phase of laminitis do not seem to influence activity in sensory nerve fibers of the hoof. Histologic data suggest that the disruption of the dermal-epidermal laminar bond is initially confined to the noninnervated basement membrane and epidermal lamellae (grade 1 histologic laminitis).[4,21] Because sensory nerve terminals are located primarily at the base of the dermal lamellae, at this stage of the disease they are likely too distant to the site of MMP action to be affected, and SEL cell injury and local inflammation are not severe enough to cause activation through neurochemical signaling. Lacking pain or discomfort, the developmental phase of laminitis often goes unnoted and therefore treatment is not initiated even though aggressive medication with nonsteroidal antiinflammatory drugs (NSAIDs) has been claimed to be indicated.[7,8]

Unless resolving on their own, histologic changes at the dermal-epidermal interface progress further causing (within 24 to 72 hours) the BM to retract so much from SEL that SDL connective tissue and SDL capillaries are injured by tension and shear force (grade 2 histologic laminitis),[4] likely provoking activation of perivascular sensory nerve terminals near the base of the dermal lamellae. At this point the developmental phase transitions into the acute phase of laminitis, which is hallmarked by classical signs of inflammation, such as bounding digital pulses and increased hoof temperature.[3–5] Nociception is most often recognized by lameness or the characteristic stance of the animal and rapidly increasing sensitivity to hoof testers.[3,5] Even though evidence for a marked increase in COX-2 enzyme activity could not be found in the acute phase of experimentally induced laminitis,[8] concentrations of other vasoactive degradation products of arachidonic acid (eg, isoprostanes) are elevated during the acute phase of experimentally induced laminitis.[9] In addition, extensive necrosis of the SEL and edema with separation of the dermal-epidermal junction has been noted in the acute phase of experimentally induced laminitis.[21] Thus, it is most likely that sensitization (peripheral hyperalgesia) develops secondary to the action of a variety of locally released inflammatory products.[15,16,22] As described in other situations of tissue damage, changes in the local environment (eg, tissue pH and local electrolyte [K^+] concentrations, accumulation of membrane degradation products, cytokines, chemokines, and growth factors from invading inflammatory cells) and upregulated enzyme systems may collectively activate expressed and silent nociceptors and sensitize them to noxious and even non-noxious stimuli.[22] Furthermore, activated sensory nerve fibers in the dermal papillary layer release neuropeptides (eg, CGRP) that target receptors on blood vessels and provoke neurogenic inflammation by causing vasodilation, plasma extravasation, and leucocyte attraction.[18,19] Even during the acute phase of laminitis, persistent afferent nociceptive signaling will initiate neural processes (addressed later in detail) that eventually create a state of central potentiation of nociceptive input to the brain (central hyperalgesia)[22] mediated in part by spinal release of excitatory amino acids, tachykinins, prostanoids, and cytokines.[16] Some of these products reflect the activation of not only neurons but also nonneuronal cells (astrocytes and microglia) that contribute to the release of products (eg, prostaglandins) that in turn increase excitability of dorsal horn neurons.[16,22] Peripheral and early central hyperalgesia may explain the rapidly worsening pain horses and ponies experience in the acute phase of laminitis.

Animals may pass through the acute phase of mild and moderate laminitis without having developed any gross structural changes to the dermal-epidermal lamellar apparatus, allowing for complete recovery from all symptoms, including pain. If not, within 2 to 3 days they enter the chronic phase of laminitis that begins with separation of the distal phalanx from the hoof wall and subsequent mechanical collapse of the foot.[3–5] It can be subdivided into three subphases: early chronic, chronic stable, and active chronic laminitis.[23] It is during the early chronic or active chronic phase of the disease process that relenting pain may develop, which is often difficult to control with traditional antiinflammatory and analgesic drug treatment.[24] However, some animals may pass the early chronic phase rather rapidly without showing severe symptoms and enter the stage of chronic stable laminitis. At this stage they may not display any significant lameness allowing even athletic performance despite unequivocal radiographic evidence of displacement of the distal phalanx.[21]

The pain animals with chronic laminitis suffer is multifactorial and greatly variable. The pathophysiological sequela occurring after structural failure of the lamellar suspensory apparatus in one animal may or may not occur to the same extent in another, and the type and scope of tissue repair and remodeling varies among individual horses.[21] A major component determining the degree of nociception is the extent of mechanical/structural failure of the foot's submural tissues, with global distal displacement of the digital phalanx (sinking) probably representing the worst scenario. Tearing of the dermal-epidermal lamellar bond with rotation or sinking of the coffin bone results in widespread injury to C and A_δ fibers in the dermal layers. Damaged sensory neurons produce spontaneous impulse discharges that lead to sustained levels of excitability.[22] These ectopic discharges begin to cross talk with adjacent uninjured nerve fibers, resulting in amplification of the response to noxious stimulation as part of the peripheral hyperalgesia that develops in the injured tissue. Distal phalanx displacement also leads to increased submural pressure from the edema that accompanies inflammation or hemorrhage.[21] Loss of digital stability with significant shifts in the distribution of strain and stress forces within the hoof capsule contribute to mechano- (A_β) and nociceptor (A_δ, C) activities, as does elevated pressure on the coffin bone caused by greater and longer lasting contact between the internal surface of the sole and the distal phalanx during locomotion.[21] Elevated eicosanoid (PgE_2, LTB_4) concentrations have not been detected in digital venous blood of horses in pain during chronic laminitis.[25] Nevertheless, it appears that inflammatory mediators released throughout all phases of laminitis play a dominant role in the pain perception during early and active chronic laminitis.[2,15,16,19] Furthermore, digital ischemia resulting from the tearing of SDL arterioles, vasoconstriction (primarily venoconstriction) in response to inflammatory mediators, arteriovenous blood shunting, thrombosis, and compression of the solar vascular bed after digital collapse may contribute important causative factors for pain.[3–5,22,24,26] Also dilation of hoof vessels in response to the release of neuropeptides (eg, CGRP) from activated sensory nerve terminals leads to a rapid increase in pressure within the hoof capsule (similar to the situation within the skull after vasodilation), thereby exacerbating foot pain.[19,20]

The previously mentioned factors only partially explain why many animals with chronic laminitis experience persistent and often times worsening pain that is refractory to therapy, whereas other animals are spared or recover. Although not studied in detail in horses with laminitis, data obtained with laboratory animal models and clinical observations in human patients with severe tissue injury indicate that lesions to peripheral somatosensory neurons can trigger a complex series of events that eventually alter peripheral nerve impulse signaling and central nervous sensory input processing. These processes result in a pain state commonly referred to as neuropathic pain (ie, pain that has its origin in a lesion or dysfunction of the sensory transmission pathways in the peripheral or central nervous system itself) and thus is considered a pathologic condition in and of itself.[15,16,23,27–30] The changes may include but are not limited to: (1) large increases in spontaneous (ectopic) activity in injured afferent nerve fibers and dorsal root ganglia (DRG) cell bodies; (2) ectopic activity in nociceptors resulting from local increase in sodium channel expression and enhanced sensitivity to excitatory products released from local inflammatory cells; (3) facilitation of synaptic neurotransmission in the dorsal horn through increased release of, or response to, excitatory neurotransmitters (eg, NMDA, glutamate) or increased ion channel conductance; (4) loss of dorsal horn inhibition otherwise mediated by spinal γ-aminobutyric acid (GABA) or glycinergic interneurons; (5) reduced sensitivity of primary sensory afferents and dorsal horn neurons toward the effects of μ-opioid agonists; (6) sprouting of central sympathetic nerve fiber terminals into layers of the dorsal horn where they can make abnormal contacts with ascending sensory neurons causing sympathetically maintained pain; (7) loss of synaptic connectivity and formation of new synaptic contacts between low-threshold A_β fibers and ascending sensory neurons that normally receive input only from nociceptive A_δ and C fibers, causing allodynia (**Table 1**); (8) activation of astrocytes and microglia leading to an increased spinal expression of pro-excitatory products, including prostanoids; and (9) neuroimmune interactions, including actions of MMPs 9 and 2 capable of inducing neuropathic pain through microglial and astrocyte activation.[15,27–31] Ectopic neural firing activity occurs within 12 to 48 hours after nerve injury, whereas sensitization and gene expression changes in spinal and maybe supraspinal neural networks begin later. Neural

Table 1	
Sensory symptoms and signs associated with neuropathic pain	
Symptom or Sign	**Description**
Allodynia	Pain due to non-noxious stimuli (eg, light touch) when applied to the affected area. May be mechanical (eg, caused by light pressure), dynamic (caused by non-painful movement of a stimulus), or thermal (caused by non-painful warm, or cool stimulus).
Anesthesia	Loss of normal sensation to the affected region.
Hyperalgesia	Exaggerated response to a mildly noxious stimulus applied to the affected region.
Hyperpathia	Delayed and explosive response to a noxious stimulus applied to the affected region
Referred pain	Occurs in a region remote from the source of stimulation.

From Galluzzi KE. Management of neuropathic pain. J Am Osteopath Assoc 2005;105(9):S12–9. *Reprinted from* JAOA—The Journal of the American Osteopathic Association Supplement. Copyright © 2005 American Osteopathic Association; with permission.

lesions alone may not be sufficient to generate neuropathic pain and other predisposing factors are of importance.[29] Nevertheless, Jones and collaborators[24] found in horses suffering from recurrent and treatment refractory laminitis, neuromorphological changes and altered gene expression that are strikingly similar to those changes observed in animal models of peripheral nerve injury or in humans with neuropathic pain (eg, from arthritis, osteosarcoma, or diabetes).[16] The nerve fiber composition of digital nerves harvested from affected animals was abnormal with significantly lower numbers of unmyelinated (43.2%) and myelinated fibers (34.6%) compared with nerves collected from normal horses.[24] Furthermore, upregulated expression of activating transcription factor-3 (ATF3), a classical marker of peripheral nerve injury, was found in DRG cells of large and small afferents. Also, neuropeptide Y (NPY) expression was increased in DRG cells of large myelinated fibers innervating the laminitic hoof. The abundant presence of MMPs 2 and 9 from the developmental phase onwards may yet be another factor contributing to the development of neuropathic neural injury.[4,31] Thus, it appears that mechanisms of peripheral and central sensitization and neuropathic remodeling previously described can play a central role in the development of the unrelenting pain experienced by so many horses during chronic laminitis.[16,29,30] In this pain state, mildly noxious or subthreshold stimuli (transmitted by small A_δ and C afferents) produce an exaggerated pain response caused by amplified pre- and postsynaptic neuronal sensitivity and activity.[24] Normally innocuous mechanical stimuli such as those activating the lamellated corpuscles and low threshold A_β fibers in the heel area when the foot touches the ground during locomotion may then be perceived as painful (tactile or mechanical *allodynia*).[27,30] This may explain the frequent limb shifting and high sensitivity to the hoof tester.

GRADING PAIN IN LAMINITIS

Various scoring systems employing either behavioral characteristics only or both behavioral and physiologic parameters have been developed to monitor pain in horses.[32] Obel[33] was among the first to describe a grading system for lameness in horses affected by laminitis. Both the Obel Grading System and the later developed graded lameness scale (0–5) of the American Association of Equine Practitioners[34] are subject to high inter-observer variability, do not fully account for the complexity of equine pain behaviors, and are somewhat limited when assessing clinically relevant changes in nociception and responses to therapy. Dutton and colleagues[35] recently applied a modified composite multifactorial pain scoring system that includes components of the Obel Grading System and the Glasgow composite pain scale in a horse suffering from severe persistent foot pain (**Table 2**). As the authors emphasize multiple observers produced consistently similar scores when assessing the pain state in the horse and changes in scores tightly followed responses to analgesic treatment and progress in the disease process. To objectively assess and quantify pain (lameness) in acute and chronic laminitis, force plate systems have been used for measuring ground reaction forces and other force parameters and to identify changes in limb-load distribution pattern that reflect changes in the disease process and responses to treatment.[36,37]

PAIN THERAPY IN LAMINITIS: MODIFYING THE APPROACH

Until very recently pain therapy in acute and chronic laminitis has largely been based on the proposed etiopathogenetic mechanisms underlying the disease (ie, vascular or thromboembolic ischemia; inflammatory; metabolic; enzymatic and biomechanical mechanisms) and consisted predominantly of anti-inflammatory drug administration.[38–48] In the acute phase this therapy was often combined with other medications (eg, acepromazine, pentoxifylline, isoxuprine, heparin, acetyl salicylic acid, nitroglycerin, dimethyl sulfoxide) addressing suspected ischemia and reperfusion injury

Table 2 Modified composite pain score	
Dynamic score: Modified Obel Grading System	
Grade	Descriptor
1	Frequent shifting of weight between the feet with no discernible lameness at the walk.
2	Does not resist having a foreleg lifted, is not reluctant to walk, but does show lameness at the walk.
3	Resists having a foreleg lifted and is reluctant to walk.
4	Walks only if forced.
Static score: Modified from Glasgow composite scale	
Score	Descriptor
1	No pain or distress: normal behavior.
2	Mild pain: irritable, restless, decreased appetite.
3	Mild pain: 2 plus resists handling.
4	Mild-moderate pain: 3 plus standing in back of stall or with back to stall door.
5	Moderate pain: 4 plus camped-out legs, increased digital pulses.
6	Moderate-severe pain: 5 plus frequent recumbency, HR >44 beats/min, and/or RR >24 breaths/min.
7	Moderate-severe pain: 6 plus sweating, muscle fasciculation, head-tossing.
8	Severe pain: 7 plus unwilling to move.
9	Severe-extreme pain: 8 plus not weight bearing when standing.
10	Extreme pain: 9 or entirely recumbent, bordering on agonal.

Maximum possible score: 14.
From Dutton DW, Lashnits KJ, Wegner K. Managing severe hoof pain in a horse using multimodal analgesia and a modified composite pain score. Equine Vet Educ 2009;21:37–43; with permission.

(oxidative damage) in the dermal-epidermal lamellae, yet with conflicting results.[39–48] This traditional approach failed to control the multifactorial pain in horses with chronic laminitis, because pain has been considered only a symptom of laminitis rather than a pathologic entity in itself. It is the abnormal neural signal processing due to damage to tissues (inflammatory pain) and nervous structures (neuropathic pain), and/or abnormal function of the nervous system as a whole (functional pain) that over the course of the disease process causes a state of nociception that is commonly referred to as pathologic or *maladaptive pain*.[30,49] Conventional NSAIDs and other medications may not or only partially target the neuropathophysiological mechanisms described in detail above.[15,16,29,32] Therefore, shifting the focus toward a more holistic strategy aimed at preventing maladaptive pain or at least reducing the risk of its occurrence appears to be more indicated.[28,32,35] This concept follows the notion that i) events leading to acute pain, peripheral and central hyperalgesia, neuropathic pain, with or without allodynia occur simultaneously and are interrelated; ii) drugs may exhibit a specific activity against only certain components of the pain syndrome; iii) early integration of drugs with anti-hyperalgesic or anti-neuropathic pain activity into the treatment plan promises to reduce the risk of maladaptive pain development; and iv) loco-regional analgesia techniques help suppressing the occurrence of hyperalgesia and neuropathic pain.[32] Accordingly, effective pain management in horses with laminitis favors a *multi-modal* approach that involves, from the beginning, a combination of drugs with different pharmacologic mechanisms of action and different target sites within the somatosensory neural conduit (**Fig. 1**). This concept may also include podiatric care, electrotherapy, tenotomy or botulinum toxin-induced relaxation of the deep digital flexor tendon, physical therapy, and other complementary modalities of treatment, most of them aimed at altering biomechanical forces on the affected digit with decreased foot pain perception and improved recovery.[32,35,41–45,50–54]

To have sustainable success pain therapy in the horse with chronic laminitis has to accomplish multiple goals: i) reduction of nociceptive signal generation in sensory nerve terminals (NSAIDs, podiatric care); ii) suppression of peripheral hyperalgesia (NSAIDs, local anesthesia and analgesia); iii) Inhibition/prevention of afferent nociceptive signal transmission to the central nervous system (loco-regional analgesia); iv) inhibition of spinal nociceptive signal transmission and central hyperalgesia development ([epidural/spinal: local anesthetics, opioids, α_2-agonists], [systemic: opioids, α_2-agonists, ketamine, NSAIDs, gabapentin, pregabalin]) and v) prevention and/or inhibition of neuropathic pain (systemic lidocaine, opioids, NSAIDS, gabapentin, pregabalin). *Multi-modal* pain therapy is mechanism driven and should be evidence based. It represents a concept that is very open and allows new drugs and techniques to be included as they become available.

As mentioned before, neither pathologic mechanisms leading to nor treatment of sensory hyperalgesia and neuropathic pain have yet been studied in detail in horses. At this stage, the equine veterinarian must rely primarily on experimental animal data and experiences in human medical practice when developing an analgesic regimen for the horse with chronic foot pain. There are a number of lessons to be learnt from experiences with neuropathic pain therapy in the human patient: i) symptoms described by patients are many, including those listed in **Table 1**, and therefore the diagnosis of neuropathic pain is often challenging and diagnostic criteria are still evolving; ii) rarely, if ever, can one single pathophysiological mechanism be claimed responsible for generating and maintaining the symptoms of neuropathic pain; iii) individual variation in the response to anti-neuropathic pain medications is substantial and unpredictable, thus favoring a stepwise process intended to identify the medication (or medication combination) that provides the greatest pain relief and fewest side effects while

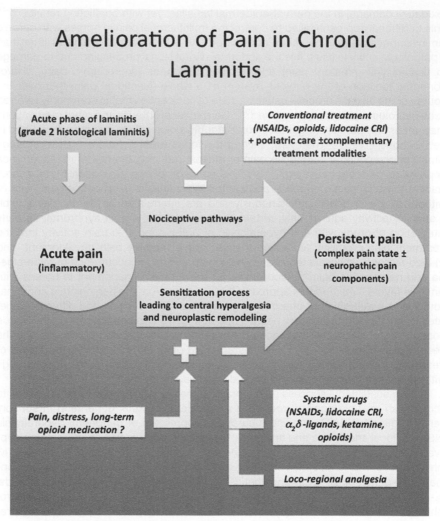

Fig. 1. Multimodal approach to pain management in the horse with chronic laminitis (see text for more detail).

discontinuing drugs lacking an analgesic effect; iv) currently first line medications for neuropathic pain cannot be ranked by degree of efficacy; v) no more than 40%–60% of patients with neuropathic pain will respond favorably to pharmacologic treatments.[55–59]

Whatever pharmacologic or other approach and technique is chosen in an individual *multi-modal* protocol, the ultimate objective is to achieve optimum pain control during each phase of laminitis, while at the same time minimizing the risk of negatively affecting the disease process itself or causing side effects of drug therapy.[32]

CONVENTIONAL SYSTEMIC ANALGESICS

Three different pharmacologic classes of drugs are commonly administered systemically to treat pain in horses affected with laminitis: NSAIDs, opioids and lidocaine. As described later in more detail, these drugs have also the potential to ameliorate nociceptive processes involved in the development of hyperalgesia and neuropathic pain.

NSAIDs

The backbone of any pharmacologic pain therapy in laminitis has been and continues to be treatment with NSAIDs (Table 3). Evidence of increased cyclooxygenase (primarily COX-2) expression, leucocyte migration, and cytokine production in the developmental and acute phases of laminitis as outlined above indicated a role for these agents, optimally before the onset of lameness. However, there is increasing evidence to suggest that commonly administered NSAIDs such as phenylbutazone, flunixine meglumine, ketoprofen, and naproxen do not mediate their effects through antiinflammatory action (ie, prostanoid synthesis inhibition) in the affected dermoepidermal hoof tissues but instead produce analgesia primarily by inhibition of central sensory neurons through COX-dependent and other independent mechanisms.[40,43,46,60] First, administration of NSAIDs during the developmental stage, when COX-2 expression is up-regulated, does not seem to prevent acute laminitis or alter the course of the disease arguing against a dominant antiinflammatory action.[61] Second, increased prostaglandin activity has not been detected in the acute and chronic phases of laminitis despite evidence for ongoing inflammation,[8,9,21,25] supporting the notion that if NSAIDS exhibit antiinflammatory activity at high doses this effect may not be related to inhibition of prostanoid synthesis.[43,46] Third, unlike

Table 3
Doses of commonly used nonsteroidal antiinflammatory drugs (NSAIDs) in horses

Non-Steroidal Anti-Inflammatory Drug	Dose, Route & Interval of Drug Administration[a]	Comments	References
Non-selective COX-1 & 2 inhibitors			
Phenylbutazone	2.2–4.4 (up to 6) mg/kg IV/PO SID-BID	Highest toxicity among NSAIDs	[43,47,55,62,64,68,73]
Flunixine meglumine	1.1 mg/kg IV/PO SID-BID	Cases of muscle necrosis reported with IM injection	[47,68,73]
Ketoprofen	2.2–3.6 mg/kg IV/IM SID-QID	Only parenteral administration	[55,64,68,73]
Vedaprofen	1–2 mg/kg IV/PO SID-BID	Limited experience	[73,74]
Eltenac	0.5–1 mg/kg IV SID	Limited experience	[68,73,74]
Naproxen	5 mg/kg IV 10 mg/kg PO SID	Initially slow IV bolus, then PO	[73]
Preferential or selective COX-2 inhibitors			
Meloxicam	0.6 mg/kg IV/PO SID-BID		[68,73,74]
Etodolac	10–20 mg/kg IV/PO SID-BID	Limited experience	[68,73]
Firocoxib	0.1 mg/kg PO SID	May require 0.3 mg/kg on 1st day of administration	[69,70,73]

Routes and intervals of drug administration: IV, intravenous; IM, intramuscular; PO, per os; SID, once daily; BID, twice daily; TID, three times daily.
[a] *Caution*: More rapid metabolism and elimination of most NSAIDs in mules and donkeys may require more frequent dosing.[62]

in peripheral tissues, where COX-1 is constitutively present for tissue homeostasis and COX-2 is inducible by inflammation,[62] both COX isoforms are constitutively present in the CNS but with functionally different roles.[63,64]

While NSAID administration in higher doses with antiinflammatory activity may be desirable in the very early (developmental) stage of laminitis, in the acute phase persistent and very effective pain relief from NSAIDs must be balanced against the risks of exacerbated structural damage due to excessive movement and limb loading of the horse,[40,47] and thus the dose should be titrated based on the comfort level of the animal. In horses with chronic laminitis, effective analgesia frequently calls for high doses of NSAIDs and an effect may still not be seen for up to 3 days after initiation of treatment.[40] This must be considered when assessing the clinical response to NSAIDs.

The previously held belief that more COX-2 preferential (meloxicam, Metacam; etodolac, Etogesic) or even COX-2 selective NSAIDS (firocoxib, Equioxx) are therapeutically superior has been challenged recently.[65–67] New laboratory data indicate that suppression of inflammation-evoked central nociceptive activity and hyperalgesia by NSAIDs may be related to the selectivity for COX isoforms since COX-2 seems to be only involved in the initiation but not necessarily the maintenance of nociceptive spinal neuron activation, which may largely depend on COX-1.[64] In contrast, in the absence of peripheral inflammation spinally initiated hyperalgesia has been shown to be mediated exclusively by constitutive COX-2 likely localized within the spinal cord dorsal horn, which argues for a prominent indication of selective COX-2 inhibitors as antihyperalgesic agents under circumstances of non-inflammation dependent central nociceptive sensitization.[63] Under the premise of inflammation being the common pathologic denominator[2] and hence the trigger for increased spinal sensory nerve excitability in all forms of laminitis, these laboratory findings suggest the use of non-selective NSAIDs as more effective candidates for analgesic therapy in laminitis. This idea is supported by two observations: i) among clinicians the non-selective COX inhibitor phenylbutazone is considered the most potent and most consistent pain relieving NSAID in laminitis;[46,60,67] and ii) only ketoprofen (3.63 mg/kg), a slightly COX-1 preferential NSAID,[68] may reduce foot pain to a greater extent than phenylbutazone (2.2 mg/kg).[69] Interestingly, the stereoisomers of ketoprofen are known to exert antinociceptive actions also through mechanisms other than COX inhibition. The R(-)-enantiomer of ketoprofen suppresses tactile allodynia via a yet to be defined mechanism of action and the S(+)-enantiomer produces analgesia through mechanisms involving serotoninergic pathways both at the spinal and supraspinal level.[70,71] In addition, ketoprofen has been demonstrated to exert antihyperalgesic activity in dairy cows suffering from unilateral hindlimb lameness.[72]

A risk of toxicity must be anticipated in animals receiving protracted courses of NSAID treatment.[65,67,73] Of interest, NSAIDs have been shown in-vitro to slightly potentiate MMP activation,[47] which cautions against an indiscriminate use in the early stages of laminitis. Currently most widely used NSAIDs are non-selective and may cause multiple adverse effects (ie, right dorsal colitis, gastric ulceration, and renal tubular necrosis) through inhibition of COX-1. This applies particularly to phenylbutazone which has a longer elimination half life and thus accumulates more extensively in tissues than other non-selective NSAIDs.[43,73] Therefore, their use may need to be restricted in horses with compromised gastro-intestinal or renal functions or in dehydrated animals, and in ponies that are more susceptible to toxic effects of NSAIDs.[43,46,74] In those cases COX-2 preferential/selective agents and ketoprofen, that have a more favorable side effect profile compared with phenylbutazone and flunixine meglumine, may be better choices to treat persistent pain in laminitis.[75,76]

OPIOIDS

Opioids (**Table 4**) are generally indicated in moderate to severe pain, however, their analgesic efficacy in horses compared with other species is less well defined, especially when used in clinically common doses.[60,77,78] At higher doses known to produce significant analgesia or antinociception (eg, butorphanol, methadone, or morphine $\geq$ 0.1 mg/kg) opioids commonly provoke central excitatory responses, requiring combination with sedatives such as acepromazine or α_2-agonists (see **Table 4**).[60,77,78] In, addition, they decrease gastrointestinal motility and cause colon impaction, thus limiting their long-term use in animals with chronic laminitis. Combining lower doses of μ-opioids with low doses of α_2-agonists (preferably in the form of a constant rate infusion [CRI]) may help achieve a desired level of analgesia by making use of the well known analgesic synergism between the two drug classes, while avoiding the profound CNS stimulatory effects of the opioids and hemodynamic effects of the α_2-agonists (see **Table 4**).[78] However, impaired intestinal motility, caused by both opioids and α_2-agonists, remains a concern with long-term treatment. Whether opioids elicit less CNS stimulatory effects and are therapeutically more effective in horses experiencing severe pain is controversial because scientific evidence is lacking.[79] Controlled trials in human patients revealed efficacy of opioids against peripheral neuropathic pain and some components of central neuropathic pain.[56,57]

Table 4
Doses of opioids and co-administered sedatives in horses

Drug	Dose, Route & Interval of Drug Administration	References
Opioids		
Morphine	0.1–0.2 mg/kg IV/IM every 4–6 hrs	73,74
Methadone	0.1–0.2 mg/kg IV/IM every 4–6 hrs	73,74
Butorphanol	0.01–0. 4 mg/kg IV, IM every 2–4 hrs[a] Bolus of 18 µg/kg bolus followed by IV CRI at 13–24 µg•kg^{-1}•hr^{-1}	55,72,74,79,80
Buprenorphine	5–20 µg/kg IV/IM TID 6 µg/kg sublingual BID	73,84,85
Fentanyl	2–3 10 mg (100 µg/hr) patches to be changed every 3 days	81–83
Co-administered phenothiazine and/or α_2 agonist sedative/analgesic		
Acepromazine[c]	0.01–0.08 mg/kg IV/IM/SC BID/TID or CRI at 2–4 µg•kg^{-1}•hr^{-1}	41,47,48
Detomidine	10–40 µg/kg IM/IV every 2–4 hrs Bolus[b] of 5–10 µg/kg IV followed by CRI at 24–36 µg•kg^{-1}•hr^{-1}	32,73,74
Medetomidine	5–7 µg/kg IM/IV every 2–4 hrs Bolus[b] of 3–7 µg/kg IV followed by CRI at 1.5–3.6 µg•kg^{-1}•hr^{-1}	32,73,74
Dexmedetomidine	Bolus[b] of 1.5–3.0 µg/kg IV followed by CRI at 0.75–1.8 µg•kg^{-1}•hr^{-1}	

Routes and intervals of drug administration: IV, intravenous; IM, intramuscular; SC, subcutaneously; SID, once daily; BID, twice daily; TID, three times daily; CRI, constant rate infusion.
  [a] Significant central excitatory responses to be expected from doses of >0.05 mg/kg onwards.
  [b] A bolus administration is optional but not always necessary, dependent on opioid dose and route of administration.
  [c] Acepromazine has also been employed to improve perfusion of the hoof,[41,46,48] even though recent studies have questioned the magnitude of such an effect.[153]

However, there is also laboratory animal and human clinical evidence that long-term use of μ-opioid agonists such as morphine can trigger the development of a state of opioid induced hyperalgesia (OIH) whereby a subject receiving opioids for the treatment of pain may actually become more sensitive to pain.[80–82] This potentially profound adverse effect should be considered when prescribing long-term opioid therapy in horses with chronic laminitis, even if the mechanisms leading to OIH and its clinical relevance are still being debated, and the phenomenon is not described in horses.[83]

Butorphanol (Torbugesic), a κ-opioid receptor agonist and μ-receptor antagonist, is probably the most widely used opioid in horses. The drug's short half-life limits its use as analgesic in laminitis, calling for a CRI to achieve persistent analgesia.[84,85] Transdermal administration of fentanyl (Duragesic), a potent but very short-acting synthetic μ-opioid receptor agonist, has been found to not consistently alleviate musculoskeletal pain.[86,87] If fentanyl patches were to be used as part of the multimodal pain management one should probably apply at least as many patches as necessary to achieve plasma fentanyl levels generally considered to be analgesic in other species (ie, $\geq$ 1 ng/mL).[88] Buprenorphine (Buprenex) is a μ-opioid-agonist and κ-opioid-antagonist, which has been claimed to have a ceiling effect.[77] When applied as a sole analgesic agent in horses, measurable antinociception has been reported to occur at doses of 10 μg/kg or higher but significant excitement and hemodynamic stimulation were noted as well.[89] Walker[90] reported recently about experience with a 5-day administration of buprenorphine in a filly with severe head and neck trauma choosing the sublingual/buccal mucosal route. The drug provided clinically effective analgesia, when given twice daily, without provoking signs of excitement.

SYSTEMIC LIDOCAINE

The clinical use of systemic lidocaine for pain treatment in humans was first reported almost five decades ago,[91] and during the past 10 years has gained much popularity also in equine practice.[32,78,92–95] The drug must be administered as CRI due to its short half-life.[96] A loading dose of 1.3 to 1.5 mg/kg administered IV over 15 minutes (min) followed by a CRI of 50–100 μg•kg^{-1}•min^{-1} is most commonly used.[78,79] Data regarding the immediate analgesic effect of lidocaine on spontaneous (not evoked) pain in animals or patients are somewhat inconsistent when infused at clinically common doses,[78,91,97–99] and higher doses carry the risk of cardio- and neurotoxicity.[86,94] Since plasma concentrations achieved during long-term infusion vary widely among horses and may accumulate over time,[78,95,96,100,101] monitoring of plasma levels (via a lidocaine ELISA kit; Neogen Corporation, Lansing, MI 48912, USA) is recommended, not only to avoid toxicity but also to ensure that concentrations known to reduce neuropathic pain behaviors (1.2–2.1 μg/mL)[91,95] are being achieved.

Information available to date indicates that the analgesic action of IV lidocaine is far more complex than previously thought. Besides its well studied local anesthetic actions (ie, Na$^+$ channel blockade) in the peripheral and central nervous system, it also exerts multiple other mechanisms of action that target the nociceptive system (spinal and supraspinal).[102–104] Both laboratory animal and controlled clinical trials in humans have found IV lidocaine to suppress development of peripheral hyperalgesia as well as central nociceptive sensitization and allodynia.[103–107] Its efficacy as an analgesic and anti-neuropathic agent has recently been demonstrated in adult patients suffering from chronic pain with tactile hyperalgesia and/or mechanical allodynia for more than 3 months as a result of a peripheral nerve injury.[98] In this trial[98] IV lidocaine failed to produce an alleviation of the spontaneous pain the patients were suffering from the nerve injury, similar to findings in a previous study from the same investigator group.[97] However it is also reported elsewhere that systemic lidocaine inhibits spontaneous pain.[91,107]

In addition to its analgesic and antihyperalgesic/anti-neuropathic properties described above lidocaine also has inflammation modifying effects and has been shown to protect tissues against ischemic and reperfusion injuries in various species including the horse.[108–113] Whether and at which plasma concentrations those effects may have a direct or indirect impact on the laminitis disease process and thus related nociceptive mechanisms and pain perception remains unclear. A most recent study indicates that in the black walnut extract model of laminitis lidocaine at plasma concentrations below 1 µg/mL does not inhibit inflammatory events in either the laminae or skin.[114]

NONCONVENTIONAL SYSTEMIC ANALGESICS WITH ANTIHYPERALGESIC AND ANTINEUROPATHIC PAIN ACTIVITY

Three evidence-based consensus guidelines for the pharmacologic treatment of neuropathic pain have been published recently in the human medical literature.[57–59] These guidelines all recommend tricyclic antidepressants (not tested in the equine species) and calcium channel $\alpha_2\delta$-ligands (gabapentin, pregabalin) as first-line treatments for patients with neuropathic pain. They suggest reserving opioid analgesics and N-methyl-D-aspartate (NMDA) receptor antagonists as second- or third-line options in most cases, despite evidence of efficacy in certain forms of hyperalgesia and neuropathic pain.[58] In two of the guidelines topical lidocaine was recommended as a first-line treatment for patients with localized peripheral neuropathic pain.[57–59]

CALCIUM CHANNEL $\alpha_2\delta$-LIGANDS (GABAPENTIN, PREGABALIN)

The anticonvulsant drugs gabapentin and pregabalin both bind with high affinity to the $\alpha_2\delta$-1 subunit of voltage-gated calcium channels in the spinal cord and brain.[115] As a result neuronal calcium currents are inhibited, ultimately causing a change in the release of neurotransmitters within the CNS such as glutamate, GABA, norepinephrine, and SP; these actions account for much of the analgesic activity of these compounds.[116,117] The expression of the $\alpha_2\delta$-1 subunit has been shown to increase in chronic pain states, as well as in both afferent sensory neurons and in the spinal cord dorsal horn in experimental neuropathic pain models.[118,119] This correlates well with the observation that gabapentin exerts analgesic properties primarily in sensitized or hyperalgesic states.[120–122] More recently gabapentin and pregabalin have been used clinically in humans to treat a variety of neuropathic pain states and early post-surgical pain, often but not always with success.[55–59,123] These drugs appear especially effective in patients with paroxysmal pain (lancinating/shooting pain), brush-induced allodynia and cold-induced allodynia/hyperalgesia, in whom it significantly lowers pain scores.[124] Laboratory animal data suggest the $\alpha_2\delta$-ligands also have activity against opioid-induced hyperalgesia.[125]

Documented therapeutic use in horses refers only to oral (PO) administration of gabapentin (Neurontin) in two animals which were thought to exhibit signs of neuropathic pain, one in conjunction with acute femoral nerve injury post-surgery and one with a history of white line disease and chronic laminitis.[35,126] Lacking information on pharmacokinetic properties of the drug in the equine at that time, gabapentin doses were extrapolated from use in other species (2.5 mg/kg at intervals of 8, 12 or 24 hrs;[125] 2.0–3.3 mg/kg at intervals of 8 or 12 hrs[35]). In the meantime two studies have been conducted in horses investigating the drug's pharmacokinetic properties as well as behavioral and cardiovascular parameters after IV and PO administration.[127,128] After IV (over 30 min) and PO administration of gabapentin (20 mg/kg), the median elimination half-lives were 8.5 and 7.7 hrs, respectively which correspond well with data in other species.[127] After IV administration plasma gabapentin concentrations remained above the 3–4 μg/mL range for approximately 15 hrs, similar to the dose associated with significant analgesic effects in adult human volunteers.[129] In the horse, oral bioavailability of gabapentin is relatively poor (~ 16 %) and therefore plasma gabapentin concentrations decreased much more rapidly than after IV drug administration (ie, within 2–3 hrs) below the analgesic threshold. Neither route of gabapentin administration was associated with effects on heart rate, rhythm or blood pressure, nor pronounced central nervous effects, which concurs in other species.[128] Further research is required to establish a dosage that will provide effective analgesia in horses with chronic laminitis and to determine if combinations with other agents create an enhanced effect.

KETAMINE

Peripheral sensory nerve stimulation leads to activation of the ligand-gated ion channel complex known as N-methyl-D-aspartate (NMDA) receptors on the postsynaptic membrane in the dorsal horn of the spinal cord. Release of NMDA, a modulating neurotransmitter, is coupled with subsequent release of the excitatory neurotransmitter glutamate.[22] The resultant extended depolarization of sensory neurons produces much larger than usual postsynaptic potentials, known as synaptic potentiation, a key component of central hyperalgesia as well as synaptic plasticity leading to chronic pain.[22,130,131]

Ketamine is an NMDA receptor antagonist.[132,133] At subanesthetic doses (100–150 μg/kg as initial bolus followed by a CRI of 60–120 μg•kg^{-1}•hr^{-1}) it blocks NMDA receptors, thereby modulating central sensitization induced both by tissue damage.[134–138] Ketamine exhibits synergism with classical analgesics such as opioids, NSAIDs, local anesthetics and $α_2$-agonists; therefore it reduces opioid analgesic consumption and increases analgesic quality.[136–138] Ketamine is used primarily as an antihyperalgesic and anti-allodynic compound in human patients at risk of developing maladaptive pain after major tissue damage and not primarily as an analgesic agent per se.[139]

Clinical effects of subanesthetic ketamine infusion (400 and 800 μg•kg^{-1}•hr^{-1}) have been studied in awake horses.[140] During or following the 12 hr infusion no analgesic effects could be demonstrated and no signs of excitement or significant changes in measured physiologic variables occurred. A CRI of 400–1500 μg•kg^{-1}•hr^{-1} has been used safely in conscious horses.[141] However, with both infusion regimens the measured plasma ketamine concentrations were about 10 times below concentrations (2–4 μg/mL) associated with measurable acute antinociceptive effects.[142] Matthews and colleagues[143] administered ketamine via infusion (400 and 800 μg•kg^{-1}•hr^{-1}) for up to 5 days in eight horses with osteomyelitis, septic joint disease, burns, or colic in a search for possible analgesic effects. Responses to ketamine varied substantially with some showing any or only slight improvements of pain symptoms, while others appeared to be markedly more comfortable within 6 to 12 hrs of the start of drug infusion. Thus, in horses as in humans, low dose ketamine infusion should be considered an adjunctive therapy for treating central hyperalgesia.

LOCO-REGIONAL ANESTHESIA AND ANALGESIA

The neuropathophysiological processes leading to the development of central hyperalgesia, neuropathic pain and allodynia are primarily triggered by increased spontaneous firing activity in ascending sensory nerve fibers during the first 4–5 days following peripheral nerve injuries.[144–146] Experimental evidence and clinical experiences in human medicine indicate that central hyperalgesia can be obliterated by no other treatment modality as effectively as by loco-regional anesthesia and analgesia aimed at interrupting or diminishing impulse trafficking from the site of tissue injury to the CNS and within the dorsal horn of the spinal cord.[56,59,78,144–149] Those techniques may include wound infiltration or joint injections with local anesthetics, topical local anesthetic application using lidocaine patches, repetitive or even better continuous peripheral nerve blocks, and epidural or intrathecal anesthesia and analgesia.

Continuous peripheral nerve blockade (CPNB) is a treatment modality that has been long introduced in human medicine and is currently widely applied in orthopedic and trauma surgery. The technique entails continuous or intermittent low-dose administration of local anesthetics via catheters placed along peripheral nerves, thus providing persistent pain control while reducing the need of systemic medications.[149] A technique for percutaneous placement of catheters along the palmar nerves in the standing, sedated horse was recently developed and provides a method for repeated or continuous perineural administration of low concentrated local anesthetic solutions (eg, bupivacaine or ropivacaine 0.125–0.25 %) over a period of multiple days.[149,150] The therapy can continue for longer periods by exchange catheters every 4–8 days. With this technique significant pain relief can be obtained in horses refractory to systemic analgesic therapy and therefore suffering from unrelenting pain during a period of early or active chronic laminitis.[151] The technique offers the advantage of titrating the analgesic effect by adjusting the concentration of the local anesthetic solution and/or the rate of drug administration to a desired level of comfort without causing complete sensory blockade. The CPNB catheters can also be placed more proximal on the limb in close proximity of the ulnar and median nerves.[151] This technique may serve as an alternative for providing significant reduction of pain perception in the distal forelimb.[151] However, the use of either CPNB technique in the acute phase of laminitis is controversial and warrants further clinical study. A pronounced nociceptive blockade of the affected limb will allow the horse to increase the load on the foot and potentially exacerbate the disruption of the lamellar dermal-epidermal bond.

In horses experiencing severe pain due to chronic laminitis in their hindlimb(s) caudal epidural administration of analgesics such as opioids (eg, morphine 0.1–0.2 mg/kg), α_2-agonists (eg, xylazine 0.17 mg/kg; detomidine 20–30 µg/kg) or a combination thereof with or without low (ie, motor function not compromising) doses of local anesthetic (eg, bupivacaine or ropivacaine 0.125–0.25%) provides long-term pain control.[152] To allow repeated drug administration it is recommended to place an epidural catheter.[152] Medications may be administered in form of intermittent boluses (15–30 mL) or as an infusion (0.5–3.0 mL/hr). As with the CPNB techniques similar restrictions apply to the use of epidural analgesia in the acute phase of laminitis.

SUMMARY

Managing pain in horses with chronic laminitis is often challenging as the disease process triggers a cascade of events that turns the somatosensory nervous system into a state of nociceptive hyperactivity with abnormal impulse processing often unresponsive to classic anti-inflammatory drug treatment. Appreciating this maladaptive pain state as the product of complex neuropathological processes affecting both the peripheral and central somatosensory nervous system is crucial when devising a treatment plan for horses afflicted by chronic laminitis. Effective analgesia calls from the outset for a multi-modal approach that involves a combination of agents with different pharmacologic mechanisms of action targeting different sites within the nociceptive system and requires both systemic and local/regional drug administration. A pain grading system should be applied that allows for objective pain assessment and close monitoring of changes in nociception as a result of disease progress and/ or response to analgesic therapy.

REFERENCES

1. Moore RM. Laminitis vision: 20/20 by 2020. In: Proceedings of the Fifth International Equine Conference on Laminitis and Diseases of the Foot. Palm Beach (FL); 2009. p. 15–20.
2. Orsini J, Galantino-Homer H, Pollitt CC. Laminitis in horses: through the lens of systems theory. J Equine Vet Sci 2009;29(2):105–14.
3. Hood DM. Laminitis in the horse. Vet Clin North Am Equine Pract 1999;15(2): 287–94.
4. Pollitt CC. Equine laminitis. Clin Tech Equine Pract 2004;3(1):34–44.
5. Rendle D. Equine laminitis 1. Management in the acute stage. In Pract 2006;28: 434–43.
6. Fontaine GL, Belknap JK, Allen D, et al. Expression of interleukin-1β in the digital laminae of horses in the prodromal stage of experimentally induced laminitis. Am J Vet Res 2001;62(5):714–20.
7. Waguespack RW, Cochran A, Belknap JK. Expression of the cyclooxygenase isoforms in the prodromal stage of black walnut-induced laminitis in horses. Am J Vet Res 2004;65(12):1724–9.
8. Blikslager AT, Yin CL, Cochran AM, et al. Cyclooxygenase expression in the early stages of equine laminitis: a cytologic study. J Vet Intern Med 2006; 20(5):1191–6.
9. Noschka E, Moore JN, Peroni JF, et al. Thromboxane and isoprostanes as inflammatory and vasoactive mediators in black walnut heartwood extract induced equine laminitis. Vet Immunol Immunopathol 2009;129(3/4):200–10.
10. Pollitt CC. Basement membrane pathology: a feature of acute equine laminitis. Equine Vet J 1996;28(1):38–46.
11. Pollitt CC, Daradka M. Equine laminitis basement membrane pathology: loss of type IV collagen, type VII collagen and laminin immunostaining. Equine Vet J Suppl 1998;26:139–44.
12. Johnson PJ, Tyagi SC, Katwa LC, et al. Activation of extracellular matrix metalloproteinases in equine laminitis. Vet Rec 1998;14(2):392–6.
13. Johnson PJ, Kreeger JM, Keeler M, et al. Serum markers of lamellar basement membrane degradation and lamellar histopathological changes in horses affected with laminitis. Equine vet J 2000;32(6):462–8.
14. Kyaw-Tanner M, Pollitt CC. Equine laminitis: increased transcription of matrix metalloproteinase-2 (MMP-2) occurs during the developmental phase. Equine vet J 2004;36(3):221–5.
15. Yaksh TL. Pain Management I: basic mechanisms in pain processing. In: Proceedings of the Fifth International Equine Conference on Laminitis and Diseases of the Foot. Palm Beach (FL); 2009. p. 84–5.
16. Yaksh TL. Pain Management II: current thinking on the mechanisms underlying laminitic pain. In: Proceedings of the Fifth International Equine Conference on Laminitis and Diseases of the Foot. Palm Beach (FL); 2009. p. 86–8.

17. Bowker RM, Brewer AM, Vex KBA, et al. Sensory receptors in the equine foot. Am J Vet Res 1993;54(11):1840–4.
18. Van Wulfen KK, Bowker RM. Evaluation of tachykinins and their receptors to determine sensory innervation in the dorsal hoof wall and insertion of the distal sesamoidean impar ligament and deep digital flexor tendon on the distal phalanx in healthy feet of horses. Am J Vet Res 2002;63(2):222–8.
19. Buda S, Budras KD. Segment specific nerve supply of the equine hoof. Pferdeheilkunde 2005;21(4):280–4.
20. Molyneux GS, Haller CJ, Mogg K, et al. The structure, innervation and location of arteriovenous anastomoses in the equine foot. Equine vet J 1994;26(4):305–12.
21. Morgan SJ, Grosenbaugh DA, Hood DM. The pathophysiology of chronic laminitis. Vet Clin North Am Equine Pract 1999;15(2):395–417.
22. Giordano J. The neurobiology of pain. In: Weiner RS, editor. Pain management: a practical guide for clinicians. 6th edition. Boca Raton (FL): CRC Press; 2001. p. 1089–100.
23. Orsini JA, Galantino-Homer H, Pollitt CC. Hot topics at the fourth international equine conference on laminitis and diseases of the foot. In: Large animal proceedings of the North American Veterinary Conference. Orlando (FL); 2009. p. 216–7.
24. Jones E, Viñuela-Fernandez I, Eager RA, et al. Neuropathic changes in equine laminitis pain. Pain 2007;132:321–31.
25. Owens JG, Kamerling SG, Keowen ML. Eicosanoid concentrations in digital venous blood from horses with chronic laminitis. Am J Vet Res 1995;56(4):507–10.
26. Moore JN, Allen D. The pathophysiology of acute laminitis. Vet Med 1996;10:936–9.
27. Doubell TP, Mannion RJ, Wolf CJ. The dorsal horn: state dependent sensory processing, plasticity, and the generation of pain. In: Wall PD, Melzak R, editors. Textbook of pain. 4th edition. New York: Churchill-Livingstone; 1999. p. 165–82.
28. Klusakova I, Dubovy P. Experimental models of peripheral neuropathic pain based on traumatic nerve injuries - an anatomical perspective. Ann Anat 2009;191(3):248–59.
29. Costigan M, Scholz J, Woolf CJ. Neuropathic pain: a maladaptive response of the nervous system to damage. Annu Rev Neurosci 2009;32:1–32.
30. Driessen B. Pain: from sign to disease. Clin Tech Equine Pract 2007;6(2):120–5.
31. Kawasaki Y, Xu ZZ, Wang X, et al. Distinct roles of matrix metalloproteases in the early- and late-phase development of neuropathic pain. Nat Med 2008;14(3):331–6.
32. Driessen B, Zarucco L. Pain: from diagnosis to effective treatment. Clin Tech Equine Pract 2007;6(2):126–34.
33. Obel N. Studies on the histopathology of acute laminitis. Uppsala (Sweden): Almqvist and Wiksells Boktryckteri AK; 1948 [dissertation].
34. American Association of Equine Practioners. Definition and classification of lameness. In: American Association of Equine Practioners: guide for veterinary service and judging of equestrian events. 4th edition. Lexington (KY); 1991. p. 19.
35. Dutton DW, Lashnits KJ, Wegner K. Managing severe hoof pain in a horse using multimodal analgesia and a modified composite pain score. Equine Vet Educ 2009;21:37–43.
36. Aviad AD. The use of the standing force plate as a quantitative measure of equine lameness. J Equine Vet Sci 1988;8:460–2.

37. Hood DM, Wagner IP, Taylor DD, et al. Voluntary limb-load distribution in horses with acute and chronic laminitis. Am J Vet Res 2001;66(9):1393–8.

38. Hunt RJ. Diagnosing and treating chronic laminitis in horses. Vet Med 1996; 91(11):1025–32.

39. Brumbaugh GW, Sumano Lopez H, Hoyos Sepulveda ML. The pharmacologic basis for the treatment of developmental and acute laminitis. Vet Clin North Am Equine Pract 1999;15(2):345–62.

40. Sumano Lopez H, Hoyos Sepulveda ML, Brumbaugh GW. Pharmacologic and alternative therapies for the horse with chronic laminitis. Vet Clin North Am Equine Pract 1999;15(2):495–516.

41. Parks AH. Treatment of acute laminitis. Equine vet Educ 2003;15(5):273–80.

42. Parks A, O'Grady SE. Chronic laminitis: current treatment strategies. Vet Clin North Am Equine Pract 2003;19(2):393–416.

43. Belknap JK. Treatment of the acute laminitis case. In: Large animal proceedings of the North American Veterinary Conference. Orlando (FL); 2006. p. 76–80.

44. Belknap JK. Treatment of the chronic laminitis case. In: Large animal proceedings of the North American Veterinary Conference. Orlando (FL); 2006. p. 79–80.

45. Piccot-Crezollet C, Olive J, Cadore JL. Diagnostic and therapeutic approaches in the face of acute laminitis in horses. Le Nouveau Praticien Veterinaire – Equine 2008;5(17):17–23.

46. Moore RM. Evidence-based treatment for laminitis - what works? J Equine Vet Sci 2008;28(3):176–9.

47. Moyer W, Schumacher J, Schumacher J, et al. Are drugs effective treatment for horses with acute laminitis? In: Proceedings of the 54th Annual Convention of the American Association of Equine Practioners, San Diego (CA); 2008. p. 337–40.

48. Divers TJ. Medical treatment of acute laminitis. In: Large animal proceedings of the North American Veterinary Conference. Orlando (FL); 2009. p. 174.

49. Siddall PJ, Cousins MJ. Persistent pain as a disease entity: implications for clinical management. Anesth Analg 2004;99:510–20.

50. Hansen N, Buchner F, Haller J, et al. Evaluation using hoof wall strain gauges of a therapeutic shoe and a hoof cast with a heel wedge as potential supportive therapy for horses with laminitis. Vet Surg 2005;34:630–6.

51. Morrison S. Rehabilitating the laminitic foot. In: Large animal proceedings of the North American Veterinary Conference. Orlando (FL); 2008. p. 186–9.

52. Hunt RJ, Allen D, Baxter GM, et al. Mid-metacarpal deep digital flexor tenotomy in the management of refractor laminitis in horses. Vet Surg 1991;20(1):15–20.

53. Vasko KA, Spauchus A, Lowry M. Laminitis treatment with electrotherapy. Equine Pract 1986;8(4):28–31.

54. Carter DW, Renfroe JB. A novel approach to the treatment and prevention of laminitis: botulinum toxin type A for the treatment of laminitis. J Equine Vet Sci 2009;29(7):595–600.

55. Galluzzi KE. Management of neuropathic pain. J Am Osteopath Assoc 2005; 105(9):S12–9.

56. Finnerup NB, Otto M, McQuay HJ, et al. Algorithm for neuropathic pain treatment: an evidence based proposal. Pain 2005;118(3):289–305.

57. Dworkin RH, O'Connor AB, Backonja M, et al. Pharmacologic management of neuropathic pain: evidence-based recommendations. Pain 2007;132(3): 237–51.

58. O'Connor AB, Dworkin RH. Treatment of neuropathic pain: an overview of recent guidelines. Am J Med 2009;122(Suppl 10):S22–32.

59. McGeeney BE. Pharmacological management of neuropathic pain in older adults: an update on peripherally and centrally acting agents. J Pain Symptom Manage 2009;38(Suppl 2):S15–27.
60. Clark JO, Clark TP. Analgesia. Vet Clin North Am Equine Pract 1999;15(3): 705–23.
61. Pollitt CC. Medical therapy of laminitis. In: Ross MW, Dyson SJ, editors. Diagnosis and management of lameness in the horse. St. Louis (MO): Saunders; 2003. p. 329–32.
62. Rouzer CA, Marnett LJ. Structural and functional differences between cyclooxygenases: fatty acid oxygenases with a critical role in cell signaling. Biochem Biophys Res Commun 2005;338(1):34–44.
63. Yaksh TL, Dirig DM, Conway CM, et al. The acute antihyperalgesic action of nonsteroidal, anti-inflammatory drugs and release of spinal prostaglandin E_2 is mediated by the inhibition of constitutive spinal cyclooxygenase-2 (COX-2) but not COX-1. J Neurosci 2001;21(6):5847–53.
64. Urdaneta A, Siso A, Urdaneta B, et al. Lack of correlation between the central anti-nociceptive and peripheral anti-inflammatory effects of selective COX-2 inhibitor parecoxib. Brain Res Bull 2009;80(1–2):56–61.
65. Simon LS. Biology and toxic effects of nonsteroidal anti-inflammatory drugs. Curr Opin Rheumatol 1998;10(3):153–8.
66. Blikslager A. Role of NSAIDs in the management of pain in horses. In: Proceedings of the American Association of Equine Practioners-Focus Meeting. Raleigh (NC); 2009. p. 218–23.
67. Divers TJ. COX inhibitors: Making the best choice for the laminitic case. J Equine Vet Sci 2008;28(6):367–9.
68. Cryer B, Feldman M. Cyclooxygenase-1 and cyclooxygenase-2 selectivity of widely used nonsteroidal anti-inflammatory drugs. Am J Med 1998;104(5): 413–21.
69. Owens JG, Kamerling SG, Stanton SR, et al. Effects of ketoprofen and phenylbutazone on chronic hoof pain and lameness in the horse. Equine Vet J 1995; 27(4):296–300.
70. Ossipov MH, Jerussi TP, Ren K, et al. Differential effects of spinal (R)-ketoprofen and (S)-ketoprofen against signs of neuropathic pain and tonic nociception: evidence for a novel mechanism of action of (R)-ketoprofen against tactile allodynia. Pain 2000;87(2):193–9.
71. Diaz-Reval MI, Ventura-Martinez R, Deciga-Campos M, et al. Evidence for a central mechanism of action of S-(+)-ketoprofen. Eur J Pharmacol 2004; 483(2–3):241–8.
72. Whay HR, Webster AJF, Waterman-Pearson AE. Role of ketoprofen in the modulation of hyperalgesia associated with lameness in dairy cattle. Vet Rec 2005; 157(23):729–33.
73. Moses VS, Bertone AL. Nonsteroidal anti-inflammatory drugs. Vet Clin North Am Equine Pract 2002;18(1):21–37.
74. Snow DH, Douglas TA, Thompson H, et al. Phenylbutazone toxicosis in equidae: a biochemical and pathophysiological study. Am J Vet Res 1981;42(10):1754–9.
75. Doucet MY, Bertone AL, Hendrickson D, et al. Comparison of efficacy and safety of paste formulations of firocoxib and phenylbutazone in horses with naturally occurring osteoarthritis. J Am Vet Med Assoc 2008;232(1):91–7.
76. MacAllister CG, Morgan SJ, Borne AT, et al. Comparison of adverse effects of phenylbutazone, flunixin meglumine, and ketoprofen in horses. J Am Vet Med Assoc 1993;202(1):71–7.

77. Bennett RC, Steffey EP. Use of opioids for pain and anesthetic management in horses. Vet Clin North Am Equine Pract 2002;18(1):46–60.
78. Driessen B. Pain: systemic and local/regional drug therapy. Clin Tech Equine Pract 2007;6(2):135–44.
79. Valverde A, Gunkel C. Pain management in horses and farm animals. J Vet Emerg Crit Care 2005;15(4):295–307.
80. Angst MS. Opioid-induced hyperalgesia: a qualitative systematic review. Anesthesiology 2006;104(3):570–87.
81. Chu LF, Angst MS, Clark D. Opioid-induced hyperalgesia in humans: molecular mechanisms and clinical considerations. Clin J Pain 2008;24(6):479–96.
82. Silverman SM. Opioid induced hyperalgesia: clinical implications for the pain practitioner. Pain Physician 2009;12(3):679–84.
83. Fishbain DAA. Do opioids induce hyperalgesia in humans? An evidence-based structured review. Pain Med 2009;10(5):829–39.
84. Sellon DC, Monroe VL, Roberts MC, et al. Pharmacokinetics and adverse effects of butorphanol administered by single intravenous injection or continuous intravenous infusion in horses. Am J Vet Res 2001;62(2):183–9.
85. Sellon DC, Roberts MC, Blikslager AT, et al. Effects of continuous rate intravenous infusion of butorphanol on physiologic and outcome variables in horses after celiotomy. J Vet Intern Med 2004;18(4):555–63.
86. Wegner K, Franklin RP, Long MT, et al. How to use fentanyl transdermal patches for analgesia in horses. In: Proceedings of the 48th Annual Convention of the American Association of Equine Practitioners. Orlando (FL); 2002. p. 291–4.
87. Thomasy SM, Slovis N, Maxwell LK, et al. Transdermal fentanyl combined with non-steroidal anti-inflammatory drugs for analgesia in horses. J Vet Intern Med 2004;18(4):550–4.
88. Orsini JA, Moate PJ, Kuersten K, et al. Pharmacokinetics of fentanyl delivered transdermally in healthy adult horses – variability among horses and its clinical implications. J Vet Pharmacol Ther 2006;29(6):539–46.
89. Carregaro AB, Luna SP, Mataqueiro MI, et al. Effects of buprenorphine on nociception and spontaneous locomotor activity in horses. Am J Vet Res 2007;68(3):246–50.
90. Walker AF. Sublingual administration of buprenorphine for long-term analgesia in the horse. Vet Rec 2007;160(23):808–9.
91. Mao J, Chen LL. Systemic lidocaine for neuropathic pain relief. Pain 2000;87(1):7–17.
92. Malone E, Graham L. Management of gastrointestinal pain. Vet Clin Equine Pract 2002;18(1):133–58.
93. Driessen B. Intravenous lidocaine infusion in balanced anaesthesia for abdominal surgery: update and clinical experiences. Pferdeheilkunde 2005;21(2):133–41.
94. Murrell JC, White KL, Johnson CB, et al. Investigation of the EEG effects of intravenous lidocaine during halothane anaesthesia in ponies. Vet Anaesth Analg 2005;32(4):212–21.
95. Robertson SA, Sanchez LC, Merritt AM, et al. Effect of systemic lidocaine on visceral and somatic nociception in conscious horses. Equine vet J 2005;37(2):122–7.
96. Feary DJ, Mama KR, Wagner AE, et al. Influence of general anaesthesia on pharmacokinetics of intravenous lidocaine infusion in horses. Am J Vet Res 2005;66(4):574–80.

97. Gottrup H, Bach FW, Juhl G, et al. Differential effect of ketamine and lidocaine on spontaneous and mechanical evoked pain in patients with nerve injury pain. Anesthesiology 2006;104(3):527–36.

98. Gormsen L, Finnerup NB, Almqvist PM, et al. The efficacy of the AMPA receptor antagonist NS1209 and lidocaine in nerve injury pain: a randomized, double-blind, placebo-controlled, three-way crossover study. Anesth Analg 2009; 108(4):1311–9.

99. Meyer GA, Lin HC, Hanson RR, et al. Effects of intravenous lidocaine overdose on cardiac electrical activity and blood pressure in the horse. Equine vet J 2001; 33(5):434–7.

100. De Solis CN, McKenzie HC 3rd. Serum concentrations of lidocaine and its metabolites MEGX and GX during and after prolonged intravenous infusion of lidocaine in horses after colic surgery. J Equine Vet Sci 2007;27(9):398–404.

101. Dickey EJ, McKenzie HC 3rd, Brown KA, et al. Serum concentrations of lidocaine and its metabolites after prolonged infusion in healthy horses. Equine vet J 2008;40(4):348–52.

102. Woolf CJ, Wiesenfeld-Hallin Z. The systemic administration of local anaesthetics produces a selective depression of C-afferent fibre evoked activity in the spinal cord. Pain 1985;23(4):361–74.

103. Ness T. Intravenous lidocaine inhibits visceral nociceptive reflexes and spinal neurons in the rat. Anesthesiology 2000;92(6):1685–91.

104. Lauretti GR. Mechanisms of analgesia of intravenous lidocaine. Revista Brasileira de Anestesiologia 2008;58(3):280–6.

105. Abram SE, Yaksh TL. Systemic lidocaine blocks nerve injury-induced hyperalgesia and nociceptor-driven spinal sensitization in the rat. Anesthesiology 1994; 80(2):383–91.

106. Koppert W, Dern SK, Sittl R, et al. New model of electrically evoked pain and hyperalgesia in human skin: the effects of intravenous alfentanil, S(+)-ketamine, and lidocaine. Anesthesiology 2001;95(2):395–402.

107. Attal N, Rouaud J, Brasseur L, et al. Systemic lidocaine in pain due to peripheral nerve injury and predictors of response. Neurology 2004;62(2):218–25.

108. Taniguchi T, Shibata K, Yamamoto K, et al. Lidocaine attenuates the hypotensive and inflammatory responses to endotoxemia in rabbits. Crit Care Med 1996; 24(4):642–6.

109. Hollmann MW, Durieux ME. Local anesthetics and the inflammatory response: a new therapeutic indication? Anesthesiology 2000;93(3):858–75.

110. Brianceau P, Chevalier H, Karas A, et al. Intravenous lidocaine and small-intestinal size, abdominal fluid, and outcome after colic surgery in horses. J Vet Intern Med 2002;16(6):736–41.

111. Cook VL, Jones Shults J, McDowell MR, et al. Attenuation of ischaemic injury in the equine jejunum by administration of systemic lidocaine. Equine vet J 2008; 40(4):353–7.

112. Cook VL, Jones Shults J, McDowell MR, et al. Anti-inflammatory effects of intravenously administered lidocaine hydrochloride on ischemia-injured jejunum in horses. Am J Vet Res 2009;70(10):1259–68.

113. Cook VL, Neuder LE, Blikslager AT, et al. The effect of lidocaine on in vitro adhesion and migration of equine neutrophils. Vet Immunol Immunopathol 2010; 129(1–2):137–42.

114. Williams JM, Lin YJ, Loftus JP, et al. Effect of intravenous lidocaine administration on laminar inflammation in the black walnut extract model of laminitis. Equine Vet J 2010;42(3):261–9.

115. Taylor CP. The biology and pharmacology of calcium channel α_2-δ proteins. CNS Drug Rev 2004;10(2):183–8.

116. Dixit RK, Bhargava VK. Neurotransmitter mechanisms in gabapentin antinociception. Pharmacology 2002;65(4):198–203.

117. Sills GJ. The mechanisms of action of gabapentin and pregabalin. Curr Opin Pharmacol 2006;6:108–13.

118. Luo ZD, Chaplan SR, Higuera ES, et al. Upregulation of dorsal root ganglion $\alpha 2\delta$ calcium channel subunit and its correlation with allodynia in spinal nerve-injured rats. J Neurosci 2001;21(6):1868–75.

119. Newton RA, Bingham S, Case PC, et al. Dorsal root ganglion neurons show increased expression of the calcium channel $\alpha 2\delta$ - 1 subunit following partial sciatic nerve injury. Brain Res Mol Brain Res 2001;95(1–2):1–8.

120. Manouf YP, Luo ZD, Lee K. $\alpha 2\delta$ and the mechanism of action of gabapentin in the treatment of pain. Semin Cell Dev Biol 2006;17(5):565–70.

121. Harding LM, Kristensen JD, Baranowski AP. Differential effects of neuropathic analgesics on wind-up-like pain and somatosensory function in healthy volunteers. Clin J Pain 2005;21(2):127–32.

122. Arendt-Nielsen L, Brøndum Frøkjær J, Staahl C, et al. Effects of gabapentin on experimental somatic pain and temporal summation. Reg Anesth Pain Med 2007;32(5):382–8.

123. Gilron I. Gabapentin and pregabalin for chronic neuropathic and early postsurgical pain: current evidence and future directions. Curr Opin Anesthesiol 2007; 20:456–72.

124. Ripamonti C, Dickerson ED. Strategies for the treatment of cancer pain in the new millennium. Drugs 2001;61(7):955–77.

125. Van Elstraete AC, Sitbon P, Mazoit JX, et al. Gabapentin prevents delayed and long-lasting hyperalgesia induced by fentanyl in rats. Anesthesiology 2008; 108(3):484–94.

126. Davis JL, Posner LP, Elce Y. Gabapentin for the treatment of neuropathic pain in a pregnant horse. J Am Vet Med Assoc 2007;231(5):755–8.

127. Dirikolu L, Dafalla A, Ely KJ, et al. Pharmacokinetics of gabapentin in horses. J Vet Pharmacol Ther 2008;31(2):175–7.

128. Terry R, McDonnell SM, van Eps AW, et al. Pharmacokinetic profile and behavioral effects of gabapentin in the horse. J Vet Pharmacol Ther, in press.

129. Eckhardt K, Ammon S, Hofmann U, et al. Gabapentin enhances the analgesic effect of morphine in healthy volunteers. Anesth Analg 2000;91(1):185–91.

130. Rison RA, Stanton PK. Long-term potentiation and N-methyl-D-aspartate receptors: foundations of memory and neurologic disease? Neurosci Biobehav Rev 1995;19(4):533–52.

131. Mori H, Mishina M. Structure and function of the NMDA receptor channel. Neuropharmacol 1995;34(10):1219–37.

132. Orser BA, Pennefather PS, MacDonald JF. Multiple mechanisms of ketamine blockade of N-methyl-D-aspartate receptors. Anesthesiology 1997;86(4): 903–17.

133. Wong CS, Cherng CH, Ho ST. Clinical applications of excitatory amino acid antagonists in pain management. Acta Anaesthesiol Sin 1995;33(4):227–32.

134. Schmid RL, Sandler AN, Katz J. Use and efficacy of low-dose ketamine in the management of acute postoperative pain: a review of current techniques and outcomes. Pain 1999;82(2):111–25.

135. Hocking G, Cousins MJ. Ketamine in chronic pain management: an evidence-based review. Anesth Analg 2003;97(6):1730–9.

136. Richebe P, Rivat C, Rivalan B. Low doses ketamine: antihyperalgesic drug, non-analgesic. Ann Fr Anesth Reanim 2005;24(11–12):1349–59.
137. Strigo IA, Duncan GH, Bushnell C, et al. The effects of racemic ketamine on painful stimulation of skin and viscera in human subjects. Pain 2005;113(3):255–64.
138. De Kock MF, Lavand'homme PM. The clinical role of NMDA receptor antagonists for the treatment of postoperative pain. Best Pract Res Clin Anaesthesiol 2007;21(1):85–98.
139. Visser E, Schug SA. The role of ketamine in pain management. Biomed Pharmacother 2006;60(7):341–8.
140. Fielding CL, Brumbaugh GW, Matthews NS, et al. Pharmacokinetics and clinical effects of a subanesthetic continuous rate infusion of ketamine in awake horses. Am J Vet Res 2006;67(9):1484–90.
141. Lankveld DPK, Driessen B, Soma LR, et al. Pharmacodynamic effects and pharmacokinetic profile of a long-term continuous rate infusion of racemic ketamine in healthy conscious horses. J Vet Pharmacol Therap 2006;29(6):477–88.
142. Levionnois OL, Menge M, Thormann W. Effect of ketamine on the limb withdrawal reflex evoked by transcutaneous electrical stimulation in ponies anaesthetised with isoflurane. Vet J, in press [Available online September 12, 2009].
143. Matthews NS, Fielding CI, Swinebroad E. How to use a ketamine constant rate infusion in horses for analgesia. In: Proceedings of the 50th Annual Convention of the American Association of Equine Practitioners. Denver (CO); 2004. p. 1431.
144. Suter MR, Papaloizos M, Berde CB, et al. Development of neuropathic pain in the rat spared nerve injury model is not prevented by a peripheral nerve block. Anesthesiology 2003;99(6):1402–8.
145. Xie W, Strong JA, Meij JT, et al. Neuropathic pain: early spontaneous afferent activity is the trigger. Pain 2005;116(3):243–56.
146. Reuben SS, Buvanendran A. Preventing the development of chronic pain after orthopaedic surgery with preventive multimodal analgesic techniques. J Bone Joint Surg Am 2007;89(6):1343–58.
147. Beloeil H, Gentili M, Benhamou D, et al. The effect of a peripheral block on inflammation-induced prostaglandin E_2 and cyclooxygenase expression in rats. Anesth Analg 2009;109(3):943–50.
148. Estebe JP, Gentili ME, Le Corre P, et al. Sciatic nerve block with bupivacaine-loaded microspheres prevents hyperalgesia in an inflammatory animal model. Can J Anaesth 2002;49(7):690–3.
149. Driessen B, Scandella M, Zarucco L. Development of a technique for continuous perineural blockade of the palmar nerves in the distal equine thoracic limb. Vet Anaesth Analg 2008;35:432–48.
150. Zarucco L, Driessen B, Scandella M, et al. Continuous perineural block of the palmar nerves: a new technique for pain relief in the distal equine forelimb. Clin Tech Equine Pract 2007;6(2):154–64.
151. Zarucco L, Scandella M, Seco O, et al. Ultrasound-guided technique for continuous ulnar and median nerve blockade in the horse. Vet Surg 2008;37(6):E34.
152. Natalini CC, Driessen B. Epidural and spinal anesthesia and analgesia in the equine. Clin Tech Equine Pract 2007;6(2):144–53.
153. Leise BS, Fugler LA, Stokes AM, et al. Effects of intramuscular administration of acepromazine on palmar digital blood flow, palmar digital arterial pressure, transverse facial arterial pressure, and packed cell volume in clinically healthy, conscious horses. Vet Surg 2007;36(8):717–23.

Digital Venography in Horses and Its Clinical Application in Europe

Lorenzo D'Arpe, DVM, PhD*, Daniele Bernardini, DVM, PhD

KEYWORDS

- Digital venography • Laminitis • Venocompression
- Equine foot

Venography is a useful diagnostic tool that allows radiographic visualization of the veins in the equine foot after an injection of radiopaque contrast liquid into the digital palmar or plantar vein (**Fig. 1**).

The technique is repeatable and is useful as a diagnostic procedure to clinically evaluate the severity of the vascular changes in laminitis, or other foot pathologies, in the standing horse. With a tourniquet applied, the circulation in the foot is closed and sometimes arteries are also visible because of retrograde filling of the arterial circulation.[1] Venography provides the equine veterinarian with important information regarding the clinical evaluation of the vascular changes of the laminitic foot (**Fig. 2**).[2] The procedure can be easily and safely performed in the standing, sedated horse with an abaxial sesamoidean nerve block and tourniquet applied; only routine radiographic equipment is required and complications are minimal. The venographic examination continues to evolve since its introduction 18 years ago.

HISTORY OF DIGITAL VENOGRAPHY

Using cadaver limbs, with a tourniquet applied proximal to the injection site, Pollitt[1] in 1992 showed retrograde filling of digital veins when radiopaque contrast fluid was injected into the lateral digital vein. Later, in 1992, Redden and Pollitt collaborated and developed a reliable technique for the standing horse because a great need existed then to better understand the effect of laminitis on the digital circulation. Thereafter, Redden[3,4] standardized the digital venographic technique and used it extensively as a diagnostic tool in clinical practice. Rucker[5,6] has described normal

Department of Veterinary Clinical Sciences, University of Padua, Agripolis, V.le dell'Università n. 16, 35020 Legnaro (Padova), Italy
* Corresponding author.
E-mail address: lorenzodarpe@tiscali.it

Vet Clin Equine 26 (2010) 339–359
doi:10.1016/j.cveq.2010.06.006
0749-0739/10/$ – see front matter © 2010 Elsevier Inc. All rights reserved.

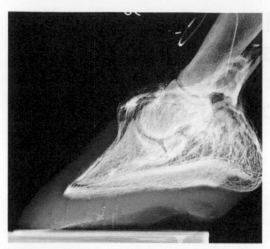

Fig. 1. Venogram of a normal foot.

aspects and artifacts of the digital venogram, and D'Arpe and Bernardini and others have described modifications to the venography technique exploring the biomechanical influence of foot loading on the vascular network during quasistatic movement.[7,8] The authors have studied and used the technique to assess the chronology of laminitis development to provide basic guidelines for the interpretation of sequential venograms. Furthermore, the authors have used venography to investigate the physiology and biomechanics of the "hydrovolumetric foot-heart pump."

COMPARING DIGITAL BLOOD FLOW DIAGNOSTIC TECHNIQUES

Various in vivo and in vitro methods have been used to gauge blood flow in the feet of laminitic horses. They include angiography by way of the digital artery, thermography,

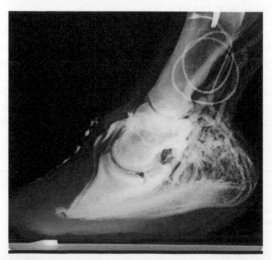

Fig. 2. Venogram of a foot affected by chronic laminitis.

scintigraphy, infrared spectroscopy, magnetic resonance imaging, ultrasound, and laser Doppler fluxometry. Some of these techniques are non-invasive. Angiography, however, calls for general anesthesia and lateral recumbency and can cause arterial spasms, which may affect the results.[3,4,9] These techniques are not readily available in clinical practice and, in the authors' experience, are not predictive of tissue damage because none allows visualization of venocompression because of pathology (permanent) or the dynamic forces of foot loading (temporary).[10] Venography helps the veterinarian in the clinical evaluation of foot perfusion in the standing, conscious horse. Venography has a predictive potential thanks to the visualization of venocompression; this enables the clinician to anticipate tissue necrosis instead of detecting it after it occurs.[11]

PODIATRY RADIOGRAPHIC TECHNIQUE AND HOW IT DIFFERS FROM TRADITIONAL ORTHOPEDIC PROCEDURES

The equine foot is the anatomic region most frequently examined using radiographs because many horse gait abnormalities result from foot problems.[12] Many scientific studies on radiologic foot measurements exist, but they were not performed using a positioning technique standardized for foot venography.[13,14] A few techniques have been standardized for postmortem studies.[12,15] When the x-ray beam is focused on the distal interphalangeal joint (DIP), the image obtained shows superimposition of the condyles of the middle phalanx and lateromedial imbalance. The palmar angle (PA) of the distal phalanx is also distorted (PA is the angle between the palmar processes of the distal phalanx and the ground surface).[16] The authors conducted a study evaluating the "magnification effect" related to the focus-film distance and the "distortion effect" related to the height of the block used to position the foot. It was concluded that an 80-cm focus-film distance was a good compromise between quality images and radiation safety.[17]

When the foot was radiographed without the foot placed on a wooden block, the x-ray focus was on the proximal interphalangeal joint, with a 50-mm woodblock the x-ray focus was on the DIP, and with a 90-mm woodblock the x-ray focus was on the middle of the solar aspect of the distal phalanx. Distortion caused by the height effect did not influence the coronary band–extensor process distance (CE). There was a remarkable variation, however, in the PA and lateromedial imbalance. Lastly, sole depth (SD) measurements were compromised if a shoe or the wooden block were superimposed on the image.[17] An evaluation of distortion caused by the height of the foot positioning block is shown in **Fig. 3**.

Centering the beam is particularly important for venography because one of the main goals of digital venography is to properly visualize, without distortion or magnification, the papillae or fimbriae of the solear dermis (fimbriae = fringe in Latin). Solear papillae can be obscured by superimposition of the palmar processes or a shoe. The length, direction, and compression of the solear papillae are clinically correlated to foot pathology and to biomechanical forces acting on the foot (**Fig. 4**).[18]

DIGITAL VENOGRAPHY PROCEDURE IN THE STANDING HORSE

The anatomic structures detected with venography are soft tissues that are undetectable with plain radiographs (**Fig. 5**). The authors perform the technique according to Redden[4] and Rucker[5,6] with some modifications, such as a screw-on injection site on the butterfly needle tubing (**Fig. 6**) to avoid blood contamination of equipment and the operator's hands. Additional radiographs are acquired at 90 and 160 seconds.

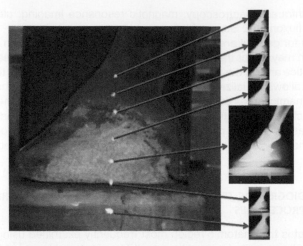

Fig. 3. The distortion effect caused by X-ray beam angle can cause errors when measuring the PA and lateral medial imbalance (LMU).[18] For every barium dot on the digit there is an arrow that shows the corresponding radiograph. A postmortem study determined which X-ray examination technique gave the most realistic measurements of the SD, CE, PA, and LMU. (*Data from* D'Arpe L, Coppola LM, Bernardini D. Radiographic imaging of the equine foot. International Laminitis Symposium Proceedings, Berlin; 2008.)

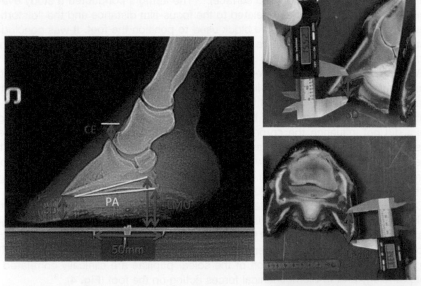

Fig. 4. Comparing radiographic and anatomic measurements. Red arrows show the measurements on the radiograph compared with the corresponding anatomic measurement. The study was performed on shod and barefoot horses taking several images at different heights of the X-ray beam; the SD, PA, lateral medial imbalance (LMU), and CE were calculated for each image. We confirmed that measurements of the SD, PA, CE, and LMU using a standardized, podiatry X-ray technique and derived when the X-ray beam was aligned with the palmar surface of the distal phalanx corresponded closely to postmortem measurements. Measurements were corrected for magnification error using a magnification correction coefficient with an 80-cm film/focus distance.

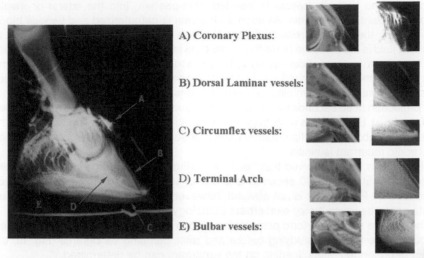

A) Coronary Plexus:

B) Dorsal Laminar vessels:

C) Circumflex vessels:

D) Terminal Arch

E) Bulbar vessels:

Fig. 5. Normal anatomic structures detected by venography. (A) Coronary venous plexus. (B) Dorsal sublamellar veins. (C) Circumflex vessels. (D) Terminal arch. (E) Bulbar vessels.

The horse is sedated with detomidine and the foot desensitized with a subcutaneous injection of 2% lidocaine, abaxially, to the medial and lateral palmar nerves at the apex of the proximal sesamoid bones (abaxial sesamoidean nerve block). The shoe is removed and the foot is cleaned thoroughly. An adhesive bandage is placed around the fetlock to secure the tourniquet when it is applied. The foot is placed on the foot

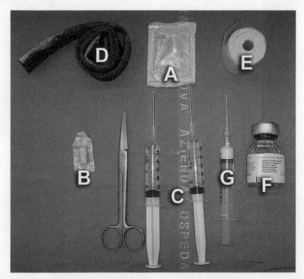

Fig. 6. Venography materials. (A) A 21-gauge butterfly needle with 30-cm tubing. (B) Sterile screw-on injection cap. (C) Two to three syringes containing 10–12 mL radiopaque intravascular contrast medium, sodium diatrizoate. (D) Tourniquet (or Esmarch bandage). (E) Elastikon (Ethicon USA, Sommerville, NJ, USA) 10 cm (or other adhesive bandage). (F) Detomidine (or other sedative). (G) Barium sulfate paste.

block and the butterfly needle is inserted, mid-pastern, into the lateral or medial palmar or plantar digital vein. As soon as the vein is catheterized and venous blood flows freely, the cap is screwed in place to close the tube. After the 20 to 25 mL of contrast fluid is injected, the butterfly needle tube is secured to the bandage that holds the tourniquet in place. Four radiographs are acquired (two lateromedial views and two dorsopalmar 0-degree views) in 40 to 50 seconds, so as to obtain optimal images before the contrast medium diffuses from the veins. We then take one more lateromedial projection at 90 seconds to visualize and evaluate the rate of perivascular diffusion and, lastly, at 120 seconds a 65-degree dorsopalmar oblique projection to detect the presence or absence of inflammatory edema or seroma that may be present in acute or chronic recurrent laminitis.

The authors have observed that "pumping" (**Fig. 7**) between the second and third radiographs at 10 and 30 seconds is a useful variation on the original technique described by Redden.[4] It is not advised, however, for clinical venography of severe acute cases because it may exacerbate pathology.

The authors usually perform pumping on normal and low-risk cases. By completely unloading the foot and studying before and after pumping venograms (**Fig. 8**), the effect of prolonged, static loading on the venogram can be determined.[19]

Routinely, the authors unlock the carpus during injection of the contrast agent to slightly unload the foot and relieve the tension of the deep digital flexor tendon (DDFT). This achieves filling of the dorsal laminae.[4] The foot is unloaded while injecting the second syringe of contrast medium to ensure lamellar perfusion. Lamellar perfusion is compromised when the foot is weight-bearing (loaded).[3,4] In venograms of a normal foot, vascular filling in the dorsal laminae can be substantially reduced[4] by venocompression if the foot is weight-bearing and immobile for a prolonged period

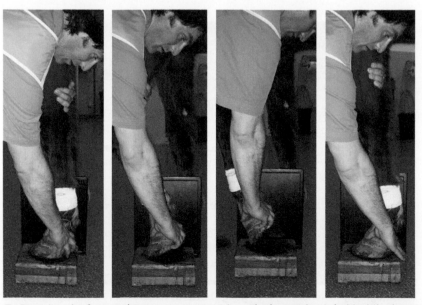

Fig. 7. Pumping the foot to detect venocompression. The horse's leg is held while the operator's shoulder is in contact with the dorsal forearm of the horse; one hand pulls the deep digital flexor tendon muscle to pick up the foot while the other hand replaces the foot to its original place.

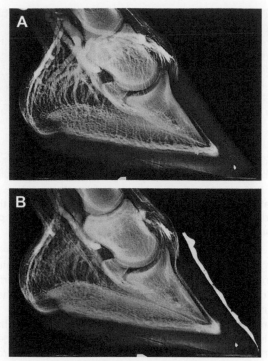

Fig. 8. The before (*A*) and after (*B*) effects of "pumping." There is more complete filling of coronary and sublamellar vessels after pumping.

of time (see **Fig. 8**A). Also, if normal horses stand still on the radiograph blocks for more than 10 minutes, and the procedure is then started, a lack of contrast in the dorsal lamellar vessels is observed. This is the normal effect of static venocompression caused by prolonged weight-bearing.

ARTIFACTS

In normal venograms, retrograde venous infusion of radiopaque contrast material should fill the venous vessels and sometimes the arteries. In abnormal venograms, retrograde venous infusion of radiopaque contrast material fails to completely fill the vessels of the foot. This can be temporary (caused by prolonged weight-bearing) or permanent (caused by advanced lamellar pathology and necrosis or by technique failure).[10–20]

Perivascular infiltration of contrast medium is the most frequent artifact found in the venographic technique.[5] If perivascular leakage has occurred, a large pool of contrast medium is evident on both the lateromedial and dorsopalmar views, at the needle insertion site, in the palmar or plantar digital vein (**Fig. 9**). The quantity of leaked contrast must be taken into consideration because it may result in inadequate venous filling of the foot.[7,21]

An inadequate volume of contrast medium results from perivascular leakage; syringes coming loose from catheters; loosened catheter clamps (if used); or from incorrect calculations of the volume needed for the venogram. Contrast volume varies with foot size: 20 to 25 ml is the range for the foot of a small horse (300–450 kg body weight, 9–12 cm diameter at the widest part of the foot) and 25 to 30 mL is adequate

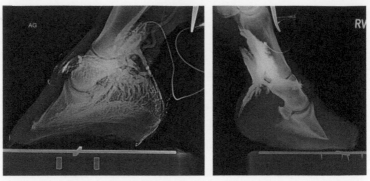

Fig. 9. Perivascular leakage of contrast material can occur if the vein is punctured during catheterization. It also occurs if the horse moves during the process, or the catheter comes out of the vein during foot manipulation, or if the digital palmar vein pressure is so high that the liquid escapes from the vein.

for the foot of a large horse (450–700 kg body weight, 12–15 cm diameter at the widest part of the foot). Inadequate volume can be confused with poor perfusion. A characteristic narrowing of the blood vessels and lack of perfusion in the heels indicate that volume is inadequate (**Fig. 10**).[5,21]

Tourniquet failure can also result in inadequate filling. Radiographs reveal contrast medium proximal to the tourniquet (**Fig. 11**). Elastic adhesive bandage (Elastikon; Ethicon USA, Sommerville, NJ, USA) placed beneath the tourniquet to prevent it from slipping is recommended, but using too much Elastikon to pad the vessels can impair tourniquet function.[5,7,21]

In the authors' experience, use of the tourniquet at mid-cannon, as described for the retrograde venous antibiotic perfusion technique, makes it more difficult to achieve an adequate volume of contrast medium and is more likely to cause tourniquet failure.

VENOGRAPHIC STUDIES OF THE QUASISTATIC BIOMECHANICS OF THE FOOT

Shearing and compressive forces within the hoof capsule caused by downward displacement of the laminitic distal phalanx contribute to mechanical circulatory collapse, hoof lamellar and solear pathology, and impact directly on varying degrees of inflammation and lysis of the distal phalanx.[3,4] The authors have used venography

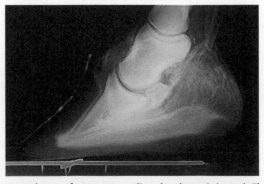

Fig. 10. An inadequate volume of contrast medium has been injected. There is lack of perfusion in heel veins and blood vessels appear narrow (compare with **Fig. 1**).

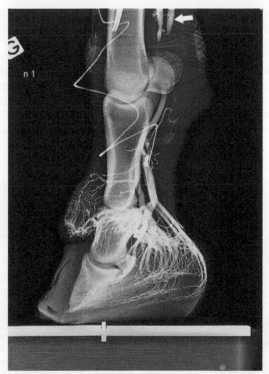

Fig. 11. Failure of the tourniquet. There is contrast proximal to the tourniquet (*arrow*). (*Courtesy of* Richard Corde, Boissy St Leger, France.)

to visualize and evaluate how in vivo venocompression is influenced by weight-bearing forces. In the authors' opinion this is a clinically important factor in the laminitis process. The weight-bearing force is transmitted through the skeletal axis to the ground at one application point: the static center of pressure (SCP) as described by Leveillard.[22] The SCP can be easily detected and its position varies depending on whether the horse is in the quadripedal or tripedal stance. Differences in weight-bearing load and balance regulation influence tension in the DDFT musculotendinous unit and can modify the venographic appearance of the digital vascular bed (**Fig. 12**).[23]

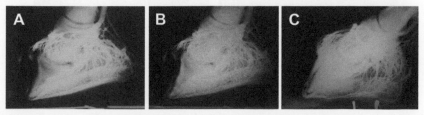

Fig. 12. Venograms of a club foot loaded (*A*), unloaded (*B*), and after deep digital flexor tendon tenotomy (*C*) at mid cannon. A change in tension in the deep digital flexor tendon musculotendinous unit has modified the venographic appearance of the digital vascular bed; there is increased venous filling after tenotomy. (*Courtesy of* Ric Redden, Versailles, KY, USA.)

The PA of the foot, and consequently the flexion-extension of the phalangeal joints, can modify the appearance of the venogram in the same horse, in the same time frame, even under constant overloading (tripedal stance).[24,25] In an in vivo study we used a dynamic PA iron and wood block called the D'Arpe-Moreau block (built for research purposes only). The aim was to visualize the vascular bed while the PA of the weight-bearing foot varied (**Fig. 13**). Using our standardized technique contrast medium was injected with the foot at 0 degrees. After injecting the contrast liquid, the contralateral foot was picked up to induce a tripedal stance. The foot was then progressively moved from −15 degrees to +15 degrees and vice versa; the head of

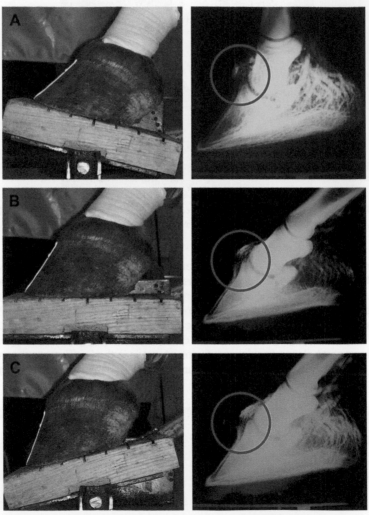

Fig. 13. A foot was prepared for venography and digital venograms were made with the D'Arpe-Moreau block at +15 degrees (*A*), 0 degrees (*B*), and −15 degrees (*C*). The contralateral limb was kept raised while the radiographs were acquired. The coronary plexus is circled in each venogram. There was less dorsal, venous filling when the toe was raised by 15 degrees (*A*).

the horse was kept in the sagittal axis to keep the weight on the foot constant. Seven radiographic images were acquired while moving the dynamic woodblock angle by 5 degrees every 30 seconds and not moving the x-ray machine from the ground.

The study showed that manipulating the PA of a loaded foot caused an alternating emptying and filling of vascular regions within the foot, suggesting that the foot, with a tourniquet applied, is an anatomically closed system. The authors concluded that the equine foot is a hydraulic pump able to develop alternating emptying and filling of blood between the hoof capsule and the distal phalanx.[40]

THE SAFETY VALVE OF THE FOOT-HEART PUMP AND THE FIVE-HEARTS THEORY

The discoveries made by the authors, using the D'Arpe-Moreau block, contradict the traditional foot pump theory. In addition, observation of the pumping action during flexion-extension of the DIP suggested a safety valve function for the coronary band. There is an interface between an abaxial flap consisting of the coronary band and the axial flap consisting of the ungual cartilages, the collateral ligaments of the DIP, and the dorsal digital extensor tendon. The latter seem to be involved in compression of the coronary venous plexus during extension and decompression during flexion, closing and opening the blood flow to the foot vascular bed in the standing quasistatic horse.[20,26]

Pollitt[1] showed in an ex vivo experiment that when the digit is loaded with a 1000-kg pressure (as on the foot of a galloping horse) and contrast medium is infused by way of the common digital artery, no arterial contrast was visible below the coronary band. The contrary occurred when the foot was not loaded; the infusion of contrast medium then filled the whole vascular network (**Fig. 14**).

Previous studies described the foot-heart pump as a hydraulic pump activated by flexion and extension of the DIP that empties and fills with blood inside the semiclosed system of the foot vascular bed. In a dynamic or quasistatic state the body weight movement over the SC induces flexion-extension of the phalanges. Tension and release in the DDFT modulates phalangeal flexion and extension and moves the SCP, biomechanically opening and closing the vascular arterial and venous safety valves. The foot pumping action, during quasistatic movement in standing horses, resembles the shifting weight behavior or paddling of laminitic horses described by Obel[27] as grade 1 laminitis in 1948. The rolling foot action has a massaging effect that moves the SCP backward and forward, even under constant overload, and without leaving the ground.

The conclusion is that the equine foot is a hydraulic pump with the coronary band acting as an anatomic safety valve, regulated by weight-bearing. In the standing horse, limb loading at low weight range less than 180 kg apparently has no appreciable effect on biomechanical venocompression. Limb loading at a medium weight range (220–330 kg) shows that the foot is able to alternately empty and fill, even under constant load, by flexion-extension of the DIJ. In the moving horse, at higher load range, the anatomic safety valve is completely closed to blood flux to protect the foot from excessive arterial pressure during full load.[1,26,28] Further investigations are required to clarify these observations.

Bouley[29] in 1851 (quoted by Bossi[30] in 1928) called the equine foot an "enclosed heart," a second "pulling and pushing vascular pump" that was biomechanically activated by the elastic properties of the foot during locomotion. Bouley underlined the important use of this pump for the horse because of the position of the foot at the most distal position of the limb where blood needs more pushing to flow in the veins and return to the heart. The authors have formulated a "five-hearts theory": "a horse

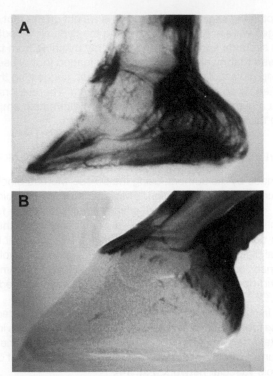

Fig. 14. Contrast medium infused by the common digital artery (*A*) fills the whole vascular network. When the foot is loaded (*B*), however, and contrast medium is infused, no arterial filling was visible below the coronet. (*Data from* Pollitt CC. Equine foot studies. Educational DVD. VideoVision, Information Technology Services. Queensland, Australia: The University of Queensland; 1992).

standing absolutely still has only 1 heart, while a moving horse has 5 hearts—one more for each foot. Nevertheless, a horse in quasi-static movement also has 5 hearts."[30]

These in vivo studies support the concept that self-adjusting PA massaging shoes[31] (Four Point Rail Shoe, Nanric USA, Versailles, KY, USA) or boots that offer a dynamic in static effect (5 Iced Heart Boots, Stilgomma Italy, Castelli Calepio, Italy) improve the foot pumping action, even during full and constant weight-bearing (**Fig. 15**A, B).

CLINICAL RELEVANCE OF VENOGRAPHY IN LAMINITIS AND OTHER SOFT TISSUE DIGITAL PATHOLOGIES

The etiology of laminitis continues to be controversial and not entirely understood. Venography offers a mean of assessing the circulatory system of the digit at various stages of laminitis development. This information helps the veterinarian and farrier develop protocols designed to mechanically and therapeutically address forces that directly restrict perfusion of the digit. It can also be used as a diagnostic tool for soft tissue lesions. Comparative, sequential venograms can become a valuable prognostic indicator along with careful clinical observations.[3,4]

Venography has shown its repeatable usefulness as a diagnostic procedure to clinically evaluate the severity of the vascular damage in laminitis or other foot pathologies

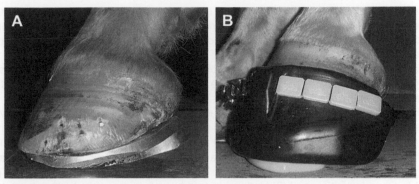

Fig. 15. A self-adjusting palmar angle shoe (A) and five Iced Hearts boot (B).

in the standing horse. The key value of venography is to check, monitor, and detect whether the examined foot is responding to therapy or is making no response and requires a different or more aggressive therapy. Sometimes pathology is irreversible with all available therapy.

In the authors' opinion the value of venography is independent of the presence or absence of pain because there is no need to walk a horse to clinically evaluate laminitis severity. This avoids the risk of forced walking inducing further mechanical trauma to the hoof lamellar dermoepidermal bond.

Venography predicts distal phalangeal displacement and the associated vascular changes.[32] This is in contrast to conventional, plain radiography, which shows distal phalanx displacement and rotation after they have already occurred. Rotation and founder distance (CE)[33] lack predictive value because they occur after the vascular damage. Detection of the continuous and rapid changes in the vascular architecture in laminitis requires venography. Venography enables clinicians to monitor vascular lesion development and to check the success of their therapeutic protocol.

Venography is relatively easy to perform, but image interpretation and data analyses are somewhat difficult. Focused experience brings timely and accurate diagnostic validity to the venographic examination. Venograms on 10 horses designated for euthanasia for non–foot related reasons showed no lesions that could be attributed to venography when compared with untreated controls.[5] Venography seems to be a clinically safe technique.

LAMINITIS PHASES: CHRONOLOGY AND SEVERITY SCORE

Understanding the time line of disease development is very important in the clinical evaluation of laminitis. It enables improved treatment and monitoring. Clinically, the authors observe two main events that predict catastrophic laminitis: the first at around 72 hours (inflammatory laminitis) and the second at 3 to 6 weeks (load-induced laminitis) from onset of the first pain event. The authors have pinpointed these two events as indicative of the passage from the developmental-acute to the chronic phase of laminitis.

Developmental laminitis mechanisms are, according to Kyaw-Tanner and Pollitt,[34] related to increased lamellar metalloproteinase activity and perturbed glucose metabolism that produce histologic and ultrastructural lesions that already exist before the onset of the visible pain. Insulin resistance and an attendant hyperinsulinemia are also associated with inflammatory laminitis development because there is an essential need for glucose by hoof lamellar hemidesmosomes. In supporting limb (contralateral or load-induced) laminitis (SLL) the failure of glucose to enter hoof lamellae compromises hemidesmosome metabolism and contributes to lamellar dermoepidermal separation and downward displacement of the distal phalanx. The time from onset of symptoms (pain, digital pulse, heat in the coronets) to the development of the initial catastrophic event is around 72 hours.

The mechanism responsible for load-induced laminitis is, from the authors' observations, constant overload and immobility of the foot. This causes prolonged ischemia because of the inefficient action of the foot hydraulic pump and biomechanical venocompression.[20,23,35] Pain is unpredictable and may not appear until the constant weight-bearing and the associated lamellar hypoxia has resulted in laminitis.[23,35] The load-induced laminitis event (SLL), when extant and clinically evident with intractable pain, is rarely reversible with therapy and euthanasia is often the necessary outcome.[35]

Laminitis can be manifest in varying degrees of severity and venography can help differentiate what is normal or mild from what is potentially catastrophic. The authors recognize developmental; acute (72 hours); subacute intermediate (until 3–6 weeks); and chronic laminitis (after 60 days). The latter can eventually lead to (1) restitutio ad integrum (return to normality); (2) life-long chronic asymptomatic laminitis with a clinically compensated lamellar pathology; or (3) symptomatic laminitis with clinically uncompensated lamellar pathology. It is the authors' observation that clinical compensation is often related to sole depth (SD), a parameter easily measured with a podiatry radiograph.

The Normal Foot

The range of normality is very broad because the vascular network can be influenced by different factors: weight of the horse, normal anatomic variations, and other organic or apparatus-induced pathologic variations. Because the starting point is different for each foot, each case must be approached with an eye to the structural characteristics of that particular foot.[23] Structural integrity of the foot is important and SLL or load laminitis is more likely to develop in a foot with a thin sole, low heel, negative PA, hoof wall defects, or other structural abnormalities absent in a healthy foot. SLL is also manifest earlier in a weak foot than in a stronger one and is more difficult to manage successfully.[23] In most horses with healthy feet and strong heels, the PA is in the range of 3 to 5 degrees.[36] Papillae of the solar corium are often not evident on a thin-soled horse.[5] Although such horses may not be lame, inadequate SD and an implied lack of blood supply are far from ideal.

In our retrospective study of 54 cases with loss of performance, horses with a SD of less than 15 mm were more inclined to palmar foot pain and pathology. Front feet radiographs were made of all horses and 14 horses underwent venography. The radiographs showed no vertical dislocation or rotation of the distal phalanx but SD was less than 15 mm. Venography showed compression of the solar papillae or fimbriae (**Fig. 16**).[37] Horses with a SD of less than 15 mm were more inclined to inflammation of the solar corium.[38] SD is, at present, the best measurement for quickly and easily summarizing a guideline reference for foot health.

Developmental laminitis

This phase begins with exposure to one of the long list of primary causes or predisposing factors and ends when clinical signs of pain appear. During the laminitis developmental phase, there may be few clinical signs and laminitis is subclinical; occasionally there are increased digital pulses and warm coronets. Horses often show no

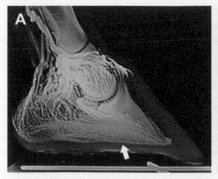 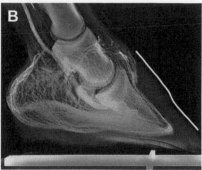

Fig. 16. Horses with a sole depth of less than 15 mm, a thin sole, a low heel, negative or zero palmar angle (*A*) were more inclined to palmar foot pain and pathology. There is compression of the solar papillae (*arrow*) and terminal papillae are directed forward. Horses with a sole depth greater than 15 mm, with strong heels, and a palmar angle in the range of 3–5 degrees (*B*) were considered low-risk and healthy.

symptoms, but venography reveals mild alterations. The authors observed that the time span of this phase is variable (hours, days, weeks, or indefinitely) depending on previous foot health and biomechanical foot management.

Acute Inflammatory Laminitis

This phase begins with the onset of typical clinical signs of pain and ends at 72 hours with the first venographic evidence of an irreversible venocompression of the papillae of the dorsal third of the solear dermis. The authors interpret this as evidence of pressure necrosis onset and correlate it to the development of primary dermal lamellar hemorrhage that has weakened the suspensory apparatus of the distal phalanx.[11] Dermoepidermal separation and vertical dislocation of the distal phalanx are events that follow the appearance of the irreversible, solear venocompression. During this phase there is a marked digital pulse, warm coronets, the characteristic laminitic stance, and lameness. In this phase it is possible to clinically score the damage using venography. The risk of causing further mechanical damage by walking or trotting the horse is thus avoided.

Low-severity damage

Venography shows the dorsal lamellar vessels are present. There is little compression of the circumflex vessels and papillae are distorted dorsally. There is normal perfusion of the terminal arch and the coronary plexus appears close to normal.

Medium-severity damage

The dorsal lamellar vessels are absent. Dorsal circumflex vessels are compressed because of downward dislocation of the distal phalanx. There is normal perfusion of the terminal arch. The coronary plexus is compressed at the extensor process, but intact in the pulvinis coronae. The damage is visible in the first few hours with a venogram and before plain radiographs show an increase in CE distance, an increase in distance between outer hoof wall and dorsal distal phalanx, and decreased SD.

High-severity damage

Dorsal lamellar vessels are absent and there is vertical dislocation of the distal phalanx apex that prolapses below the dorsal circumflex vessels. The coronary plexus is void of contrast medium at the extensor process. In cases of particular severity, the coronary band seems to act as a tourniquet. Plain radiographs show a further increase in CE distance, an increase in the thickness of dorsal horn-lamellar zone, and a progressive decrease in SD.

Supporting Limb (Load) Laminitis

This condition develops during a period of abnormal, prolonged weight-bearing on a single limb and becomes clinically evident when pain is present. Clinical signs are often less evident than in the development of other types of laminitis and this fact too often gives the clinician a false sense of security concerning the supporting foot: "if the horse is not showing signs of discomfort, then there is no problem."[23] According to Redden,[23] lamellar degeneration in the supporting foot likely begins within a few hours of constant loading, although the clinical manifestations of SLL appear around 4 to 6 weeks postinjury.

Clinically, these horses often show mild or absent pain during the development phase despite the presence of venographic filling deficits. Sometimes, around 3 to 6 weeks, without any clinical indications, an unpredictable, catastrophic painful event occurs revealing lesions that are already well developed and, unfortunately, often irreversible.

Horses may pass through the developmental and acute phases and, either because the inciting condition was mild or therapy was successful, their symptoms become subclinical. They can be considered restitutio ad integrum (restored to normality).

The authors have observed restitutio ad integrum after applying prolonged cryotherapy to horses with early, severe acute laminitis. The feet were monitored by venography for 60 days and with plain radiographs every month thereafter. With prolonged cryotherapy and quasistatic massaging the damage and risk severity scores remained low during all the laminitis phases described previously. Furthermore, there was less need for surgically aggressive interventions, such as DDFT tenotomy, wall ablation, and transcortical casting as is usual in the clinical handling of these cases.[39,40]

When the foot returns to apparent normality the potential remains for it again to develop clinical signs of laminitis. As mentioned previously, a thin-soled foot with a negative PA is more prone to redeveloping laminitis than it was the first time.

Chronic Recurring, Uncompensated Laminitis

This phase starts 6 weeks after the acute phase and ends when the horse is pain-free. The distal phalanx damage is irreversible but bone remodeling speed can be slowed by biomechanical manipulation and increased sole protection. Horses may continue to show intermittent, life-long pain that correlates to SD and damage to circumflex vessels because of vertical dislocation of the distal phalanx. Rotation is, in the authors' experience, a helpful but not significant parameter for prognosis. Biomechanical therapy and prolonged cryotherapy may prevent the rotation process and the associated pathology but in some cases the speed at which dorsal lamellar vessel damage occurs and the degree of lamellar dermoepidermal pathology makes rotation irreversible.

Low-severity damage

In this phase dorsal, sublamellar vessels are present but only in the distal third. There is mild compression of the circumflex vessels and terminal papillae are distorted dorsally. There is normal perfusion of the terminal arch and the dorsal coronary plexus is close to normal. Venography confirms distal phalanx rotation without vertical dislocation. A seroma is sometimes present.

Medium-severity damage

Dorsal sublamellar vessels are present but reduced in density and present only in the distal third. Circumflex vessels are compressed with a typical long stretched appearance proximal to the apex of the distal phalanx. There is normal perfusion of the terminal arch but the coronary plexus is compressed and void of contrast.

High-severity damage

Dorsal sublamellar vessels are absent but sometimes visible after pumping. Circumflex vessels are absent or compressed and dislocated above the apex of the distal phalanx. The coronary plexus is compressed and dislocated distally inside the hoof capsule. The terminal arch is poorly perfused and the semilunar canal of the distal phalanx is enlarged because of remodeling and is abnormally close to the distal margin of the distal phalanx. The vascular damage detected with venography predicts a major problem.

Very high-severity damage

Bone remodeling and extensive osteolysis has removed most of the semilunar canal and the terminal arch is no longer protected within it.

CONSIDERATIONS AND CONCLUSIONS

The technique of venography is relatively easy to perform; however, image interpretation and data analysis require a large number of cases and daily practice before the technique has precise diagnostic value. Because of the many variables found among breeds, conformation, environmental influences, and foot health and management, the authors encourage colleagues to become competent with the procedure and to develop a specialized working knowledge of normal feet before attempting to use venography in clinical practice.

When a tourniquet is in place, the vascular bed of the foot is an anatomically closed system; the vessels are enclosed between the hoof capsule and the distal phalanx. The authors interpret the studies of Pollitt[1] to suggest that the coronary band and ungual cartilages act as a safety valve for the foot by closing arterial blood and opening venous flow when the foot is loaded. With the horse in the tripedal stance and one foot overloaded it is still possible to create variations in pressure and volume by manipulating the PA and changing the distribution of the weight-bearing load and the location of the SCP. These results tend to confirm Redden's observation[23] that raising the heels to produce a positive PA preserves vascular perfusion of the dorsal laminae even during full weight-bearing. It follows that contralateral limb laminitis may be preventable in at-risk patients by mechanically supporting the weight-bearing foot in a way that preserves dorsal lamellar perfusion during full loading.

The five-hearts theory opposes the traditional concept that the foot pump depends on digital cushion compression and the relative enlargement of the hoof capsule during the load phase. Instead, the authors propose that the action of the foot-heart pump is attributable to flexion and extension of the DIP emptying and filling the vascular bed enclosed between the hoof capsule and the distal phalanx. Furthermore, quasistatic movement opens and closes blood flow to the foot by its action on the coronary band and the ungular cartilages. Compression of the coronary plexus (venous blood flow out) occurs during extension (negative PA) and relaxation (arterial blood flow in) occurs during flexion (positive PA).

Besides its documented usefulness in laminitis diagnosis and prognosis, venography may also have some therapeutic action, because the clinical condition of severely laminitic horses undergoing venography tends to improve.[41] This suggestion requires confirmation by scientific study. Nevertheless, the authors have seen clinical improvement in feet that have undergone venography. Perhaps the hyperosmotic contrast medium, by reducing interstitial edema, alleviates pain.

The authors suggest that venography is superior to plain radiography because the destructive changes in vascular architecture, associated with laminitis, can be detected early and can be continuously monitored. Vascular compromise, as evidenced by venography, appears on the laminitis time line days or weeks before vertical dislocation and rotation of the distal phalanx. Venography enables clinicians to treat laminitis proactively and prevent the pathologic consequences of prolonged vasocompression and ischemia. A clinician performing venograms on horse feet detects and treats the laminitis pathology earlier and more effectively than one relying on plain radiography.

The key to minimizing the destructive potential of laminitis is to support the weight-bearing foot in a way that maintains lamellar perfusion and reduces the biomechanical impact of lamellar dermoepidermal separation.

SUMMARY

Clinical diagnostic venography allows in vivo visualization of the digital venous system and the effects of venocompression related to foot load and laminitis pathology. Venography has predictive potential and helps the clinician anticipate and treat laminitis tissue damage before it is detectable by plain radiography.

The authors describe the podiatry radiographic technique to correctly perform digital venography and the modifications they have developed. In addition, venography has been applied to investigate the anatomy and physiology of the hydrovolumetric foot-heart pump and its quasistatic biomechanical properties. Using a dynamic PA iron-wood block called the D'arpe-Moreau block, the effects of manipulating the PA on the vascular bed were studied. The results contradict the theory of the foot pump being attributable to frog, cushion, and hoof capsule enlargement during loading and unloading of the foot, which can be valid only in a moving horse with very high values of weight. Instead, they attribute foot-heart pumping to the action of the DDFT modulating flexion and extension movements of the DIP. This produces emptying and filling of the foot vascular bed, enclosed between the hoof capsule and the distal phalanx, even during quasistatic overload. The authors support the existence of a biomechanical safety valve, anatomically constituted by the coronary band that is an interface between the pulvinus coronae and dorsal exstensor tendon completed caudally by the collateral ligaments and the ungual cartilages.

The authors provide guidelines for the interpretation of laminitis venograms in the context of laminitis chronology. These are presented as horses that are normal, whereas those with developmental, acute, subacute, or life-long chronic asymptomatic or symptomatic laminitis are differentiated. Frequent venographic monitoring of laminitis helps clinicians understand the sometimes puzzling chronology of the disease process and improves therapeutic outcome.

ACKNOWLEDGMENTS

The authors acknowledge the assistance of R.F. Redden, A. Rucker, D. Mansmann, and A. Spadari in the preparation of this article and L.M. Coppola, X. Moreau, S. Masiero, P. Vigini, M. Pavan, D. Leveillard, and H. Castelijns for technical support. The first author is the inventor and principal developer of the "5 Iced Heart Boot System," Stilgomma Italy, srl., Castelli Calepio, Italy.

REFERENCES

1. Pollitt CC. Equine foot studies. Educational DVD, VideoVision. Queensland (Australia): Information Technology Services, The University of Queensland; 1992.
2. D'arpe L. The Importance of the venogram in laminitis. The European Farriers Journal 2003;100:22–35.
3. Redden RF. The use of the venogram as a diagnostic tool. In: Abstracts of the 7th Bluegrass Laminitis Symposium. Louisville (KY); 1993.
4. Redden RF. A technique for performing digital venography in the standing horse. Equine Vet Educ 2001;3:172–8.
5. Rucker A. Aspects of the normal digital venogram: anatomy, parameters and variations. In: Abstract of the 16th Bluegrass, Laminitis Symposium. Louisville (KY); 2003.
6. Rucker A. Performing digital venograms. In: Abstract of the 16th Bluegrass, Laminitis Symposium. Louisville (KY); 2003. p. 114–8.
7. D'arpe L. Comment faire une Veinographie digitale chez le cheval Fourbu. In: Abstract of the Annual Congress AVEF. Pau; 2004. p. 452–4.
8. Hood DM, Taylor D, Wagner IP. Effects of ground surface deformability, trimming, and shoeing on quasistatic hoof loading patterns in horses. Am J Vet Res 2001; 62:895–900.
9. Rosenstein DS, Robert MS, Bowker M, et al. Digital angiography of the feet of horses. Am J Vet Res 2000;61:255–9.
10. D'Arpe L, Bernardini D. The digital venography exam: a diagnostic and prognostic tool in equine laminitis. In: Proceedings of the Annual Congress of the Italian Equine Veterinary Medicine Association. Turin; 2008. p. 41–9.
11. Hood DM. The pathophysiology of developmental and acute laminitis. Vet Clin North Am Equine Pract 1999;15:321–43.
12. Kummer M, Lischer C, Ohlerth S, et al. Evaluation of standardised radiografic technique for equine hoof. Schweiz Arch Tierheilkd 2004;146:507–14.
13. Lindford RL, O'Brien TR, Trout DR. Qualitative and morphometric radiographic findings in the distal phalanx and digital soft tissues of sound thoroughbred racehorses. Am J Vet Res 1993;54(1):38–51.
14. Vershooten F, Roels J, Lampo P, et al. Radiographic measurement from the lateromedial projection of the equine foot with navicular disease. Res Vet Sci 1989;46: 15–21.
15. Tacchio G, Davies HM, Morgante M, et al. A radiographic technique to assess the longitudinal balance in front hooves. Equine Vet J Suppl 2002;34:368–72.
16. Redden RF. Radiographic imaging of the equine foot. Vet Clin Equine 2003;19: 379–92.
17. D'Arpe L, Coppola LM, Guidi V, et al. Evaluation of the magnification effect related to the focus film distance and the distortion effect related to the highness of foot positioning blocks in the normal radiology of the equine foot (preliminary study).

In: Presented at the Veterinary European Equine Meeting of the year 2008. XIII AVEF/FEEVA. Versailles, 2006.

18. D'Arpe L, Coppola LM, Bernardini D. Radiographic imaging of the equine foot. In: International Laminitis Symposium Proceedings. Berlin; 2008.

19. D'Arpe L, Coppola LM, Bernardini D. Last modifications to digital venography procedure in the standing horse. In: Presented at the International Laminitis Symposium. Berlin, 2008.

20. D'Arpe L, Bernardini D. Interpreting contrast venography in horses with contro-lateral laminitis. In: Abstract of ESVOT Annual Conference, Munich; 2008. p. 34–9.

21. Rucker A. Interpreting venograms: normal or abnormal artifacts that may be mis-interpreted. In: Abstract of the 16th Bluegrass, Laminitis Symposium. Louisville (KY); 2003.

22. Leveillard D. Parer les pieds en fonction des aplombs et de la conformation du chev-al. In: Presented at the V International Podiatry Congress. Rimini, 2006. p. 43–9.

23. Redden RF. Preventing laminitis in the contralateral limb of horses with non-weight-bearing lameness. Clin Tech Equine Pract 2004;3:57–63.

24. D'arpe L. Relationships between the palmar angle and venography. The European Farriers Journal 2003;105:8–22.

25. D'Arpe L, Coppola LM, Bernardini D. Equine digital venogram in relation to the biomechanics of the foot. In: Proceedings of the 10th Congress of Equine Medi-cine and Surgery. Geneva; 2007.

26. D'arpe L, Moreau X, Vigini P, et al. La theorie des cinq coers du cheval. In: Abstract of the 13th podiatry congress Michel Vaillant. Cluses; 2009.

27. Obel N. Studies on the histopathology of acute laminitis. Almquist and Wiksells Boktyckeri AB; 1948.

28. Olivier A, Hood M, Jenkins W, et al. Effect of weight loading on the coronary band interstitial fluid pressure in horses. Am J Vet Res 1989;50(8):1198–201.

29. Bouley H. Traite du pied du cheval: La structure, des fonctions et des maladies de cet organe, Labe by Horses, 1st edition; 1851.

30. Bossi V. Trattato di mascalcia. 1st edition. Milan (Italy): Vallardi; 1928.

31. Redden RF. How to use self-adjusting palmar angle to treat heel pain. In: Proceedings of the 16th Bluegrass, Laminitis Symposium. Louisville (KY); 2003.

32. Hood DM. The mechanism and consequences of structural failure of the foot. Vet Clin North Am Equine Pract 1999;15:437–61.

33. Cripps PJ, Eustace RA. Factors involved in the prognosis of equine laminitis in the UK. Equine Vet J 1999;31:433–42.

34. Kyaw-Tanner M, Pollitt CC. Equine laminitis: increased transcription of matrix metalloproteinase-2 (MMP-2) occurs during the developmental phase. Equine Vet J 2004;36:221–5.

35. D'Arpe L, Xavier M, Coppola LM, et al. Equine digital venogram in relation to the biomechanics of the foot. In: Abstract of the International Laminitis Symposium. Berlin; 2008.

36. Redden RF. Manipulating the palmar angle. In: Proceedings of the 16th bluegrass Laminitis symposium. Louisville (KY); 2003.

37. D'arpe L, Mascia A, Bernardini D. Loss of performance caused by inflammation of the dermal fimbriae of the sole: retrospective study of 54 pedal pathology cases. In: Abstract of the European Congress of the Year SIVE. Bologna; 2009. p. 104–5.

38. D'Arpe L, Mascia A, Coppola LM, et al. Is laminitis still a valid term to describe this disease or we should better distinguish between laminar and solar corionitis? In: Proceedings of the international laminitis symposium. Berlin; 2008.

39. van Eps AW, Pollitt CC. Equine laminitis: cryotherapy reduces the severity of the acute lesions. Equine Vet J 2004;36:255-60.
40. D'Arpe L, Hetzmann A, Rossignol F, et al. Marechalerie et fourbure chez le cheval. Le nouveau. Pract Vet Equine 2008;5(17):29-33.
41. Redden RF. Possible therapeutic value of digital venography in two laminitic horses. Equine Vet Educ 2001;13:125-7.

Pasture Management to Minimize the Risk of Equine Laminitis

Kathryn Watts, BS

KEYWORDS

• Equine • Laminitis • Grass • Pasture • Carbohydrates

Grass breeders have historically developed improved cultivars with an increased ability to accumulate high concentrations of sugar, starch, and fructan, collectively known as nonstructural carbohydrates (NSC).[1,2] Grasses high in NSC have increased calories, stimulate microbial fermentation, and increase use of excess nitrogen in the rumen of cattle.[3] Higher NSC concentrations lead to increased animal intake and subsequent increased animal daily gain.[4] Although these increases in carbohydrate content of forages have benefited meat and milk producers, they have not necessarily been good for domesticated equids.

If animal managers better understand the effects of environmental conditions and cultural practices, they are in a better position to successfully manage horses prone to laminitis. Most horses that have recovered well from a bout of laminitis can tolerate some grazing if the pasture is properly managed, and horses are removed to a dirt paddock during times when NSC peak as a result of uncontrollable environmental conditions. These same conditions also affect the NSC of hay, so avoidance of green grass does not always prevent a relapse.

FACTORS AFFECTING NSC CONTENT OF GRASS

Concentrations of NSC are highly dependent on environment, plant species, and stage of development. Cool-season grasses grown in cool temperatures accumulate sugars, starch, and fructan.[5] Warm-season grasses accumulate only sugars and starch. Accumulation of NSC in grass occurs in response to stress, allowing those that accumulate the most to have a competitive advantage when the stress is over. Cool-season grasses that evolved in climates with severe cold or frequent drought tend to be highest in the ability to accumulate NSC. Many warm-season grasses go completely dormant under severe stress and therefore do not need to fuel long periods of low level metabolism to survive winter. NSC concentrations have been shown to vary over time, being low in the morning and high in the afternoon.[6] Temperatures

This work was funded by the Animal Health Foundation, Pacific, MO.
Rocky Mountain Research & Consulting, Inc, 0491 West CR 8 North, Center, CO 81125, USA
E-mail address: katygrasslady@gmail.com

Vet Clin Equine 26 (2010) 361–369
doi:10.1016/j.cveq.2010.04.007
0749-0739/10/$ – see front matter © 2010 Elsevier Inc. All rights reserved.

at 10°C or less caused increased water-soluble carbohydrate (WSC) concentrations in perennial ryegrass.[7] (WSC = sugar + fructan; sugar = all mono- and disaccharides, eg, glucose, fructose, and sucrose; fructan = all polysaccharides with a fructosyl bond; starch is not assayed in a WSC analysis; NSC = WSC + starch.) Perennial ryegrass with increased WSC levels are more competitive in mixed stands, more persistent after grazing with increased regrowth rates than perennial ryegrasses lower in WSC.[8] In orchardgrass, water-soluble carbohydrates increased by 40% of dry matter (dm) as drought stress increased.[9]

Species

A study to compare NSC concentration of various grass selections was conducted in Colorado, USA, in a high mountain valley where the sunny cool climate creates optimum conditions for accumulation of NSC. Four replications of 24 species in randomized blocks were sampled in the late afternoon for maximum daily NSC concentration. The site was cut twice per season to simulate hay production. Plots were fertilized 3 times per growing season and irrigated to simulate optimum commercial production. Samples were analyzed by a modified Megazyme method that included acid hydrolysis to better quantify the long-chain fructan inherent to grass. The varieties grown commercially in the area contained between 17% and 22% NSC on a dm basis when averaged over 8 harvests throughout the growing season. Perennial ryegrass (*Lolium perenne*)>Timothy (*Phleum pretense*)>crested wheatgrass (*Agropyron cristatum*)>tall fescue (*Festuca arundinacea*)>orchard (*Dactylis glomerata*)>redtop (*Agrostis alba*)>Garrison meadow foxtail (*Alopecurus pratensis*)>Kentucky bluegrass (*Poa pretense*)>meadow brome (*Bromus riparius*)>smooth brome (*Bromus inermis*)>blue and Sideoats grama (*Bouteloua gracilis* and *B curtipendula*). The 5 lowest in NSC out of 24 were species native to the region, and had not gone through any selection programs for increased nutritional density or increased production. The 2 grama grasses both averaged less than 10% NSC dm (**Fig. 1**).

There is a tendency to incorrectly assume that NSC concentration is inherent to a species of grass. It is more correct to view NSC content as genetic potential that must be triggered by appropriate conditioning before the characteristic is expressed. Grass grown under one set of conditions can vary widely in carbohydrate content when grown in a different environment. Perennial ryegrasses, known for being high in sugar in the United Kingdom, were found to be only average when grown in New Zealand's warmer climate.[7] Most improved species of grass, common in pastures

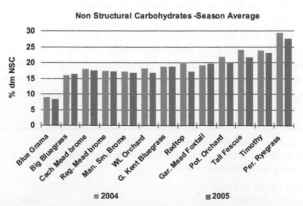

Fig. 1. NSC of some selected grass species averaged over 8 harvests, 2 consecutive years.

and hay fields around the world, are capable of accumulating levels of NSC that are inappropriate for laminitic horses under certain conditions but may be safe under other conditions. When seeking low sugar forage, it is best to focus on conditions that do not trigger high sugar traits.

Temperature

Temperature has a great effect on NSC content of pasture plants. Amount of fructan accumulated is greatly influenced by day/night temperatures, particularly just before harvest. The enzymes that facilitate respiration of sugars slow at less than 5°C and cease below freezing. When grown for 4 weeks under controlled conditions, leaf tissue from cool-season grasses subjected to 10°C days and 5°C nights averaged 3 times higher in NSC compared with 25°C days and 15°C nights.[10] Grasses grown under cool conditions accumulate sugars, which in turn triggers the formation of storage carbohydrates. Under cool conditions fructan formation will commence in most cool-season grasses and certain broadleaf weeds, whereas starch will accumulate in warm-season grasses and clover. Even mature high-fiber grasses can contain high levels of NSC when subjected to cold temperatures as long as some green tissue remains.[11] The same respiratory enzymes become more efficient under the influence of warm temperatures. Sugars may be rapidly metabolized in hot weather, making C3, cool-season grasses in summer much lower in NSC, especially if other inputs such as water and nutrients are not limiting growth.

This is demonstrated by the data in **Fig. 2**, which were generated from the same study mentioned previously. Kentucky bluegrass (*Poa pratensis*) averaged 25% dm NSC in early spring, decreased to 15% under optimum growing conditions during summer, and NSC returned to 20% after the onset of freezing temperatures in the fall. The average NSC dm across 24 species was approximately 21% in spring, 13% in summer, and 18% in early fall. The highest total NSC at any harvest date was 37.8% dm in perennial ryegrass during late fall after repeated freezes and desiccating winds. Perennial ryegrass is not sustainable in the region where this study was conducted, and was probably under more stress than the better adapted species.

Conversely, C4 warm-season grasses commonly grown in tropical regions may peak in starch with up to 19% in leaf tissue, when conditions are sunny and hot.[12] C4 grasses have a different morphology and metabolism than C3 grasses. Tropical regions often have a cloudy rainy season and a season of drought when grass goes dormant. Plants that evolve there must be able to make better use of sunlight when it is available during the wet season. C4 grasses native to temperate regions, such as the grama grasses in the intermountain region of the United States, grow very quickly in response to warm soil and summer rains and go dormant after the soil dries or cold weather returns. These grasses have no need to accumulate NSC. As illustrated by the data in **Fig. 2** the grama grass remained low in NSC throughout its life cycle. C4 grasses do not grow during cold weather; therefore data were missing for periods when C3 grasses were peaking in NSC.

Stage of Growth

Hay growers try to cut just as grass starts to develop seed heads. This is when grass has maximum yield, but before nutritional quality starts to decrease. In pastures, this is when NSC per acre and per bite are at maximum. In temperate regions this occurs in late spring (harvest 3 in **Fig. 2**), which often coincides with increased incidence of laminitis. Horses are known to selectively graze emerging seed heads. Horses prone to laminitis must not be allowed to graze seed heads. Mowing or grazing by cattle, sheep, or low-risk horses in a rotational grazing program removes the NSC-rich heads.

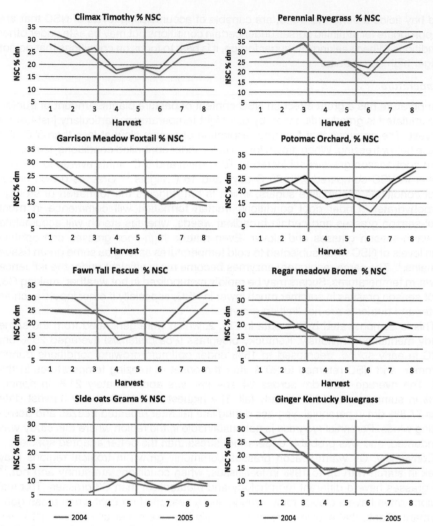

Fig. 2. Seasonal variation of NSC in grasses grown in Colorado, USA. The green vertical lines represent removal of hay crop, and application of nitrogen fertilizer. Harvest 1, 2, 3, May; harvest 4, July; harvest 5, August; harvest 6, September; harvest 7, October; harvest 8, November.

Leafy regrowth after mowing is lowest in all components of NSC, especially if it occurs during warm weather. However, rapidly growing grass in overgrazed pastures may represent a significant increase in NSC per acre, removing limitations to intake, and representing a sudden change in dietary components.

Rate of Growth

Frequently people think that fast-growing grass is higher in NSC, although this contradicts our basic understanding of plant physiology. Rapidly growing fertilized grass after grazing or mowing is lowest in NSC concentration (see **Fig 2**, harvests 4–6) because sugars are used by the plant as quickly as they are formed to make fiber, protein, and energy. Researchers of grazing management warn against grazing new, low NSC regrowth before the plant has an opportunity to replenish reserves, as depletion of NSC at this vulnerable stage reduces the ability of grass to survive subsequent environmental stress.[13] Nitrogen availability is the most common limiting factor to growth in grass. Nutrient deficiency is another plant stress that limits growth and causes NSC to accumulate. Increasing amounts of applied nitrogen, expressed as crude protein in grass was inversely related to WSC (sugar + fructan) content in perennial ryegrass.[14]

Native Species

Native species are often, but not always, lower in NSC than those species that have been improved for higher nutrient density and production. They are generally less productive and may only grow in those environments to which they are perfectly adapted. Native grasses are less competitive and may be taken over by sod forming invasive species such as fescue or Kentucky bluegrass that come up from seed lying dormant in the soil. Native grass seed is expensive, and may take 2 years to completely establish before it is strong enough to survive grazing or harvesting for hay. As most native grasses have low tolerance for overgrazing, they require sophisticated, intensive management programs for sustainable production. Native grass production is not within the budget, ability, or patience level of the average horse owner. Managing the existing stand of grass to minimize stress and lower overall NSC concentration is more likely to be successful for most horse owners than trying to grow low NSC species of native grass.

MANAGEMENT TO MINIMIZE NSC CONTENT

Large seasonal variations in NSC concentration per mouthful and amount of NSC per acre occur in pastures. Understanding the environmental effects on NSC in grass can allow caretakers to limit grass intake for high-risk horses and ponies during times when either NSC concentration or NSC/acre peaks in their particular climate. The worst season for laminitis cases varies globally depending on climate, and may vary from one year to the next in the same region because of variations in weather. The times most apt to trigger laminitis are when temperatures are less than 5°C for 2 to 3 weeks during the night, coupled with grass in such excess that horses have the opportunity to overeat. In many climates, maximum NSC concentration and NSC per acre coincide in late spring, when nights are still cool and grass is just starting to head out. In areas with summer drought, the onset of drought stress may create high NSC pastures. In areas with fall rains, the combination of cool temperatures and increase in biomass may trigger laminitis. In regions with marine climates, such as the United Kingdom, mild winters allow grass to remain green and fructan concentrations to peak in midwinter.[15]

Prevent Heading

Grass has 2 types of reproduction: seed production or vegetative reproduction from new sprouts called tillers. If developing seed heads are removed before head emergence, grass switches its reproductive strategy and develops more tillers from crowns or stolons (underground stems). Mowing or intensive grazing by cattle or sheep have similar effects and there is an optimum stage for mowing (**Fig 3**).

Set equipment height just low enough to remove embryonic seed heads still within the stem. Mowing any closer to the ground is not necessary. Timely mowing or grazing can keep grass in a vegetative stage. As long as grass is not heading out, additional

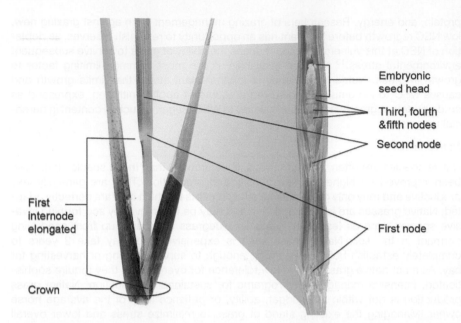

Fig. 3. A grass plant with the first stem internode elongated, raising the developing seed head above the level of the crown. Lengthening of the remaining nodes will raise the seed head above the rest of the plant. Unelongated nodes and the undeveloped seed head are meristematic tissues, comparable with embryonic tissue in the animal world. They await hormonal signals to trigger growth and development. *From* Watts KA, Pollitt CC. Managing pasture to minimise the risk of laminitis in horses. RIRDC publication no. 10/063. https://rirdc.infoservices.com.au/collections/hor; with permission.

mowing is not necessary, and may be counterproductive to producing grass with lower sugar concentration. Tall thick grass is self-shading. Only the top portions of the plant have potential for maximum photosynthetic rate. Short thin grass has every blade in a position to make use of any light available to make sugar.

Graze in Shade

Light intensity has a direct effect on the ability of plants to produce sugar. Grass grown in shade is lower in sugar[16,17] When possible, use existing shade in woodlots or adjacent to hedges or buildings (**Fig. 4**).

Fast-growing trees may be planted to create more shade in desired areas. Make sure to give shaded grass a rest period from grazing to prevent killing the grass from depletion of limited NSC resources.

Control High Sugar Weeds

Many broadleaf weeds contain high levels of sugars and inulin under the same conditions that cause NSC to accumulate in grass: cold and drought stress. Dandelion (*Taraxacum officinale*) (**Fig 5**), plantain (*Plantago* sp) and members of the thistle families (*Cirsium* and *Sonchus* sp) may contain high levels of fructooligosaccharides and sugars.

Cold treatment caused concentration of NSC in plantain (*Plantago lanceolata* L.) to increase from 135 to 230 mg/g dm.[18] These weeds may escape control by mowing

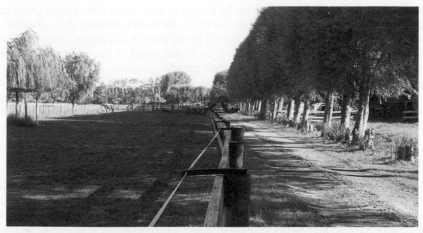

Fig. 4. Pasture in paddocks shaded from direct sunlight produces less NSC. *From* Watts KA, Pollitt CC. Managing pasture to minimise the risk of laminitis in horses. RIRDC publication no. 10/063. https://rirdc.infoservices.com.au/collections/hor; with permission.

because of their low growth habit, but are easily controlled with appropriate herbicides.

Limiting Intake of Grass

When environmental stress occurs that may increase the NSC in pasture, monitoring of susceptible animals on a daily basis for subtle signs of lameness is advisable. The progress of mild laminitis may often be halted by moving the animal from the pasture to a bare dirt paddock at the first sign of lameness, and feeding tested hay lower than

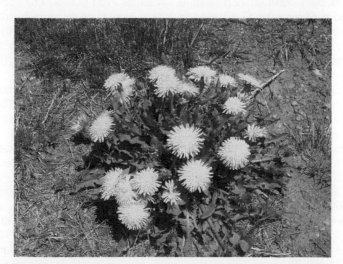

Fig. 5. Dandelion (*Taraxacum officinale*), a palatable pasture weed may contain up to 25% sugars and fructans as dm in its above-ground leaves and stem. *From* Watts KA, Pollitt CC. Managing pasture to minimise the risk of laminitis in horses. RIRDC publication no. 10/063. https://rirdc.infoservices.com.au/collections/hor; with permission.

average (<11% dm) in NSC. No access to weeds or even short overgrazed grass can be allowed for horses in acute stage laminitis. Proactive owners may choose to remove high-risk animals completely during times when NSC peaks, such as when nighttime temperatures are less than 5°C or at the onset of severe drought. When the environmental stress is over, and grass growth resumes, sugar concentrations begin to diminish, although NSC per acre may increase because of increased biomass. Availability of excess grass may warrant some means to limit intake, depending on the tolerance of individual animals. This may be accomplished using grazing muzzles, limiting grazing time, or strip or cell grazing.

SUMMARY

The sugar, starch, and fructan content (collectively referred to as NSC) of pasture plants is dependent on the environmental conditions under which they have grown. Pasture that is stressed by cold, drought, or lack of nutrients can be 2 to 3 times higher in NSC than pasture that grows quickly in warm weather and is adequately watered and fertilized. Horses at risk for laminitis should have access to pasture limited or be removed completely when environmental conditions are conducive to high levels of NSC accumulation.

REFERENCES

1. Smith K, Reed K, Foot J. An assessment of the relative importance of specific traits for the genetic improvement of nutritive value in dairy pasture. Grass Forage Sci 1997;52:167–75.
2. Humphreys M, Yadav R, Cairns A, et al. Review: a changing climate for grassland research. New Phytol 2006;169:9–26.
3. Trevaskis LM, Fulkerson WJ. The relationship between various animal and management factors and milk urea, and its association with reproductive performance of dairy cows grazing pasture. Livestock Prod Sci 1999;57:255–65.
4. Mayland H, Shewmaker G, Chatterton J, et al. Nonstructural carbohydrates in tall fescue cultivars: relationship to animal preference. Agron J 2000;92(6):1203–6.
5. Housley TL, Pollock CJ. The metabolism of fructan in higher plants. In: Suzuki M, Chatterton NJ, editors. Science and technology of fructans. Boca Raton (FL): CRC Press; 1993. p. 191–225.
6. Fisher DS, Mayland HF, Burns JC. Variation in ruminants' preference for tall fescue hays cut either at sundown or at sunup. J Anim Sci 1999;77:762–8.
7. Parsons A, Rasmussen S, Xue H, et al. Some 'high sugar grasses' don't like it hot. Proc New Zealand Grassland Assoc 2004;66:265–71.
8. Donaghy D, Fulkerson W. The importance of water-soluble carbohydrate reserves on regrowth and root growth of Lolium perenne (L.). Grass Forage Sci 1997;52: 401–7.
9. Volaire F, Lelievre F. Production, persistence, and water-soluble carbohydrate accumulation in 21 contrasting populations of Dactylis glomerata L. subjected to severe drought in the south of France. Aust J Agric Res 1997;48:933–44.
10. Chatterton N, Harris P, Bennett J, et al. Carbohydrate partitioning in 185 accessions of Gramineae grown under warm and cool temperatures. J Plant Physiol 1989;134:169–79.
11. Watts K. Carbohydrates in forage: what is safe grass?. In: Pagan J, editor. Advances in equine nutrition. 4th edition. Nottingham (UK): Nottingham University Press; 2009. p. 29–42.

12. Wilson JR, Ford CW. Temperature influences on the growth, digestibility, and carbohydrate composition of two tropical grasses, *Panicum maximum* var. *trichoglume* and *Setaria sphacelata*, and two cultivars of the temperate grass *Lolium perenne*. Aust J Agric Res 1971;22:563–71.
13. Fulkerson W, Donaghy D. Plant-soluble carbohydrate reserves and senescence – key criteria for developing an effective grazing management system for ryegrass-based pastures: a review. Aust J Exp Agric 2001;41:261–75.
14. Lovett DK, Bortolozzo A, Conaghan P, et al. In vitro total and methane gas production as influenced by rate of nitrogen application, season of harvest and perennial ryegrass cultivar. Grass Forage Sci 2004;59:227–32.
15. Pollock CJ, Jones T. Seasonal patterns of fructan metabolism in forage grasses. New Phytol 1979;83(1):9–15.
16. Smith D. Nonstructural carbohydrates. In: Butler GW, Bailey RW, editors. Chemistry and biochemistry of herbage. London: Academic Press; 1973. p. 147–8.
17. Burner DM, Belesky DP. Diurnal effects on nutritive value of alley-cropped orchardgrass herbage. Crop Sci 2004;44:1776–80.
18. Skinner HR. Cultivar and environmental effects on freezing tolerance of narrow-leaf plantain. Crop Sci 2005;45:2330–6.

Endocrinopathic Laminitis: Reducing the Risk Through Diet and Exercise

Nicola J. Menzies-Gow, MA, VetMB, PhD, CertEM(Int.med), MRCVS

KEYWORDS

• Laminitis • Insulin resistance • Obesity • Diet • Exercise

Although it is important to be able to recognize and treat laminitis, ideally it is better to prevent the condition from occurring in the first place. To do this, we need to understand why the disease occurs in certain individual animals at certain times of the year.

Certain individual animals appear predisposed to recurrent pasture-associated laminitis, but the exact mechanisms underlying their predisposition remain a fundamental question in laminitis research. It seems likely that there are certain phenotypic traits common to these individuals. Multiple variables have been evaluated as risk factors for laminitis, with the findings generally being inconsistent between studies. An association between the occurrence of laminitis and (1) being a pony, (2) the spring and summer months,[1] (3) being female, (4) increased age,[2] and (5) obesity[3,4] have been demonstrated in some studies. The most likely endocrinologic disorders that may play a role in this predisposition are those associated with excess glucocorticoids, specifically pituitary pars intermedia dysfunction, and those associated with insulin resistance (IR).[4] Thus, more recently, research has concentrated on the role of IR in individual predisposition to recurrent laminitis, because identification of ponies at a risk of this condition may allow preventive measures to be taken.

Animals at greatest risk of pasture-associated laminitis have a metabolic phenotype, including obesity and IR, similar to that seen in human metabolic syndrome (HMS).[5] Thus, the same pathologic mechanisms that underlie the cardiovascular disease associated with HMS, including changes in insulin signaling, inflammatory cytokines, and endothelial dysfunction, could contribute to laminitis.

REDUCING THE RISK

If endocrinopathic laminitis is a consequence of IR and chronic inflammation, then the risk for an individual animal to be affected may be reduced if steps are taken to improve insulin sensitivity and reduce inflammation. Exercise has been shown to

Department of Veterinary Clinical Science, Royal Veterinary College, Hawkshead Lane, North Mymms, Hertfordshire, AL9 7TA, UK
E-mail address: nmenziesgow@rvc.ac.uk

Vet Clin Equine 26 (2010) 371–378
doi:10.1016/j.cveq.2010.04.005
0749-0739/10/$ – see front matter © 2010 Elsevier Inc. All rights reserved.

reduce IR and suppress inflammation, and dietary manipulation can significantly affect insulin sensitivity.

EXERCISE
Effect on Insulin Sensitivity

The beneficial effect of exercise on insulin sensitivity in the horse has been demonstrated in several studies. A single bout of high-intensity treadmill exercise was sufficient to significantly decrease plasma insulin concentrations in healthy standardbred mares.[6] After 7 days of light (trotting for 30 minutes on the lunge) exercise, insulin sensitivity was improved in aged mares that were lean (insulin-sensitive) and obese (insulin-resistant).[7] Short-term (7 consecutive days) treadmill exercise for 45 minutes per day in normal standardbred horses resulted in increases in insulin sensitivity.[8] Constant moderate-intensity treadmill exercise for 8 weeks increased insulin sensitivity, glucose effectiveness, and disposition index, and decreased acute insulin response to glucose in healthy Arabian geldings.[9] In 10 hyperinsulinemic ponies, 6 weeks of exercise significantly improved their insulin sensitivity.[10]

The length of time for which the improvement in insulin sensitivity persists after the cessation of exercise varies between studies. In one study, the enhancement was still evident after 5 days of inactivity,[8] and in another, the improved insulin sensitivity was maintained for at least 6 weeks after cessation of exercise.[10] However, in one study insulin sensitivity appeared to return to pre-exercise values within 72 hours of cessation of exercise,[11] whereas in another the same occurred 9 days later.[7]

Thus, it would appear that light exercise is sufficient to improve insulin sensitivity, but that this probably needs to be maintained on a regular or possibly daily basis for the improvement to persist. It must be emphasized that this is possible only once an animal has recovered from an episode of laminitis and is sound. There should be a gradual increase in the intensity and duration of the exercise undertaken.

Effect on Inflammation

Tumor necrosis factor-α (TNF-α) is a proinflammatory cytokine secreted by the adipose tissue, which plays an important role in HMS.[12] TNF-α is implicated in IR development in HMS,[13,14] is a risk factor for increased IR in horses,[15] and is associated with laminitis predisposition.[16] In addition, it stimulates apoptotic cell death in many tissues, including epidermal epithelial cells,[4] and endothelial dysfunction.[17] The effect of exercise on the circulating concentrations of inflammatory mediators has not been investigated in the horse. However, TNF-α overexpression returned to normal levels after 1 hour of acute swimming in TNF-receptor knockout mice[18]; and chronic exercise suppressed circulating concentrations of proinflammatory factors, including TNF-α, and augmented concentrations of anti-inflammatory factors, including interleukin (IL)-4, IL-10, and adiponectin, in humans.[19] Thus, exercise may protect against TNF-α–induced IR and the consequent endothelial dysfunction and laminitis.

Additional Effects

High-intensity exercise also appears to be associated with decreases in feed intake in normal horses.[20] Thus, it may have the additional beneficial effect of aiding with weight loss through the reduction in calorie consumption.

DIET

Dietary manipulation is important for 2 main reasons: to improve insulin sensitivity in the insulin-resistant animal and to achieve weight loss in the overweight animal. Not every insulin-resistant animal is overweight, and therefore, mere weight loss may not be the answer in every case of endocrinopathic laminitis.

Improving Insulin Sensitivity

The effect of manipulating the carbohydrate, fat, and fiber contents of diet to improve insulin sensitivity in the horse has been investigated in several studies. After an 8-week adaptation to feeds that were high in sugar and starch or fat and fiber, horses that adapted to fat and fiber tended to have higher insulin sensitivity and disposition index.[9,21] Feeding a diet that was rich in nonstructural carbohydrate (NSC) to healthy adult standardbred horses for 6 weeks resulted in decreased insulin sensitivity and impaired glucose tolerance.[22] The effect of the amount of starch fed on the glycemic and insulinemic responses of horses was investigated.[23] A starch feed less than 1.1 g/kg of body weight (BW) resulted in lower glucose and insulin responses compared with a starch feed of 1.1 to 2 g/kg ($P<.01$). Thus, the investigators recommended that a starch intake of less than 1.1 g/kg of BW per meal or a meal size of 0.3 kg/100 kg of BW (starch content of 30%–40%) be used.

Fat supplementation in the form of fish oil, soybean oil,[24] or rice bran oil,[25] and the addition of purified soluble or insoluble fiber[26] to a corn meal did not affect postprandial glucose and insulin responses in healthy horses. Thus, feeding strategies should focus more on starch reduction per meal than on the addition of fat or purified fiber.

The starch content of oats, barley, and corn is approximately 45% to 55%, 60% to 65%, and 65% to 75%, respectively, and sweet feeds contain grains and molasses, with the NSC content of some of these feeds approaching 30% to 40%. At certain times of the year, the NSC content of pasture forage may approach 30% to 40% of dry matter. Thus, the common management practice of feeding starch-rich cereal grains in 2 large meals a day, unrestricted access to pasture, and feeding of NSC-rich forage may exacerbate IR and should be avoided.[27] Instead, a diet based on grass hay (or hay substitute) with low (<10%) NSC content should be fed, and cereals should be avoided.[27]

Ideally the forage should be analyzed, including directly measuring NSC content, before it is fed. An NSC content of less than 10% is recommended. If this is not undertaken, general rules include[27]:

1. Mature hay (ie, hay with visible seed heads and a high stem-to-leaf ratio) is preferred because of its lower NSC content compared with less mature hay.
2. Alfalfa hay or other legumes such as clover are less preferred because, on average, these forages have higher NSC content compared with grass hay.
3. Ensiled forages generally have lower NSC content than hay made from the same crop, but the high palatability may result in a higher total NSC intake.

Some nutritionists have recommended soaking hay in water for 30 to 60 minutes before feeding to leach water soluble carbohydrates (sugars and fructans) and therefore circumvent the need to analyze the forage. However, a recent study revealed that this does not reliably decrease the NSC content to less than 10%.[28]

Forage-only diets do not provide adequate protein, minerals, or vitamins. It is therefore recommended to supplement the forage diet with a low-calorie commercial ration balancer product that contains sources of high-quality protein and a mixture of vitamins and minerals to balance the low levels of vitamin E, vitamin, copper, zinc, selenium, and other minerals typically found in mature grass hay.[27]

If weight gain is required or the animal is undertaking a large amount of exercise, then a forage-based diet may not meet energy requirements. Caloric intake can be increased in several ways. Unmolassed, soaked sugar beet pulp, which is rich in highly digestible fiber, provides more digestible energy when compared with most hay types, and does not elicit a marked glycemic or insulinemic response, can be added to the diet at 0.2 to 0.7 kg per day.[27] Vegetable oil can be fed; 100 to 225 mL of oil fed once or twice daily (up to a maximum of 100 mL/100 kg of BW) can be gradually introduced to the diet over 7 to 10 days.[27] It should be added to a small amount of fiber-based food, for example, beet pulp, because of its low palatability. Supplemental antioxidant (vitamin E, 100–200 IU per 100 mL of added oil) should also be provided. Alternatively, a commercial feed with low starch and sugar content (<20%–25% NSC) can be fed in conjunction with the forage.

Dietary supplements
Several supplements are marketed claiming to improve insulin sensitivity, but scientific evidence of their efficacy is lacking. Many products contain magnesium, chromium, or cinnamon.

Magnesium Some human studies have demonstrated an association between magnesium status and IR in type 2 diabetes.[29,30] It is hypothesized that magnesium deficiency results in defective insulin receptor tyrosine kinase activity and exaggerated intracellular calcium concentration, which impair insulin action and worsen IR.[29] There have been several clinical trials assessing the potential benefit of magnesium supplementation in human diabetic patients that have shown mixed effects. A review of all randomized double-blind controlled trials that evaluated the effects of magnesium supplementation for 4 to 16 weeks in type 2 diabetes in humans showed that supplementation may be effective in reducing fasting plasma glucose concentrations and increasing high-density lipoprotein cholesterol levels but only in patients with actual magnesium deficiency, which is determined by the measurement of intraerythrocytic concentrations.[30]

There are no published reports of the magnesium status of insulin-resistant or laminitis-prone horses or ponies that are obese. The magnesium requirement of a mature horse at maintenance is 7.5 g per day[31]; thus, it is advisable to ensure that this is met by the diet. Studies are required to determine whether increased magnesium supplementation will affect insulin sensitivity in the horse.

Chromium Chromium is thought to potentiate insulin action by means of activation of insulin receptor kinase or inhibition of insulin receptor tyrosine phosphatase.[32,33] Suboptimal intake of chromium appears to contribute to IR in type 2 diabetes and metabolic syndrome in humans.[34] An improvement in glucose tolerance in insulin-resistant humans who were given a chromium supplement has been seen in some studies[32] but not in others.[35] Chromium supplementation has been shown to reduce blood glucose level and the time taken for glucose concentrations to return to baseline values after a glucose peak in yearling horses[36] and exercising thoroughbred horses.[37] Peak insulin responses during an oral starch tolerance test were modestly lower in overweight, hyperinsulinemic ponies supplemented with chromium for 4 weeks compared with nonsupplemented ponies.[38] Thus, supplemental chromium (2.5–5 mg/d) is often fed to insulin-resistant horses and ponies. However, further studies are required to fully determine the beneficial effects of chromium supplementation on IR in the horse.

Cinnamon Cinnamon has a long history as an antidiabetic spice, because it may have a natural insulin-sensitizing action, but trials involving cinnamon supplementation have produced contrasting results.[39,40] A review of all randomized controlled clinical trials of cinnamon that involved human patients with diabetes and those with IR concluded that although definitive conclusions cannot be drawn regarding the use of cinnamon as an antidiabetic therapy, it does possess antihyperglycemic properties and the potential to reduce postprandial blood glucose concentrations.[41] To date, there are no such published studies on equines.

Weight Loss

Obesity in the horse is associated with IR[42]; insulin sensitivity was approximately 80% lower in obese horses than in nonobese horses.[21] Thus, the primary benefit of weight loss is to improve insulin sensitivity and hence reduce the risk of laminitis. It has been demonstrated that weight loss in obese ponies through energy restriction at a rate of 1% of ideal BW per week resulted in improved insulin sensitivity.[43] In most cases, the underlying reason for the obesity is that excess energy has been stored as fat because of the animal being overfed relative to its activity level.[44] Thus, the focus should be on reducing calorie consumption to a level that promotes weight loss and then maintaining a moderate body condition score (BCS) of 4 to 6 on a 9-point scale.[45]

Strategies that can be employed depend on the present and desired body conditions and other individual circumstances. These strategies have been well reviewed by Geor and Harris.[27] Stopping pasture turnout feeding may be necessary for adequate control of dietary intake. A study in obese pony mares reported no change in BW when ponies were provided access to pasture for 12 hours per day, probably due to increased forage consumption during the restricted grazing period.[46] In another study, it was estimated that ponies could consume 40% of their daily dry matter intake during as little as 3 hours of pasture turnout.[47] Alternatively, strategies that allow turnout while minimizing forage intake include use of grazing muzzles, strip grazing behind other horses, mowing the pasture and removing cuttings, putting a deep layer of wood chips over a small paddock, or using bare paddocks or indoor arenas.

In general, the diet should be high in fiber and low in NSC. Grain and other concentrated sources of calories (eg, commercial sweet feeds, feeds containing added fats) should be totally removed from the diet, and feeding of other treats, such as carrots and apples, should be stopped.[27] Forage should be the primary, if not sole energy-providing component of the diet. In some areas, forage-based low-calorie feeds complete with vitamins and minerals are available commercially. This type of feed offers convenience and may be used as a substitute to hay or fed as a component of the ration along with hay. In a study of obese ponies that were provided an ad libitum forage diet during the summer and winter, voluntary intake (dry matter basis) was approximately 2% of BW, and the BCS was virtually unchanged during the study period.[48] Thus, hay or hay substitute should initially be provided at less than or equal to 1.5% of current BW per day, with subsequent further reductions in feed amount depending on the extent of weight loss. It is preferable not to decrease forage provision to less than 1% of target BW, because this may increase the risk for hindgut dysfunction, stereotypical behaviors, ingestion of bedding, or coprophagy.[27] The ration should be divided into 3 to 4 feedings per day, and strategies to prolong feed intake time should be considered, such as the use of hay nets with multiple small holes.[27]

SUMMARY

The risk of endocrinopathic laminitis can be reduced if steps are taken to improve insulin sensitivity and reduce inflammation using strategies based on exercise and diet. Regular, light exercise appears to improve insulin sensitivity and may reduce inflammation. A diet with NSC content of less than 10% and based mainly on forage and the avoidance of cereals prevents the exacerbation of IR. This diet can also be fed (at a lower percentage of BW) to an obese animal to promote weight loss and hence improve insulin sensitivity. To date, there is no definitive evidence that any of the numerous supplements available will additionally improve insulin sensitivity in the horse.

REFERENCES

1. Hinckley KA, Henderson IW. The epidemiology of equine laminitis in the UK. Presented at the 35th Congress of the British Equine Veterinary Association. Warwick (UK), September 9, 1996.
2. Alford P, Geller S, Richardson B, et al. A multicenter, matched case-control study of risk factors for equine laminitis. Prev Vet Med 2001;49:209–22.
3. Treiber KH, Hess TM, Kronfeld DS, et al. Insulin resistance and compensation in laminitis-predisposed ponies characterized by the Minimal Model. Presented at the Equine Nutrition Symposium, vol. 21. Hannover (Germany): Pferdeheilkunde, 2005. p. 91–2.
4. Johnson PJ, Messer NT, Slight SH, et al. Endocrinopathic laminitis in horses. Clin Tech Equine Pract 2004;3:45–56.
5. Treiber KH, Kronfeld DS, Hess TM, et al. Evaluation of genetic and metabolic predispositions and nutritional risk factors for pasture-associated laminitis in ponies. J Am Vet Med Assoc 2006;228:1538–45.
6. Gordon ME, McKeever KH, Betros CL, et al. Exercise-induced alterations in plasma concentrations of ghrelin, adiponectin, leptin, glucose, insulin, and cortisol in horses. Vet J 2007;173(3):532–40.
7. Powell DM, Reedy SE, Sessions DR, et al. Effect of short-term exercise training on insulin sensitivity in obese and lean mares. Equine Vet J Suppl 2002;34:81–4.
8. Stewart-Hunt L, Geor RJ, McCutcheon LJ. Effects of short-term training on insulin sensitivity and skeletal muscle glucose metabolism in standardbred horses. Equine Vet J Suppl 2006;36:226–32.
9. Treiber KH, Hess TM, Kronfeld DS, et al. Glucose dynamics during exercise: dietary energy sources affect minimal model parameters in trained Arabian geldings during endurance exercise. Equine Vet J Suppl 2006;36:631–6.
10. Freestone JF, Beadle R, Shoemaker K, et al. Improved insulin sensitivity in hyperinsulinaemic ponies through physical conditioning and controlled feed intake. Equine Vet J 1992;24(3):187–90.
11. de Graaf-Roelfsema E, van Ginneken ME, van Breda E, et al. The effect of long-term exercise on glucose metabolism and peripheral insulin sensitivity in standardbred horses. Equine Vet J Suppl 2006;36:221–5.
12. Picchi A, Gao X, Belmadani S, et al. Tumor necrosis factor-alpha induces endothelial dysfunction in the prediabetic metabolic syndrome. Circ Res 2006;99(1):69–77.
13. Houstis N, Rosen ED, Lander ES. Reactive oxygen species have a causal role in multiple forms of insulin resistance. Nature 2006;440(7086):944–8.
14. Nishikawa T, Kukidome D, Sonoda K, et al. Impact of mitochondrial ROS production in the pathogenesis of insulin resistance. Diabetes Res Clin Pract 2007;77(Suppl 1):S161–4.
15. Vick MM, Adams AA, Murphy BA, et al. Relationships among inflammatory cytokines, obesity, and insulin sensitivity in the horse. J Anim Sci 2007;85(5):1144–55.

16. Treiber K, Carter R, Gay L, et al. Inflammatory and redox status of ponies with a history of pasture-associated laminitis. Vet Immunol Immunopathol 2009;129: 216–20.
17. Zhang H, Park Y, Wu J, et al. Role of TNF-alpha in vascular dysfunction. Clin Sci (Lond) 2009;116(3):219–30.
18. Keller C, Keller P, Giralt M, et al. Exercise normalises overexpression of TNF-alpha in knockout mice. Biochem Biophys Res Commun 2004;321(1):179–82.
19. Bruunsgaard H. Physical activity and modulation of systemic low-level inflammation. J Leukoc Biol 2005;78(4):819–35.
20. Gordon ME, McKeever KH, Bokman S, et al. Interval exercise alters feed intake as well as leptin and ghrelin concentrations in standardbred mares. Equine Vet J Suppl 2006;36:596–605.
21. Hoffman RM, Boston RC, Stefanovski D, et al. Obesity and diet affect glucose dynamics and insulin sensitivity in thoroughbred geldings. J Anim Sci 2003;81: 2333–42.
22. Pratt SE, Geor RJ, McCutcheon LJ. Effects of dietary energy source and physical conditioning on insulin sensitivity and glucose tolerance in standardbred horses. Equine Vet J Suppl 2006;36:579–84.
23. Vervuert I, Voigt K, Hollands T, et al. Effect of feeding increasing quantities of starch on glycaemic and insulinaemic responses in healthy horses. Vet J 2009; 182(1):67–72.
24. Vervuert I, Klein S, Coenen M. Short-term effects of a moderate fish oil or soybean oil supplementation on postprandial glucose and insulin responses in healthy horses. Vet J 2009;182(1):67–72.
25. Frank N, Andrews FM, Elliott SB, et al. Effects of rice bran oil on plasma lipid concentrations, lipoprotein composition, and glucose dynamics in mares. J Anim Sci 2005;83(11):2509–18.
26. Vervuert I, Klein S, Coenen M. Effect of mixing dietary fibre (purified lignocellulose or purified pectin) and a corn meal on glucose and insulin responses in healthy horses. J Anim Physiol Anim Nutr (Berl) 2009;93(3):331–8.
27. Geor RJ, Harris P. Dietary management of obesity and insulin resistance: countering risk for laminitis. Vet Clin North Am Equine Pract 2009;25(1):51–65, vi.
28. Longland AC, Harker I, Harris PA. The loss of water-soluble carbohydrate and soluble protein from nine different hays submerged in water for up to 16 hours. Presented at the Proceedings of the Equine Science Society. Keystone Colorado, USA, May 31, 2009.
29. Barbagallo M, Dominguez LJ, Galioto A, et al. Role of magnesium in insulin action, diabetes and cardio-metabolic syndrome X. Mol Aspects Med 2003; 24(1–3):39–52.
30. Song Y, He K, Levitan EB, et al. Effects of oral magnesium supplementation on glycaemic control in Type 2 diabetes: a meta-analysis of randomized double-blind controlled trials. Diabet Med 2006;23(10):1050–6.
31. Anon. National Research Council nutrient requirements of horses. 6th revised edition. Washington, DC: National Academies Press; 2007.
32. Anderson RA. Chromium in the prevention and control of diabetes. Diabetes Metab 2000;26(1):22–7.
33. Lau FC, Bagchi M, Sen CK, et al. Nutrigenomic basis of beneficial effects of chromium(III) on obesity and diabetes. Mol Cell Biochem 2008;317(1–2):1–10.
34. Jeejeebhoy KN, Chu RC, Marliss EB, et al. Chromium deficiency, glucose intolerance, and neuropathy reversed by chromium supplementation, in a patient receiving long-term total parenteral nutrition. Am J Clin Nutr 1977;30(4):531–8.

35. Iqbal N, Cardillo S, Volger S, et al. Chromium picolinate does not improve key features of metabolic syndrome in obese nondiabetic adults. Metab Syndr Relat Disord 2009;7(2):143–50.
36. Ott EA, Kivipelto J. Influence of chromium tripicolinate on growth and glucose metabolism in yearling horses. J Anim Sci 1999;77(11):3022–30.
37. Pagan JDT. The effect of chromium supplementation on metabolic response to exercise in Thoroughbred horses. Presented at the Proceedings of 14th Equine Nutrition and Physiology Symposium. Ontario (Canada), October 10, 1995.
38. Verveurt I, Obwald B, Coenen M. Effects of chromium supplementation on metabolic profile in insulin resistant ponies. Presented at the Proceedings of the 12th Congress of the European Society for Veterinary Clinical Nutrition. Vienna, Austria, September 25, 2008.
39. Khan A, Safdar M, Ali Khan MM, et al. Cinnamon improves glucose and lipids of people with type 2 diabetes. Diabetes Care 2003;26(12):3215–8.
40. Vanschoonbeek K, Thomassen BJ, Senden JM, et al. Cinnamon supplementation does not improve glycemic control in postmenopausal type 2 diabetes patients. J Nutr 2006;136(4):977–80.
41. Kirkham S, Akilen R, Sharma S, et al. The potential of cinnamon to reduce blood glucose levels in patients with type 2 diabetes and insulin resistance. Diabetes Obes Metab 2009;11(12):1100–13.
42. Carter RA, McCutcheon LJ, George LA, et al. Effects of diet-induced weight gain on insulin sensitivity and plasma hormone and lipid concentrations in horses. Am J Vet Res 2009;70(10):1250–8.
43. Van Weyenberg S, Hesta M, Buyse J, et al. The effect of weight loss by energy restriction on metabolic profile and glucose tolerance in ponies. J Anim Physiol Anim Nutr (Berl) 2008;92(5):538–45.
44. Harris PA, Geor RJ. Nutritional countermeasures to laminitis. Presented at the 1st Waltham-Royal Veterinary College Laminitis Conference. London (UK), March 24, 2007.
45. Harris PA, Bailey SR, Elliott J, et al. Countermeasures for pasture associated laminitis in ponies and horses. J Nutr 2006;136:2114S–21S.
46. Buff PR, Johnson PJ, Wiedmeyer CE, et al. Modulation of leptin, insulin and growth hormone in obese pony mares under chronic nutritional restriction and supplementation with ractopamine hydrochloride. Vet Ther 2006;7:64–72.
47. Ince J, Longland AC, Moore-Colyer M. A pilot study to estimate the intake of grass by ponies with restricted access to pasture. Presented at the Proceedings of the British Society of Animal Science. York (England), 2005.
48. Dugdale AHA, Curtis GC, Knottenbelt DC. Changes in body condition and fat deposition in ponies offered an ad libitum chaff-based diet. Presented at the Proceedings of the 12th Congress of the European Society for Veterinary Clinical Nutrition. Vienna, Austria, September 25, 2008.

Field Treatment and Management of Endocrinopathic Laminitis in Horses and Ponies

Donald M. Walsh, BS, DVM

KEYWORDS

- Endocrinopathic laminitis • Hyperinsuliemia
- Risk evaluation • Exercise

Endocrinopathic laminitis in horses and ponies is a difficult disease to successfully treat and manage. It has the potential to cause extensive damage to the feet before clinical signs of laminitis are apparent. Early diagnosis and intervention are critical if the crippling changes that are seen in the disease are to be avoided.

This article describes the methods used at Homestead Veterinary Hospital, Pacific, Missouri, to recognize and intervene early in the disease process of endocrinopathic laminitis. My years of experience in practice have taught me the benefits of preventing laminitis rather than treating the disease in patients.

Often the affected animal is presented with a history of acute-onset lameness without ever being diagnosed with laminitis. Physical examination of the feet reveals dropped soles, abnormal growth rings on the external hoof wall, seedy toe, and radiographic evidence of an abnormal relationship between dorsal hoof wall and the distal phalanx. All of these changes are evidence of long-standing pathology. Many of these animals are obese, but that is not always the case, particularly with Cushing disease.

The early detection of these changes by veterinarians performing annual wellness examinations (an approach to health care that emphasizes preventing illness and prolonging life, as opposed to emphasizing treating diseases), before laminitis occurs, can be an important means of early intervention. People performing the hoof care of the animal, if properly educated, can also alert the owner or veterinarian that something abnormal is occurring in the feet. Veterinary clinicians should strive to have a good working relationship with all of the farriers and hoof caregivers in their area encouraging the latter to feel comfortable in contacting veterinarians to discuss their observations and concerns. Unfortunately, warnings often go unheeded by owners and sometimes veterinarians, seeing no obvious signs of clinical lameness, fail to

Homestead Veterinary Hospital, 3615 Basset Road, Pacific, MO 63069, USA
E-mail address: walshvet@gmail.com

Vet Clin Equine 26 (2010) 379–390
doi:10.1016/j.cveq.2010.05.001
0749-0739/10/$ – see front matter © 2010 Elsevier Inc. All rights reserved.

vetequine.theclinics.com

diagnose the disease process taking place until a bout of laminitic pain occurs. Blood, taken after fasting, should be analyzed for adrenocorticotropic hormone (ACTH), insulin, glucose, and thyroid hormone if any of the following are present: abnormal changes in the hoof growth pattern (especially laminitic rings); dropped or flat soles; seedy toe; laminitic pain without an apparent causative factor; and laminitic pain associated with pasture consumption. The blood sample is best obtained in the morning after an overnight fast and before feeding. If this is not possible, fasting for 4 hours in a nonstressful situation is usually satisfactory. The sample should be cooled immediately and centrifuged within 3 hours. If the schedule of the attending veterinarian prevents this, request that the owner take the cooled sample to the clinic to be centrifuged. The sample needs to be shipped to the diagnostic laboratory frozen or chilled.

The presence of elevated insulin levels in the blood of animals suffering from laminitis has been reported in a field study led by the author.[1] The study showed a significant correlation between the level of insulin and the grade of laminitis in animals suffering from endocrinopathic laminitis. This study was based on the use of a single fasting sample for insulin. A more complete evaluation of the level of insulin resistance can be done using dynamic testing, but clinical cases of laminitis associated with hyperinsulinemia invariably have insulin concentrations well above the normal range.

The goal of the clinician should be to decrease blood insulin into the normal range as quickly as possible. All too often the clinical signs of laminitis respond to nonsteroidal anti-inflammatory drug therapy and the true etiologic factor, hyperinsulinemia, goes undiagnosed. Diet restrictions and removal from grass to a dry lot quells the present episode, but in reality the disease progresses and with every recurring episode more damage occurs. Each recovery is followed by periods of deteriorating soundness until permanent lameness is present. Administering nonsteroidal anti-inflammatory drugs, without diagnosing and correcting hyperinsulinemia, is an incomplete treatment. This is the reason why it is necessary to continue monitoring blood insulin after "recovery" to ensure the disease process has abated to a subpathologic level. This is the only way to treat hyperinsulinemic laminitis successfully. The disease process associated with hyperinsulinemia is not yet completely understood. Experimental induction of laminitis in horses and ponies has been achieved with supraphysiologic doses of insulin, but the cellular pathophysiology of this form of laminitis is still unknown.[2,3] Seasonal variations and environmental conditions can influence the results of endocrine tests and make them difficult to interpret.

ADRENOCORTICOTROPIC HORMONE

ACTH is tested to diagnose equine Cushing disease. The normal range for ACTH level is 7 to 35 pg/mL, and elevations greater than 35 pg/mL are considered abnormal. Pain from laminitis may raise ACTH, but if the results are greater than 70 pg/mL Cushing disease is very probable. Normal significant elevations are seen in all horses and ponies during the months of August, September, and October, rendering the test unreliable during the autumnal season of the year.[4,5] From a practical point of view, if the test result is significantly elevated during this time and laminitis is present, the animal can be put on pergolide until the month of November, then taken off the drug for 2 weeks and retested. If the ACTH is elevated above 35 pg/mL at this time the animal is positive for Cushing disease and should remain on the pergolide treatment.

INSULIN

Normal range for fasting insulin is 10 to 40 uU/mL. Many things, such as pain, stress, flight, or any condition that results in increased blood glucose, can cause mild elevations in insulin. For this reason one must be careful when basing a diagnosis on one insulin sample. A fasting sample from a horse with laminitis that is greater than 70 uU/mL, however, suggests hyperinsulinemia is the cause of the laminitis. The mean insulin concentration of 30 cases of endocrinopathic laminitis at Homestead Veterinary Hospital was 120.5 uU/mL (unpublished data). Most cases of equine metabolic syndrome (EMS) and Cushing disease that have laminitis also have significant increases in fasting insulin levels. The problem arises when the clinician suspects EMS but the fasting insulin level is in the high normal range. Repeated high normal fasting values are very suspicious for EMS. A panel representing the American College of Veterinary Internal Medicine has released an EMS Consensus statement that suggests that a fasting insulin level greater than 20 uU/mL is abnormal. Additional dynamic glucose-insulin testing may be necessary to diagnose EMS in these cases. The combined glucose-insulin testing described by Eiler should be used to diagnose EMS if insulin levels are in the normal range.[6]

Correcting hyperinsulinemia, whatever the form of endocrinopathic laminitis, can be challenging for the clinician. Horses with a positive diagnosis of Cushing disease respond to low-dose administration of pergolide, 1 mg/day orally.[1] Insulin levels return to normal and the laminitis improves. Many of these horses are older and have pain associated with osteoarthritis in many joints. Some of these individuals continue to show symptoms of laminitis pain after insulin levels return to normal. The inflammatory processes going on in other areas of the body may be responsible for continued pain, and long-term treatment and management of the osteoarthritis helps this resolve. Other problems associated with Cushing disease, such as immunodeficiency, must also be addressed to restore a state of general health to the animal.[7]

Horses with EMS have normal ACTH levels but insulin levels above the normal range. They also may have very low thyroid levels.[1,8] Their blood glucose levels are usually on the high side of the normal range. Many of these animals suffer from chronic obesity with excess fat deposits in the nuchal crest area of the neck. Many of their episodes of laminitis are associated with an intake of grass. The long-term improvement of these animals is dependant on significant weight loss.[9] Changing the diet is helpful, but many of them are already on greatly reduced caloric intakes. Exercise helps burn fat-stored calories and at the same time stimulates the need for increased Glut4 receptors on skeletal muscle, helping to reduce insulin levels.[10] The temporary use of pain-reducing medications and the application of therapeutic foot appliances are necessary to enable affected animals to exercise in comfort. It is difficult for many owners to devote the necessary amount of time to exercise their horse or pony every day. It has been shown that 10 minutes of exercise per day was sufficient to lower insulin resistance in ponies.[11] The use of thyroid supplements to raise the metabolic rate has been shown to affect weight loss and reduce insulin resistance.[8] Some horses after initial weight loss and improvement in their feet still have elevated insulin levels when rechecked. Many owners are satisfied with their horse's progress, but careful clinical examination reveals mild pain remains. If owners can significantly increase the horse's exercise intensity and accomplish further weight loss to a body condition score of 4 (on a scale of 10) many owners describe amazing improvement. Owners report that now, while being ridden, the horse moves much better. Owners often realize that their horse's feet have been a problem for years and are now completely sound for the first time.

This leads to the question of whether the hyperinsulinemic form of laminitis is reversible. As a clinician I believe that it is, if caught early and completely corrected. Radiographic evidence and significant improvement in foot growth patterns support this observation. It has been reported that ultrastructural damage to the lamellar basement membrane in hyperinsulinemic laminitis is significantly less than in the oligofructose induction model.[12] Hyperinsulinemia induces lamellar mitogenesis causing secondary epidermal lamellae to lengthen. Perhaps when hyperinsulinemia is reversed the mitogenic effect abates and lamellae return to their normal length. This is demonstrated in radiographs of successfully recovered animals that show a decrease in the distance between dorsal hoof wall and distal phalanx. Reversibility is dependant on the extent of the laminitis-associated pathology. If major pathology is present with severe rotation of the distal phalanx, lytic lesions in the distal phalanx, and shortening of the deep digital flexor musculotendon unit, then reversal of such pathology is impossible.

The best way to combat laminitis is to try to intervene before significant problems occur. For the past 6 years, a Laminitis Risk Evaluation Form has been used at the Homestead Veterinary Hospital. Clinicians approach the owners of overweight horses and ponies considered at risk of developing laminitis. Instead of merely commenting that their horse or pony is fat and needs dietary restriction, the Laminitis Risk Evaluation Form is used to introduce the subject of a complete nutritional evaluation. This can greatly benefit the animal and also creates a new income stream for the practice. With the owner the clinician becomes involved in a combined effort to implement weight reduction. This generally leads to a discussion about possible hormone testing and radiography of the feet if this seems appropriate. By being proactive EMS and Cushing disease are detected in horses before treatment for laminitis is needed. Owners appreciate knowing about their horse's risk level, and usually, if the risk is real, take the necessary steps to try to prevent laminitis (**Fig. 1**).

Question number 3 requires an evaluation of the horse or pony's weight, diet, and exercise level (**Fig. 2**). This allows the clinician the opportunity to evaluate the metabolic status of the animal. Many owners are frustrated with their lack of success in trying to achieve weight loss in their animal and welcome the interest and assistance of professional knowledge. The form starts by using actual caloric values to calculate the dietary needs and weight-reduction goals. Few commercial horse feeds have caloric information on the bag. This information can be obtained from the company. There is also very little information regarding the carbohydrate level in the feed. Some new, lower-carbohydrate, special feeds do list the levels. The goal is to provide a diet that is low in carbohydrate that results in a minimal release of insulin when consumed. It is recommended that the hay being fed be tested and that it should be less than 10% starch and water-soluble carbohydrate. If that is not possible, soaking hay in water for 60 minutes before feeding reduces the carbohydrate level by up to 30%.[13]

During the evaluation the horse is first weighed using the tape measure formula and the owner is encouraged to weigh the horse to become familiar with the technique. After the weight is calculated the veterinarian prescribes what amount of weight needs to be lost and records the desired weight on the form.

Next, all feeds and supplements currently being fed are weighed and recorded. If the horse is allowed out on grass, the amount of time they are out is recorded. The pasture should be examined to judge the amount of grass that is available for consumption and the types of grasses that are in the pasture. Hay is sampled using a hay core drill and mailed to Equi-analytical Laboratories (730 Warren Road, Ithaca, NY 14850; E-mail: service@equi-analytical.com) for analysis.

The horse is physically examined and digital photos are taken of the horse and its feet for future reference. The results of the examination may suggest that hormone testing and radiographs of the feet are appropriate at this time. The data and the samples are taken to the clinic and analyzed. Based on the results, dietary changes and an exercise program are recommended. The complete evaluation analysis is

LAMINITIS RISK EVALUATION

Management of a horse in order to prevent laminitis first requires recognizing if your horse is at risk for the disease.

The following questionnaire is a simple and quick Laminitis Risk Evaluation form which can indicate a high-risk horse.

Assign a score in response to each question.

_____ 1.) Has your horse ever had laminitis? (yes = 10; no = 0)

_____ 2.) Is your horse overweight? Body condition scoring (0-9).
          (Body score of 6 or higher = 10; less than 6 = 0)

_____ 3.) Is your horse in a positive caloric state? This occurs when
          more calories are taken in than are required. A nutritional
          and exercise evaluation is necessary to make this
          calculation. (5000 or more calories than required = 10; 100
          to 5000 more calories than required = 5; calories do not
          exceed requirement = 0)

_____ 4.) Is your horse given access to grass pasture? (yes, all the
          time =10; yes, part of the time = 5; no = 0)

_____ 5.) Age of your horse; less than 2 yrs = minus 5; 2-18 yrs = 0;
          over 18yrs = 5)

_____ YOUR HORSES'S TOTAL

A HIGH RISK HORSE =
A TOTAL SCORE OF 25 or HIGHER

Fig. 1. A laminitis risk evaluation form to determine high-risk animals before laminitis is present.

mailed or faxed to the owner. Later, a telephone consultation is scheduled to ensure the owner understands the program. A follow-up examination is scheduled for 1 month after starting the weight loss exercise program.

Weight loss diets based on pasture (forage) and hay require vitamin and mineral supplementation to protect against deficiencies. If the horse or pony has laminitis it is removed from grass until insulin levels are normal. Then, limited exposure to grass using strip or cell grazing or a grazing muzzle can be attempted, but the animal is carefully observed and checked for any signs of foot soreness or elevated insulin levels. Grazing is not allowed during the spring and fall when stressed pasture may accumulate dangerously high levels of nonstructural carbohydrates (see the article by Kathryn Watts elsewhere in this issue for further exploration of this topic.)

Nutrition & Exercise Evaluation

Is your horse in a positive caloric state? This occurs when more calories are eaten than required. A nutritional and exercise evaluation is necessary to make this calculation. (5000 or more calories than required daily= 10; 100 to 5000 more calories then required daily= 5; calories do not exceed daily requirement= 0)

Horse's Name: _____ Date: _____ Weight: _____

Exercise Level: _____   Desired Weight: _____

Present Diet:

Feed:_____lbs/day_____X cal/lb_____=_____feed cal/day

Feed:_____lbs/day_____X cal/lb_____=_____feed cal/day

Feed:_____lbs/day_____X cal/lb_____=_____ feed cal/day

Hay:_____lbs/day_____X cal/lb_____=_____hay cal/day

Hay:_____lbs/day_____X cal/lb_____=_____hay cal/day

     Grass Hay (800 cal/lb)   *Legume Hay* (1000 cal/lb)

Pasture Grass:_____lbs/day_____X cal/lb_____=_____grass cal/day

Pasture Grass Consumption (1100 cal/lb)
Grazing Consumption (1-3hrs) = 0.33 lbs per 100Lbs. Body Weight per hour
Grazing Consumption (Over 3 hrs) = 0.10 lbs per 100Lbs. Body Weight per hour
If a grazing muzzle is used, Total Calorie Intake is reduced to 25% of the Total Grass Calories per Day.

_____**Total** cal/day

Desired Weight:_____X_____cal/lb=_____**Total** cal/day

No Work- *15cal/lb/day*, **Light Work-** *18cal/lb/day*, **Moderate Work-** *21cal/lb/day*

Heavy Work- *24cal/lb/day*, **Very Heavy-** *31cal/lb/day*

Recommended Diet Change:

    Feed:_____lbs/day_____X cal/lb_____=_____feed cal/day

    Feed:_____lbs/day_____X cal/lb_____=_____feed cal/day

    Hay:_____lbs/day_____X cal/lb_____=_____hay cal/day

Pasture Grass:_____lbs/day_____X cal/lb_____=_____grass cal/day

                Horse's New Diet:_____**Total** cal/day

                (should equal the desired caloric intake above)

Fig. 2. A nutrition and exercise evaluation form to measure the calories in the current diet and the recommended new diet.

Exercise is a critical part of the successful prevention of endinocrinopathic laminitis. Insulin resistance can be reduced with daily exercise (see the article by Nicola J. Menzies-Gow elsewhere in this issue for further exploration of this topic.)[11,14] Exercise also mobilizes and reduces the size of the large, abnormal fat depots that characterize EMS and contribute to weight loss (**Fig. 3**). If the horse or pony has suffered laminitis and has foot pain this makes significant exercise difficult. This is another good reason to advocate early intervention before laminitis strikes. Animals recovering from laminitis can be started on small amounts of exercise built up gradually. If severe foot changes have already occurred and there is bone loss and extreme rotation of

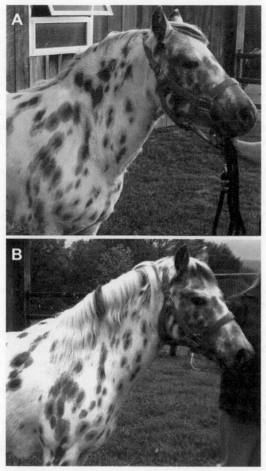

Fig. 3. A hyperinsulemic pony before (*A*) and after (*B*) being on a 6-month exercise and restricted diet prescription. Initially the pony was significantly lame but trotted freely at 6 months.

the distal phalanx, exercise may not be possible and the laminitis has now trapped the animal in its unrelenting disease process. Nevertheless, walking these animals often seems to improve their condition slightly and may diminish the rate of their deterioration.

Owner compliance with the exercise regimens is the most difficult part of the new program. I often have observed that owners who successfully implement their animal's exercise program are rewarded with weight loss for themselves. If considered appropriate this benefit may be pointed out to an owner as an additional incentive for compliance. It is important that the owner knows the weight of the animal will be checked in 1 month to evaluate the progress of the entire program. Most successful weight-reduction programs for people involve a support group to praise progress. The same is true for the owners of horses and ponies.

Another other important aspect of an exercise program is to ensure that a proper facility is available in which to perform exercise in all types of weather conditions. The need for a properly graded round pen with a good exercise surface is essential to success. Providing the names of people who can assist owners in getting this accomplished greatly increases the possibility of it happening. Many landscapers are more than happy to get involved in these projects. Meeting with them, and the farm supply people who sell panels for round pens, for a few minutes ensures that a functional exercise area is installed. Point out to the owner that the cost of this project may be much less than the cost of laminitis treatment and that it is a cost-effective investment.

If the owner really does not have the time available, supplying a list of qualified people who can be hired to exercise the horse or pony increases the chance of success. These are excellent afterschool jobs for responsible neighborhood teenagers. The relationship that occurs often provides the owner with people they can trust to care for their animals when they are out of town (**Figs. 4** and **5**).

Recovery from laminitis is fraught with complications that can make exercise painful. Foot abscesses are commonly seen after laminitis. Exacerbation of subsolar bruising and further separation of the healing lamellae can occur if exercise is too strenuous. During this initial period much care must be taken not to reinjure the horse's feet. The benefits of even small amounts of exercise, however, are significant (see **Fig. 3**).

DRUG THERAPY

The use of pergolide for the treatment of equine Cushing disease has been extremely helpful in my practice and limits the recurrence of laminitis in affected animals.[15] The dose ranges from 1 to 5 mg orally each day. Animals are started on 1 mg/day and then after 1 month the ACTH and insulin levels are rechecked. ACTH levels should be less than 70 pg/mL, but may never return to below the 35 pg/mL normal range. The purpose of treatment is to prevent very high levels from occurring and affecting blood insulin levels.

The use of metformin has been helpful in reducing insulin levels in people with type 2 diabetes. It has been tried in horses and ponies with positive reports (see the article by Andy Durham elsewhere in this issue for further exploration of this topic.)[16] Studies have shown a reduced oral bioavailability and an increased clearance rate in horses compared with humans. More studies are needed to establish efficacy and safety for its use in horses.[17]

For decades phenylbutazone has been used to diminish the pain associated with laminitis. In endocrinopathic laminitis it is often helpful to reduce pain to enable the animals to start moving around. Exercise lowers insulin levels, an important part of breaking the cycle of the disease process.

The use of laminitis risk evaluation has provided my practice with a means of early intervention in horses and ponies likely to develop laminitis. It enables the clinician to use all the tools currently available to prevent endocrinopathic laminitis. Monitoring blood insulin levels and doing periodic radiographs of the feet can track disease progress. In spite of controlling the diet, using muzzles to limit grass intake, exercise programs to reduce insulin levels, and weight reduction preventing clinical laminitis is not always successful. Owners often try advertised supplements that offer cures for laminitis. Because of labeling laws the ingredients of the product are not stated. For years magnesium and chromium supplements have been used to treat endocrinopathic laminitis with anecdotal reports of improvement. To date no controlled studies have been performed to prove an effect on lowering insulin levels or improving the laminitis. A number of products have appeared in the last few years using combinations of all the popular supplements with claims of helping laminitis victims. The extent and popularity of these products indicates that the owners of horses and ponies are frustrated with the veterinary profession's lack of understanding and inability to help.

ESTIMATING HORSE BODY WEIGHT WITH A SIMPLE FORMULA

$$\frac{(\text{Heartgirth} \times \text{Heartgirth} \times \text{Body length})}{330} = \text{Weight in pounds}$$

Note: Heartgirth and Body Length in inches

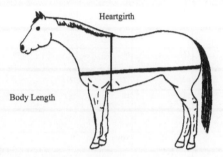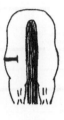

Measurements should be taken and recorded in inches with a tape that is at least 75 inches long. Plastic measuring tapes are preferred over cloth tapes because they won't stretch. Metal tapes can be used but they sometimes scare horses, making them the least preferable.

As shown in the figure, heartgirth is a measure of the circumference, taken by running the tape measure all the way around the horse, using the highest part of the withers. Body length is measured from the point of the shoulder, straight back along the horse's side, and to the point of the buttock. The rearview figure shows that the tape should go around the corner of the hip and to the actual point of the buttock, which is essentially half the distance from the corner to the tail. Two persons will be needed in taking body length measurements. (This procedure may not be highly accurate for pregnant mares or for horses with extreme conformational irregularities, especially very unbalanced horses). All in all, horse owners should be able to utilize this simple tool in better managing horses.

Courtesy of: Texas Horse Owner's Reference Guide
Texas A&M University, Department of Animal Science, Equine Sciences Program
P.G. Gibbs and D.D. Householder. Estimating Horse Body Weight With A Simple Formula

Fig. 4. A simple formula to estimate body weight in horses. *Data from* Gibbs PG, Householder DD. Texas horse owner's reference guide. TAMU, Department of Animal Science, Equine Science Program.

Equally frustrating is the knowledge that the feral horse seems to be almost completely free of laminitis. Today, many owners purchase any product that is labeled "natural" to somehow emulate the benefits of the feral lifestyle. There are major differences, however, between domestic horse husbandry and life in the feral state. In the North American winter feral horses have a significantly reduced food supply. This causes them to use stored fat depots for their caloric needs and brings them into spring in lean to thin body condition. Domestic horses and ponies are usually fed more in the winter and arrive in the spring fat. Perhaps domestic horses and ponies suffering from EMS should have their caloric intake reduced by 75% during the winter

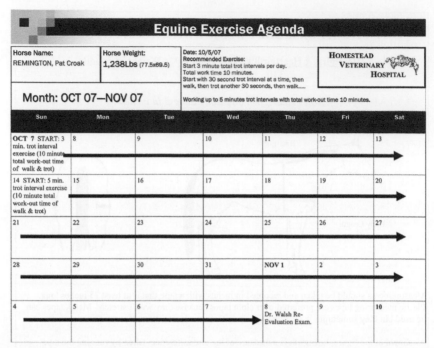

Fig. 5. This is an example of an exercise agenda for a horse recovering from laminitis. The animal has been observed at the trot and is sufficiently recovered to start exercise. The owner is advised that the animal should be evaluated each day before exercise. If the level of comfort has diminished the intensity of exercise should be reduced. If further deterioration occurs a veterinary consultation is indicated.

months. It has been speculated by Frank and colleagues[18] that long-term, continuous obesity results in the development of EMS in horses and ponies.

Genetic studies on endocrinopathic laminitis are a major hope for better detection and improved treatment and understanding of the disease. Horses and ponies that possess the "easy-keeper, thrift" genes seem able to pass these on to their offspring.[19] On certain farms, clinicians often see laminitis in multiple generations. Veterinarians could counsel the owners of animals having these genes and expressing the "laminitis high-risk phenotype" not to breed them because they are likely to produce animals similarly at risk. Many owners of laminitic horses or ponies are unaware that the endocrinopathic form of the disease has a genetic component and when informed support not passing the laminitic dilemma on to future generations. Breeders have a lot more invested in their genetic line, however, and are more difficult to convince. They suggest that the show-winning and the special redeeming characteristics of the individual makes taking the chance on laminitis acceptable. More research may enable genetic counseling to help people select and breed animals with reduced risk of developing the disease.

SUMMARY

By becoming proactive and recognizing the disease process in its earliest stage before significant damage has occurred in the feet makes the prevention of endocrinopathic laminitis is possible. Endocrinopathic laminitis should be recognized as an ongoing, slow disease, which requires constant monitoring. If detected early, correct medication and good husbandry practices regarding diet, exercise, and exposure to grass normalize abnormally high hormone levels and help manage this crippling disease. Failure to diagnose hyperinsulinemia, prevent its continuing deleterious effects, and repeated bouts of laminitis allow endocrinopathic laminitis to win repeatedly. The knowledge and the tools to work with owners to prevent this now exist. Clinicians are moving closer to freeing the horse from this disease.

REFERENCES

1. Walsh DM, McGowan CM, Mc Gowan T, et al. Correlation of plasma insulin concentration with laminitis score in a field study of equine Cushing's disease and equine metabolic syndrome. J Equine Vet Sci 2009;29:87–94.
2. Asplin KE, Sillence MN, Pollitt CC, et al. Induction of laminitis by prolonged hyperinsulinaemia in clinically normal ponies. Vet J 2007;174:530–5.
3. De Laat MA, Mc Gowan CM, Sillence MN. Equine laminitis: induced by 48 h hyperinsulinaemia in Standardbred horses. Equine Vet J 2010;42:129–35.
4. Place NJ, McGowan CM, Lamb SV, et al. Seasonal variation in serum concentrations of selected metabolic hormones in horses. J Vet Intern Med 2010;24(3): 650–4.
5. Donaldson MT, Jorgensen AJ, Beech J. Evaluation of suspected pituitary pars intermedia dysfunction in horses with laminitis. J Am Vet Med Assoc 2004;224: 1123–7.
6. Eiler H, Frank N, Andrews FM, et al. Physoilogic assessment of blood glucose homeostasis via combined intravenous glucose and insulin testing in horses. Am J Vet Res 2005;66:1598–604.
7. Schott HCII. Pituitary pars intermedia dysfunction: equine Cushing's disease. Vet Clin North Am Equine Pract 2002;18:237–70.
8. Frank N, Sommardahl CS, Eiler H, et al. Effects of oral administration of levothyroxine sodium on concentrations of plasma lipids, concentration and composition of very low density lipoproteins, and glucose dynamics in healthy adult horses. Am J Vet Res 2005;66:1032–8.
9. Johnson PJ, Wiedmeyer CE, Messer NT, et al. Medical implications of obesity in horses-lessons for human obesity. J Diabetes Sci Technol 2009;3:163–74.
10. Hawley JA. Exercise as a therapeutic intervention for the prevention and treatment of insulin resistance. Diabetes Metab Res Rev 2004;20:383–93.
11. Freestone JF, Beadle R, Shoemake K, et al. Improved insulin sensitivity in hyperinsulinaemic ponies through physical conditioning and controlled feed intake. Equine Vet J 1992;24:187–90.
12. Nourian AR, Baldwin GI, van Eps AW, et al. Equine laminitis: ultrastructural lesions detected 24–30 hours after induction with oligofructose. Equine Vet J 2007;39:360–4.
13. Cottrell E, Watts K, Ralston S. Soluble sugar content and glucose/insulin responses can be reduced by soaking chopped hay in water. Proceedings of the Nineteenth Equine Science Society Symposium. Tuscon (AZ): Equine Science Society; 2005:293–8.
14. Jeffcott LB, Field JR, McLean JG, et al. Glucose tolerance and insulin sensitivity in ponies and Standardbred horses. Equine Vet J 1986;18:97–101.
15. Donaldson MT, LaMonte BH, Morresey P, et al. Treatment with pergolide or cyproheptadine of pituitary pars intermedia dysfunction (equine Cushing's disease). J Vet Intern Med 2002;16:742–6.

16. Durham AE, Rendel DI, Newton JE. The effect of metformin on measurements of insulin sensitivity and beta cell response in 18 horses and ponies with insulin resistance. Equine Vet J 2008;40:493–500.
17. Hustace JL, Firshman AM, Mata JE. Pharmacokinetics and bioavailability of metformin in horses. Am J Vet Res 2009;70:665–8.
18. Frank N, Elliott SB, Brandt LE, et al. Physical characteristics, blood hormone concentration, and plasma lipid concentration in obese horses with insulin resistance. J Am Vet Med Assoc 2006;228:2311–21.
19. Treiber KH, Kronfeld DS, Hess TM, et al. Evaluation of genetic and metabolic predispositions and nutritional risk factors for pasture-associated laminitis in ponies. J Am Vet Med Assoc 2006;228:1538–45.

Clinical Presentation, Diagnosis, and Prognosis of Chronic Laminitis in Europe

Robert A. Eustace, BVSc, Cert EP, Cert EO, FRCVS

KEYWORDS

• Laminitis • Acute • Chronic • Founder • Horse

CLINICAL PRESENTATION AND DIAGNOSIS
Definitions and Nomenclature: Traditional

Laminitis means "idiopathic inflammation or ischaemia of the sub-mural structures of the foot".[1] This definition covers a wide range of clinical conditions, from pedal sepsis (pus in the foot) to thrombotic occlusion of the digital arterial supply causing ischemia. No mention is made of the typical stance shown by laminitis cases.

Distal displacement of the third phalanx is defined as "even movement of the distal phalanx distally within the hoof capsule in horses with laminitis such that the distal phalanx remains in alignment with the dorsal hoof wall and the phalangeal axis. Often referred to as a "sinker," as opposed to rotation of the distal phalanx."

All horses that have rotation of the distal phalanx also have a degree of distal displacement. Sinkers also experience slight rotation of the distal phalanx in relation to either the proximal phalanges or the hoof capsule; this rotation becomes more obvious over time.

Chronic laminitis is the "phase of laminitis that begins with separation of the dermal and epidermal laminae resulting in mechanical collapse of the foot. It results in displacement of the distal phalanx relative to its normal relationship with the hoof capsule".[2] However, because no case of chronic laminitis has been known to result in proximal displacement of the distal phalanx, the above definition must mean distal displacement or possibly disto-palmaro/plantaro displacement.

These definitions, if followed logically, mean that chronic laminitis only follows sinking. Therefore, how are those cases of chronic laminitis defined in which rotation of the distal phalanx is the predominant displacement? In addition, any horse that experiences displacement of the distal phalanx in relation to the hoof will be described as a chronic laminitic for the rest of its life, regardless of whether it dies soon after

The Laminitis Clinic, Mead House, Dauntsey, Chippenham, Wiltshire SN15 4JA, England, UK
E-mail address: rae@equilife.co.uk

Vet Clin Equine 26 (2010) 391–405
doi:10.1016/j.cveq.2010.06.005
0749-0739/10/$ – see front matter © 2010 Elsevier Inc. All rights reserved.

displacement or lives for another 30 years and possibly experiences episodes of clinically overt laminitis and further displacement in the interim.

Clearly a less mutually contradictory and more appropriate system of nomenclature is necessary to help clinicians dealing with chronic laminitis to identify the type of case and stage of the pathologic process.

Definitions and Nomenclature: New

A study that identified and measured statistically significant prognostic parameters for all types of laminitis cases has been undertaken and the results published.[3,4] The nomenclature used in these reports is followed, henceforth, in this article.

Laminitis
Lameness characteristic of laminitis becomes evident (strong digital pulses, toe-relieving stance, weight-shifting from one affected foot to another). Any or all feet can be affected and the severity of lameness varies from a slight shortening of stride length to recumbency and distress. The stance the animal adopts depends on the feet affected. No abnormal radiologic measurements can be detected in a first-time laminitis case.

Acute founder
In acute founder disease, the clinical signs of laminitis are present in addition to palpable supracoronary depressions that extend part way around the coronary contour. The deeper and longer the depressions, the worse the displacement. All surviving acute founder cases develop into chronic founder cases (unless effective treatments have been used soon after the onset of acute founder). It takes a minimum of 3 months before new divergent hoof horn growth rings become clinically recognizable and the case becomes defined as chronic founder. All chronic founder cases display the following clinical changes: concave dorsal hoof walls, abnormally wide dorsal white lines from quarter to quarter, and divergent growth rings on the hoof walls. The growth rings are more widely spaced at the heels than the toes, leading to relative overgrowth of the hoof wall at the heels. On visual examination, the perioplic ring is missing and the skin seems to merge directly with the hoof horn.

Sinker
A sinker does not show the characteristic toe-relieving laminitis lameness but is reluctant to move, has strong digital pulses, and supracoronary depressions that extend the entire way around the coronary contour. The feet may be abnormally cold to the touch. Surviving sinkers develop a distinct hoof wall growth ring that remains equidistant from the coronary band until it is worn or trimmed away at the ground surface of the hoof. No horses are defined as chronic sinkers; a recovered sinker is clinically indistinguishable from a normal horse.

Solar prolapse
Solar prolapse is characterized by protrusion of the solar corium through the horny sole from relative displacement between the distal phalanx and the hoof in an acute or chronic founder case, or in a sinker.

The four cardinal signs of displacement of the distal phalanx in relation to the hoof capsule after loss of lamellar cohesion are (1) lameness or reluctance to ambulate, (2) increased strength of digital arterial pulsation, (3) the presence of palpable supracoronary depressions, and (4) an increase in founder distance.

An increase in founder distance results in a reduction of the vertical distance between the center of articulation of the distal interphalangeal joint and the ground.

However, the author finds it helpful to regard this change as proximal displacement of the hoof in relation to the distal phalanx rather than distal displacement of the distal phalanx, because the term *distal displacement* tends to imply that stretching of the musculotendinous unit of the deep digital flexor muscle has occurred. No evidence suggests that increased tension in the deep digital flexor muscle and tendon is present after relative displacement.

The previous definition of chronic laminitis[1,2] is not one the author finds helpful; rather, the author believes chronic laminitis refers a patient that has experienced laminitis for an abnormally protracted time (eg, has an underlying medical or iatrogenic condition).

Before analysis of abnormal anatomy is discussed, a review of normality is appropriate.

NORMALITY
Clinical Features

A horse with ideal conformation will grow hoof horn at the same rate all the way around the coronary contour. If hoof growth rings are apparent and are caused by a change in diet, work, or environment, they will be concentric (ie, equal inter-ring distances will be present) (**Fig. 1**).

Nutrition influences horn growth rate but does so uniformly around the coronary circumference, and therefore any hoof growth rings remain concentric. Increased loading, whether constant or intermittent, reduces coronary horn growth rate; for instance, flexural contracture results in horn rings more widely spaced at the heels than the toe, whereas collapsed heels result in the converse.

The horny sole of a normal horse is somewhat concave. The degree of concavity depends on breed and hoof trimming.

The white line of a normal horse—the distance between the edge of the solar horn and the inner edge of the stratum medium of the wall—maintains the same width all the way around the sole.

Normal horses show a distinct, pale-colored ring of perioplic horn all around the coronary contour, which defines the skin from the hoof wall. No depression proximal to the perioplic ring is palpable when one runs a finger down the pastern and onto the hoof wall. However, some old horses develop abnormal supracoronary contours. The

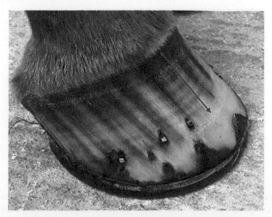

Fig. 1. A normal horse shows equal coronary horn growth at the toe and heel.

supracoronary tissues are not so palpably firm as in younger animals, perhaps because of changes in the physical characteristics of the collagen in the dermis and subcuticular tissues. These cases should not be confused with acute or chronic founder cases unless the other three cardinal signs of displacement are also present.

Radiologic Measurements

In the normal horse, the hoof wall is parallel to the dorsal surface of the distal phalanx. The three phalangeal bones have a straight axis so that the interphalangeal joints are not flexed or extended. Founder distance is less than 10 mm in the normal horse when measured while the limb is weight-bearing. Wall thickness, the distances measured perpendicularly from the mid-point of the dorsal surface of the distal phalanx to the dorsal surface of the hoof wall, highlighted by a wire marker, is less than 18.7 mm; this distance is dependent on the height and breed of the animal.[5] These are the four radiological parameters which define normality.

The normal radiologic anatomy of the hoof has been described.[5–7] Hoof trimming can alter angular measurements and wall- and sole-thickness measurements. The only radiologic hoof measurement that cannot be altered by hoof trimming or stance is founder distance (**Fig. 2**).

MEASUREMENT OF FOUNDER DISTANCE

A weight-bearing lateromedial radiograph should be taken of the affected hoof. Before exposure, a straight, stiff radiodense marker with square ends and of known length (50 mm is suitable for all breeds) should be taped to the dorsal hoof wall in the sagittal plane. The positioning of the proximal end of the marker is critical if measurements of founder distance are to be repeatable and referable to previous reports on prognosis. The proximal end of the marker should be placed where a palpable horny ridge is evident. Pressing firmly on the proximodorsal hoof wall will identify this ring of mature horn. The axis of the limb should be as close to vertical as possible, and the radiographic exposure should be obtained when the limb is weight-bearing. The founder distance is the vertical distance between two lines drawn parallel to the surface on which the horse was standing (see **Fig. 2**).

One line passes through the top of the wire marker, and the second through the proximal limit of the extensor process of the distal phalanx. This distance should be

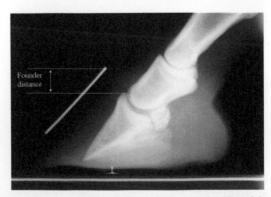

Fig. 2. Founder distance is the vertical distance between the dorsal limit of the extensor process of the distal phalanx and the ridge of palpably firm horn below the periopic ring, after correction for possible magnification errors.

corrected for any magnification errors, either automatically by the software in modern digital radiographic generators or by using the following formula;

True founder distance = measured founder distance × (true length of marker/ measured length of marker).

The placement of the dorsal wall marker is a subjective measurement and therefore vulnerable to interoperator and temporal errors. The errors involved in the measurement of founder distance have been described and subjected to statistical analysis[3]; adherence to a standard technique minimizes interoperator errors.

PROGNOSIS: ALL CASES

One study measured nine clinical and eight radiologic parameters from all types of laminitis cases at first presentation.[3,4] All cases were treated using a standard protocol at the same premises (stable confinement on a deep shavings bed, frog support, dorsal wall resection on acute founder cases, deep digital flexor tenotomy when clinically indicated, no elevation of heel height). Outcomes were recorded and statistical calculations made to identify which of the initial parameters was significant in predicting outcome. Analysis showed that the clinical ability to identify a case as a laminitic, acute founder, sinker, or chronic founder had the most prognostic significance. If the data from only acute founder and sinker cases were subjected to analysis, then founder distance was the only statistically significant parameter. A graph showing the relationship between initial founder distance and outcome for 111 acute founder cases is shown in **Fig. 3**.

The 20% success rates reported in two studies recording the results of treating sinkers[3,8] were similarly low.

Breed has a significant influence on treatment outcome for all types of cases. The failure rate of Arabs, Arab crosses, and Thoroughbreds was nearly three times higher

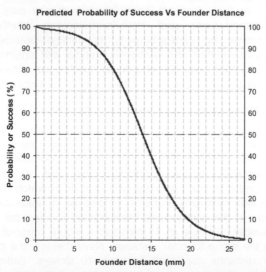

Predicted Probability of Success Vs Founder Distance

Probability or Success (%) (y-axis: 0 to 100)

Founder Distance (mm) (x-axis: 0 to 25)

Fig. 3. Graph showing founder distance as a predictor of success for horses with acute founder. Prediction obtained using binary logistic regression. Graph produced using Minitab from data obtained from 111 acute founder cases (Eustace and Cripps, unpublished data, 2010).

than for other breeds, independent of lameness grade, founder distance, or whether the cases were acute founder, sinkers or chronic founder.[3]

Lateromedial radiographs for acute founder or sinker cases showed no significant relationship was found between outcome and the difference between the angle subtended by the hoof wall to the ground and the angle of the dorsal surface of the distal phalanx to the ground. These findings do not support those of a previous study[9] reporting a significant prognostic relationship between the angle of rotation and outcome. A negative correlation between an increase in this angle and a successful outcome was only found for chronic founder cases.[3]

No significant relationship exists between outcome and the height of the animal (ie, ponies had the same prognosis as horses if the severity of clinical and radiologic abnormalities were equally severe).[3]

A significant relationship was found between outcome and the number of feet affected. Acute founder cases with one affected foot had a 33% success rate compared with those affected in two (82%) and four feet (62%).

A significant relationship was also found between grade of lameness and outcome, which is in agreement with a previous report.[10] However, the significance of lameness grade versus outcome disappeared when cases were examined within groups. Laminitis cases may show severe lameness but have no pathologic alteration to the normal digital anatomy and have an excellent prognosis. However, some acute founder cases may exhibit mild lameness yet have clinical and radiologic evidence of significant displacement of the distal phalanx and incur a bad prognosis.

A significant association was seen between prolapse of the sole and outcome. However, the recognition of group had greater prognostic significance than the presence of solar prolapse. This finding is related to founder distance again. Those cases that incurred a small founder distance but a large angle of rotation had a statistically significantly better prognosis than those that incurred a larger founder distance.

The presence of underlying medical pathology adversely affects the prognosis. The most common of these are infection, chronic liver or kidney disease, equine Cushing's disease, or the iatrogenic administration of any corticosteroid drugs. Triamcinolone, dexamethasone, and methylprednisolone, whether administered intramuscularly, intrathecally, intra-articularly, or periligamentously, seem to be the most commonly associated with iatrogenic founder and sinking. Unless a causative medical complication can be effectively treated or eliminated, continued lamellar dysadhesion and a worsening prognosis can be expected.

The Significance of Nomenclature, Supracoronary Depressions, and Founder Distance

Some might think that the differentiation between acute founder and sinker cases arises from semantic confusion. This view is not generated by the results of prognostic studies.[3] Acute founder cases, which show supracoronary depressions extending circumferentially to the quarters of the hoof, invariably have larger founder distances and a worse prognosis than cases in which the supracoronary depression is both less extensive and deep. However, a sinker develops a supracoronary depression all the way around the coronary contour contemporaneously. A sinker with a founder distance of 13 mm has a worse prognosis than an acute founder case with the same founder distance. Nevertheless, the prognostic significance of founder distance continues to apply to sinkers. Sinkers with founder distances of less than 13 mm can be successfully treated using modern therapies, if promptly applied.

Prognosis Related to Hoof Pathology in Cases of Recent Relative Displacement (Acute Founder and Sinker Cases)

Imagine the scenario in which a horse experiences an insult to the lamellae in a non–weight-bearing limb sufficient to cause dysadhesion between the dermal and epidermal lamellae in that hoof. No abnormality will be apparent clinically or radiologically until the limb is loaded, when the four cardinal signs of relative displacement become apparent.

Upon loading, the weight of the horse overcomes the cohesion between the dermal and epidermal lamellae, and relative displacement occurs between the hoof capsule and the distal phalanx. In most cases, the area of lamellar dysadhesion begins in the dorsal hoof so that a palpable depression first appears in the dorsal sagittal plane. Lamellar dysadhesion results in stretching and bending of the dorsal coronary and dorsal terminal papillae. Whether papillary distortion results in tissue necrosis or just a reduction in horn formation is proportional to the founder distance; the higher the founder distance, the more severe the effect on the vascular supply to the papillae.

Some cases also show relative displacement in both proximodistal and dorsopalmar or dorsoplantar axes. Radiologic examination of these cases shows an increased founder distance and unusually large wall thickness. The author's impression is that for a given founder distance, cases that also show displacement in a palmar or plantar direction have a poorer prognosis.

In rare cases, usually coinciding with medial-lateral foot imbalance (both sides of the hoof cannot touch the ground simultaneously without abnormal abduction or adduction of the limb by the horse), a supracoronary depression may first develop on the medial (common) or lateral (uncommon) aspect of the coronary contour. The prognosis for these cases is still significantly related to founder distance, and the treatment concept remains unaltered. Treatments must be applied to the area of the hoof below the supracoronary depression, despite it being on the side of the hoof rather than in the more usual dorsal aspect.

To continue with the imaginary scenario of a non–weight-bearing limb, the hoof of which experiences lamellar dysadhesion, no increase has occurred in the distance between the origin and the insertion of the deep digital flexor muscle. The dorsal lamellar junction has been disrupted, the focus of tension of this muscle, which has allowed the muscle to continue to contract now without counteraction. Contraction of the deep digital flexor muscle thereby causes distraction of the dorsal surface of the distal phalanx from the inner hoof wall and flexion of the distal interphalangeal joint. Whether this contraction continues when the limb is loaded, unloaded, or differentially heel-loaded in a foundering horse has not been determined, nor has the timing of contracture. Whether the flexion of the distal interphalangeal joint in an acute founder case is primarily from flexor contracture or an increase in fluid and tissue pressure forcing the dorsal surface of the distal phalanx from the dorsal hoof wall remains unclear. Through whatever means, the dorsal surface of the distal phalanx will lose parallelism with the dorsal hoof wall in all cases that founder or sink. This movement induces compression of the blood vessels in the solar corium, the circumflex artery, and vein and causes a shearing force to be applied to the surviving lamellae in the palmar/plantar part of the foot. All of these events compromise the digital circulation.

Abcessation is a common sequel during the 3 months after acute founder and sinking. The prognostic significance of abscessation entirely depends on whether an abscess discharges and drains. A supracoronary swelling appears before eruption of a submural abscess. Abscesses that erode into the distal interphalangeal joint or navicular bursa are serious sequelae and often result in the horse being euthanized.

Abscesses that become established within a bone, usually the distal phalanx, causing osteomyelitis are also often fatal.

Pedal abscesses may result in disruption of the hoof/skin junction over a variable area (splitting of the coronary band). Data from a series of 23 acute founder and sinker cases[11] that developed separation of the coronary band at least 8 cm long showed that the outcome was not related to either the chronicity of the case or the presence of concurrent solar prolapse. Outcome was significantly related to founder distance and the character of the fluid discharging from the coronary separation.

Progressive distal phalangeal osteopenia is a common sequel to acute founder cases with large founder distances. The prognostic significance of osteopenia is directly proportional to its severity. As distal phalangeal mass is resorbed, so is the area available for lamellar cohesion and suspension for the distal phalanx within the hoof.

PROGNOSIS DEPENDS ON THE TIMING AND TYPE OF TREATMENTS USED

Effective treatments are those that counteract all of the major pathologic changes that occurred within the hoof after founder or sinking.

REESTABLISHING THE NORMAL ANGULATION OF THE DORSAL CORONARY AND TERMINAL PAPILLAE

Horses that founder but incur founder distances less than 13 mm are able to realign the coronary papillae proximal to the areas of lamellar dysadhesion, with or without treatment. However, this realignment is never perfect and always leaves the papillae at a more acute angle to the ground than it was before the founder episode. The founder distances of these cases are always higher than before they foundered, because the distal tips of the papillae are trapped within the hoof wall, and their only means of realignment is to move their bases in the coronary cushion proximally. This condition can be seen clearly in hoof sections of founder cases (**Fig. 4**).

Subcoronary grooving, thinning of the horn over the coronary corium so that the horn is easily deformed by light finger pressure, often with petechial hemorrhages present through the horn and dorsal wall resection, have been used as treatments for acute founder. None of these, to the author's knowledge, has resulted in reduction of founder distance and realignment of coronary papillae.

Failure to restore parallelism between the angulation of the coronary papillae and the dorsal surface of the distal phalanx always results in a mass of horn production from the lamellae; a lamellar wedge. This results in a hoof that is functionally compromised because the distal phalanx no longer has a normal attachment to the hoof wall. These cases show an increased wall thickness. Gross separation between the stratum medium of the hoof wall and the sole leaves this area open for invasion by debris and infection, including pedal sepsis, seedy toe, and white line disease.

An imperfect reformation of interlamellar cohesion after acute founder or sinking reduces the animal's prognosis as an athlete. Factors that seem to increase the amount of abnormal, submural lamellar horn formation include an increased founder distance, abnormally high tension in the deep digital flexor tendon, and chronic hyperinsulinemia.

Raising the heels of a foundered horse is a treatment for acute founder. Some horses develop marked flexion of the distal interphalangeal joint after acute founder. This flexion is often progressive but then stops, often coincident with the appearance of solar prolapse. At this time, the angle subtended by the dorsal surface of the distal phalanx to the ground is no more than 75°, at which point the torque applied by the

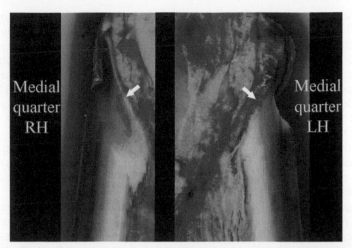

Fig. 4. Postmortem sections of the hind hooves of a case that foundered medially on both hind hooves 14 days previously. The severity of acute founder was more severe on the left (LH) than the right hind (RH). The coronary papillae have realigned in the right hind (*arrowed*), whereas in the left hind, the greater distal displacement of the distal phalanx has left the papillae (*arrowed*) distracted from the hoof wall.

deep digital flexor tendon around the distal sesamoid bone becomes negligible, as does the angular moment. Because of the lack of reports regarding treatment, whether raising the heels prevents either joint flexion or solar prolapse is unclear. If the founder distance is less than 13 mm and the horse has no metabolic condition continuing to destroy the lamellar cohesion, the horse will survive despite whether the heels are raised.

The author does not raise the heels of foundered horses despite the reports of Thomason and colleagues[13] and Hansen and colleagues.[12] If experimental in vivo reports were available of the effectiveness of raising the heels when using a plastic shoe held on by glued tabs, this may be a rational approach to treating acute founder cases, particularly if combined with a coronary peel and dorsodistal wall fenestration for severe cases. The amount of heel raising used in practice seems to be subjective. Raising the heels increases heel loading but puts the phalangeal column still further out of alignment and risks increasing the compression of the dorsal coronary papillae and shearing of the surviving dorsal lamellae, with a consequent increase in founder distance. Questions remain, such as does raising the heels prevent contracture of the deep digital flexor muscle or just mask it? What happens if the horse stabilizes and the heel heights must be reduced? If deep digital contracture occurred during the period of heel elevation, then surgery to the inferior check ligament or deep digital flexor tendon will be necessary to realign the phalangeal bones.

The only clinical situations in which the author has known foundered horses to raise their heels voluntarily by digging their toes into a deep shavings bed are when they have developed deep digital flexor contracture, are developing an abscess in the palmar or plantar parts of the hoof, or have an unprotected solar prolapse that is in contact with the bedding.

Extension of the distal interphalangeal joint can be achieved through lowering the heels, dividing the inferior check ligament or deep digital flexor tendon, or raising the toe using shoe wedges. Lowering the heels in a horse that has an unstable distal phalanx is contraindicated because it will induce increased tension in the deep digital flexor musculotendinous unit[14] and result in increased founder distance and further rotation. The distal phalanx can be deemed unstable in a horse with acute founder if the condition just developed, in the continued presence of supracoronary depressions, and if the horse is experiencing continued pain. When doubt exists, a toe-wedge test can be used. Raising the toe lowers the heels without damaging the hoof. If a toe wedge, (shaped to the hoof so it does not cause sole pressure) is placed under the toe of an acute founder case and the contralateral limb is raised, the horse will resent the procedure and the supracoronary depression will become palpably deeper. In this situation, the heels should not be lowered.

A decision to surgically divide either the inferior check ligament or deep digital flexor tendon should not be made on the clinical appearance of a horse while it is receiving analgesic drugs; these will effectively mask the clinical signs of contracture (ie, tendency to bear weight on the toe and off the heel).

The prognosis for acute founder and sinker cases in which deep digital flexor tenotomies are made depends on the founder distance, the interval between contracture and surgery, whether the phalangeal column is straightened with hoof dressing after surgery, and whether palmar or plantar extension shoes are fitted. Postoperative complications can be minimized through manual restraint of the animal until the effects of local anesthesia have dissipated and a wood shavings bed has been provided, which provides a thick area for recumbency and a less-deeply bedded area for standing.

The tissues that experience compression, stretching, bending, and vascular compromise in the horse's foot after acute founder and sinking have epithelial equivalents in the horse's intestine. The soft tissues in the foot are no more durable than those in the gut; the only difference is that horses take less time to die after gut insults (any surgical colic) than after foot insults (acute founder and sinking). With the development of improved surgical facilities for treating colic, practitioners have little hesitation in advising intervention or referral to remove devitalized regions of intestine or restore normal anatomic relationships within the abdomen. Practitioners who recognize the urgency of instituting treatment of acute founder and sinker cases have found that cases with small founder distances had similar prognosis despite whether invasive or conservative treatments were used,[15] whereas a bad prognosis prevailed for cases with large founder distances no matter what the treatment. This situation tended to reinforce their feeling of hopelessness when treating acute founder and sinker cases.

However, a recently reported technique[16] provides grounds for early intervention and an improved prognosis, even in cases with large founder distances. The technique addresses all three pathologic changes in the foundered horse. Removal of the entire coronary epidermis dependent to supracoronary depressions removes a major constriction in the proximodorsal part of the hoof, allowing distoproximal blood and lymphatic flow; removes malaligned coronary papillae; and allows the coronary tissues to remodel in a more normal relationship to the distal phalanx, with a reduction in founder distance. Fenestration of the dorsodistal hoof wall allows drainage of serosanguinous fluid from the dorsal, interlamellar space and the dorsal solar corium, and prevents compression on the dermal tissues by malaligned but still vital terminal papillae. Concurrent division of the deep flexor tendon prevents shearing of the lamellae in the palmar part of the hoof and abolishes compression on the subsolar blood vessels and epidermal structures they supply. A normal phalangeal axis is also restored. The technique results in marked reduction of pain and requires minimal postoperative analgesia.

The prompt application of the above procedure seems critical; delay (more than 14 days from onset of displacement) is likely to significantly reduce the likelihood of a successful outcome.

OTHER FACTORS THAT INFLUENCE PROGNOSIS OF ACUTE FOUNDER OR SINKER CASES
Economics and Enthusiasm of the Owner

The treatment is likely to cost more than the owner can, or is willing, to pay. This cost depends on the treatments used. The prompt application of the partial coronary epidermectomy (coronary peel), dorsodistal wall fenestration, and deep digital flexor tenotomy technique[16] results in a significantly reduced hospitalization time, reduced drug and dressings costs, and a quicker return to work. Nevertheless, despite the treatment used, a horse that has experienced acute founder or sinking should not be worked until a new hoof wall has grown down, which takes an average of 8 months. An incomplete hoof capsule means an incomplete area for supporting lamellar cohesion, and therefore exercise-induced founder is a real risk until healing is complete.

Uncontrollable, Severe Pain

When appropriate, treatments should be terminated on humane grounds. These cases may self-harm, sometimes fatally. However, in the author's experience, these cases are rare.

Anticipated Prognosis

The anticipated prognosis depends on the knowledge, attitude, experience, and skill of the attending veterinary surgeon, nurses, and farrier.

The Attitude of the Animal

Successfully treated animals have a spirit or will to live but will allow treatments, and will lie down and rest between treatments. This process is enhanced by a quiet environment for their stabling and treatments and, in some cases, the adjacent stabling of a long-time companion so they can see and hear one another.

Cases for Whom Treatments Fail

Even the most modern treatments cannot save some horses. In the author's experience, cases that received corticosteroid drugs or who experienced a delay in beginning effective treatments are those for whom treatments most commonly fail. The most significant signs of a positive response to treatment are a reduction in the palpable depth and collateral extent of supracoronary depressions; reduction in founder distance; increased comfort and resumption of a normal stance, independent of analgesics; and renewed hoof growth in the areas previously dependent to supracoronary depressions.

Religious Beliefs of the Owner

Some religions do not allow humane destruction of animals and owners may wait for the will of their God to be exerted. In cases of extreme suffering, it behoves veterinary surgeons to exert the humane will of man and euthanize instead of waiting for a God to intervene.

PROGNOSIS IN CASES OF CHRONIC RELATIVE DISTAL PHALANGEAL DISPLACEMENT (CHRONIC FOUNDER)

The treatment of chronic founder cases is generally much less challenging and thus less rewarding than acute cases. Although the tissues are amenable to reconstruction in acute cases, this is not so when the case is chronic.

The aim of treatment in these cases is to optimize, as far as is practicable, the functionality of the horse through correcting or minimizing the painful effects of the pathologic changes characteristic of chronic founder.

Prognosis for these cases is significantly related to (1) the angle subtended by the phalangeal axis and the ground, (2) grade of lameness, (3) founder distance, and (4) the extent of distal phalangeal osteopenia.[3,4]

Based on a limited number of cases, performing a coronary peel on a chronic founder case does not improve founder distance. Removal of the lamellar wedge either through hoof trimming or dorsal wall resection rarely prevents the regrowth of lamellar horn and a distorted hoof. However, if dorsal lamellar horn is not removed, a gradual loss of parallelism between the dorsal hoof wall and the dorsal surface of the distal phalanx develops, causing the distal interphalangeal joint to remain in a flexed position. This position impairs functionality, displaces the horny sole distally, and impairs digital circulation. The only way to prevent this is through regular hoof trimming to restore the parallel relationship between the remaining dorsal wall and the dorsal surface of the distal phalanx. This maintenance has the added benefit of removing the distorted horn around the white line, preventing the ingress of debris that may lead to horn infections or subsequent pedal sepsis. Depending on the amount of white line separation palmarly or plantarly, these cases demand strict hoof hygiene if horn infection at the quarters is to be avoided.

Compared with the distorted coronary papillae in the dorsal parts of the foot, palmar or plantar coronary papillae are unaffected by relative displacement of the distal phalanx. This finding results in a higher rate of heel horn growth compared with horn derived from the toe. Repeatedly removing more heel horn than toe horn will help maintain a normal phalangeal axis. Horses that experience acute founder but incur a small founder distance show the characteristic divergent growth rings for approximately 4 months after foundering. Thereafter, any growth rings that become visible may be nearly, but never perfectly, concentric (**Fig. 5**).

If the horse experiences further episodes of acute founder, each time incurring a small increase in founder distance, the divergence in hoof growth rings becomes

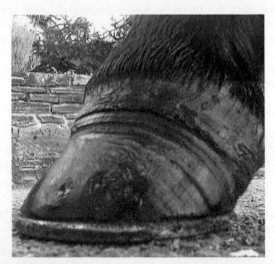

Fig. 5. The hoof of a chronic founder case after four episodes of acute founder; subsequent hoof growth, as shown by divergent rings, is never again equal.

more obvious. Each time the horse founders, an increase in founder distance and wall thickness results.

In some horses, the phalangeal axis cannot be restored with dorsal hoof wall trimming and lowering of the heels, and these cases are lamer after these changes are made. A toe-wedge test, made before lowering the heels, will identify cases that have significant deep digital flexor muscle contracture. The prognosis for these cases is at best guarded. The treatment options are either to leave the heels at a height that allows the distal interphalangeal joint to remain partly flexed but with the animal reasonably comfortable, or resection of the inferior check ligament or division of the deep digital flexor tendon (DDFT) in an attempt to realign the phalangeal column.

The decision to perform a desmotomy or tenotomy is made on clinical grounds when the animal is not receiving analgesics. If the flexure is mild, a desmotomy may be appropriate. In more severe cases, in which a large heel height would have to be removed to achieve straightening of the phalangeal column, a tenotomy may be preferred. The prognosis for these cases depends on whether a significant amount of distal phalangeal osteopenia is present and the chronicity of the case. If significant distal phalangeal bone loss, and consequent lamellar area reduction, has occurred, then it is common for the horse to founder acutely after surgery and for the DDFM to re-contract over the next 12 months. Additionally, even in longstanding cases that have experienced minimal distal phalangeal osteopenia, remodeling of the ligaments may have occurred in the palmar part of the hoof, so that even after tenotomy the middle and distal phalanges remain unable to assume normal alignment. These cases cannot be diagnosed before surgery, and the possible sequelae should be explained to the owner or keeper of the horse. DDFT tenotomy of these cases invariably results in an increase in lameness often to the point at which euthanasia is required.

Chronic founder cases remain susceptible to episodes of laminitis or acute founder. Prognostically, the clinical signs of chronic founder should be noted, because these will affect treatment choices and prognostic evaluations (**Fig. 6**).

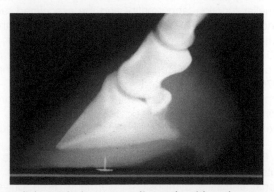

Fig. 6. This lateromedial weight-bearing radiograph, although correctly positioned for measurements relating to founder, is overexposed so that the soft tissues cannot be evaluated. The lack of a dorsal wall marker and the untrimmed drawing pin compounds the poor technique. Without clinical information relating to the presence of supracoronary depressions, this could be a case of laminitis, sinking, or acute founder. Unless information relating to the presence of divergent growth rings is provided, this film could also be from a recently trimmed chronic founder case. Without adequate clinical information, radiologic examination of these films is neither diagnostic nor prognostic.

Rather than term every case a *chronic laminitic*, clinicians should instead refer to them as a chronic founder case with laminitis or a chronic founder case having foundered again. The use of this terminology tends to clear the thinking of the clinician and allow for more accurate prognoses and more timely and appropriate treatments.

SUMMARY

Classifying cases as laminitis, acute founder, sinkers, and chronic founders based solely on clinical examination is the most statistically significant prognostic indicator yet reported. The measurement, and correction for magnification effects, of founder distance using a standardized radiographic technique enables refinement of prognosis for acute founder and sinker cases. The coronary peel, deep digital flexor tenotomy, and dorsodistal hoof wall fenestration technique treats the pathologic changes after acute founder and facilitates restoration of normal hoof anatomy, thereby improving prognosis.

REFERENCES

1. O'Grady SE, Parks AW, Redden RF, et al. Podiatry terminology. Equine Vet Educ 2007;19:263.
2. Hood DM. Laminitis in the horse. Vet Clin North Am Equine Pract 1999;15:287.
3. Cripps PJ, Eustace RA. Factors involved in the prognosis of equine laminitis in the UK. Equine Vet J 1999;31:433.
4. Eustace RA. Radiological measurements involved in the prognosis of equine laminitis [Fellowship Thesis]. London: Royal Collage of Veterinary Surgeons (RCVS); 1991.
5. Cripps PJ, Eustace RA. Radiological measurements from the feet of normal horses with relevance to laminitis. Equine Vet J 1999;31:427.
6. Bushe T, Turner TA, Poulos PW, et al. The effect of hoof angle on coffin, pastern and fetlock joint angles. In: Proceedings of the American Association of Equine Practitioners. Phoenix (Ariz): AAEP; 1987. p. 729.
7. Linford RL. A radiographic, morphometric, histological, and ultrastructural investigation of lamellar function, abnormality and the associated radiographic findings for sound and footsore thoroughbreds, and horses with experimentally induced traumatic and alimentary laminitis [dissertation]. Davis, Calif: University of California Davis; 1987.
8. Baxter GM. Equine laminitis caused by distal displacement of the distal phalanx: 12 cases (1976–1985). J Am Vet Med Assoc 1986;189:326.
9. Stick JA, Lann HW, Scott EA, et al. Pedal bone rotation as a prognostic sign in laminitis of horses. J Am Vet Med Assoc 1982;180:251.
10. Hunt RJ. A retrospective evaluation of laminitis in horses. Equine Vet J 1993; 25:61.
11. Eustace RA, Emery SL. Partial separation of the hoof at the coronary band following acute founder or sinking—a review of 23 cases. In: Proceedings of the International Laminitis Symposium. Germany: Free University of Berlin; 2008.
12. Hansen N, Buchner F, Haller J, et al. Evaluation using strain gauges of a therapeutic shoe and a hoof cast with a heel wedge as potential supportive therapy for horses with laminitis. Vet Surg 2005;34:630.
13. Thomason JJ, Biewener AA, Bertram JEA. Surface strain on the equine hoof wall in vivo: implications for the material design and functional morphology of the wall. J Exp Biol 1992;166:145.

14. Wilson AM, Eustace RA, Naylor JRJ, et al. The effect of wedge shoeing on tendon force in the equine distal limb. In: Proceedings of the Association of Equine Sports Medicine. Fallbrook, CA, March 13–16, 1993. p. 33.
15. Peremans K, Verschooten F, De Moor A, et al. Laminitis in the pony: conservative treatment vs dorsal hoof wall resection. Equine Vet J 1991;23:243.
16. Eustace RA, Emery SL. Partial coronary epidermectomy (coronary peel), dorso-distal wall fenestration and deep digital flexor tenotomy to treat severe acute founder in a Connemara pony. Equine Vet Educ 2009;21:91.

Farriery for Chronic Laminitis

Stephen E. O'Grady, DVM, MRCVS

KEYWORDS

- Chronic laminitis • Lamellae • Displacement • Realignment
- Therapeutic farriery • Wooden shoe

Laminitis is considered chronic once the distal phalanx has displaced within the hoof capsule. Chronic laminitis generally occurs as a direct sequel to acute laminitis, but at present, it is not possible to predict which horses with acute laminitis will progress to chronic laminitis let alone when it will occur or if it will happen at all. Because the bulk of laminitis research has been directed toward acute laminitis, treatment regimens for chronic laminitis are generally empirically based on the past experience of the attending clinician/farrier. The biggest challenge to the veterinarian and the farrier is to improve the morphology and function of a foot or feet that may have potential, substantial, and possibly permanent structural changes. It should be remembered from the onset that the extent of the pathologic condition of the lamellae influences not only the ability to treat a horse with laminitis but also the eventual outcome of a laminitic case.[1,2] Each case of laminitis should be approached on an individual basis, noting the predisposing cause, clinical signs, physical examination, movement, foot conformation, and structures of the foot that can be used to change the forces placed on or within the hoof capsule. These observations then suggest the overall goals of treatment that address the anatomic and functional abnormalities identified. The approaches to treatment should be based on principles aimed at restoring the form and function in a given laminitic foot rather than on any method of farriery or a product. This article presents an overview of chronic laminitis and addresses those farriery principles that can be used to treat chronic laminitis. It is imperative that medical, metabolic, environmental, and dietary issues be addressed concurrently with foot management in chronic laminitis.

CHRONIC LAMINITIS

Chronic laminitis is defined by the presence of mechanical collapse of the lamellae and displacement of the distal phalanx within the hoof capsule.[3] There are 3 manifestations of displacement of the distal phalanx: dorsal capsular rotation, distal displacement (sinking), and mediolateral rotation or asymmetric distal displacement (**Fig. 1**). A combination of all 3 forms of displacement can exist simultaneously. Lamellar

Northern Virginia Equine, PO Box 746, Marshall, VA 20116, USA
E-mail address: sogrady@look.net

Vet Clin Equine 26 (2010) 407–423
doi:10.1016/j.cveq.2010.04.008
0749-0739/10/$ – see front matter © 2010 Elsevier Inc. All rights reserved.

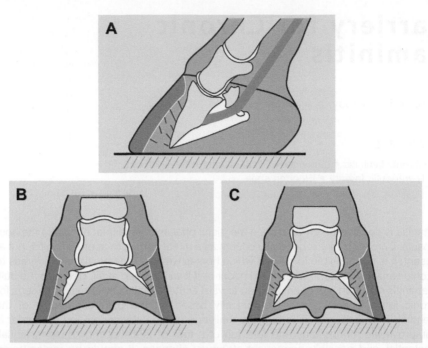

Fig. 1. (*A*) Dorsal capsular rotation, (*B*) mediolateral rotation, and (*C*) distal displacement (sinking).

separation of the distal phalanx occurs when the forces acting on the lamellae exceed their tensile strength. In simplistic terms, the acute phase is the phase of injury and chronic phases are phases of tissue repair. The eventual outcome of the treatment for horses with chronic laminitis can be divided into function and morphology. The functional outcome is most likely to dictate the difference between athletic performance, pasture soundness, and euthanasia. The morphologic outcome is more likely to determine the degree to which continued and potentially lifelong therapeutic measures are necessary. At the onset of chronic laminitis, the eventual outcome is hard to predict, but the most important indicator for survival remains to be the severity of the initial insult to the lamellae. The appearance of the initial radiographs does not necessarily correlate with either the functional or the morphologic outcome. The thickness of the sole and the angle between the solar surface of the distal phalanx and the ground appear to be better indicators of the degree of difficulty in treating horses with dorsal capsular rotation, and both the parameters appear more useful than using just the degree of rotation in successfully predicting the rehabilitation of the horse.[4] In contrast to treating horses with acute laminitis, in which medical therapy frequently assumes priority, hoof care is the most important element for success in treating horses with chronic laminitis.

PATHOPHYSIOLOGY OF CHRONIC LAMINITIS

A brief review of the pathophysiology and the mechanical events that occur in the lamellae, leading to chronic laminitis, may provide some useful insight into the principles of therapy. Separation of the lamellae is a consequence of the severity of the original pathologic processes, such as inflammation, ischemia, thrombosis, and the mechanical load placed on the lamellae. Lamellar separation at any point around the circumference of the distal phalanx is, therefore, a balance between the severity of the underlying disease processes and the magnitude of lamellar stresses. The way in which the distal phalanx displaces is related to the distribution of lamellar separation around the circumference of the distal phalanx and is therefore related to the distribution of the disease and stresses. The greatest stress imposed on the lamellae is weight bearing. Superimposed on weight bearing is the stress caused by the moment about the distal interphalangeal joint and the tension in the deep digital flexor tendon, which is opposed by tension in the dorsal lamellae. Movement of the horse alters the magnitude and position of the ground reaction force (GRF) and the tension in the deep digital flexor tendon and therefore the magnitude and distribution of load placed on the lamellae. As a horse lifts a foot off the ground, the load on the contralateral limb is doubled. Also, as a horse moves, stress or load is concentrated on the dorsal hoof wall at breakover. Circumferential lamellar loss predisposes to distal displacement (sinking) of the entire distal phalanx within the hoof capsule. In contrast, relatively greater lamellar disruption at the toe or at either quarter causes the distal phalanx to displace asymmetrically within the hoof capsule. When this loss is greatest dorsally, the result is dorsal capsular or phalangeal rotation.[5] Capsular rotation refers to deviation of the parietal surface of the distal phalanx with respect to the hoof capsule. Phalangeal rotation refers to rotation of the distal phalanx with respect to the axis of the proximal phalanges (ie, distal interphalangeal joint flexion). If 1 quarter suffers greater lamellar injury or if excessive load is placed on 1 quarter, the distal phalanx displaces unilaterally (sinks medially or laterally). This displacement is a far less-frequent scenario than dorsal capsular rotation. It is the author's clinical impression that unilateral displacement is conformationally driven such that a disproportionate amount of load is placed on 1 side of the foot. When unilateral displacement occurs, it generally involves the medial side of the foot.

Immediately after mechanical failure of the dorsal lamellae and rotation of the distal phalanx, the dorsal hoof wall is still straight and is of normal thickness, but the space created by the separation is filled due to hemorrhage and with inflamed and necrotic tissue. As the tissue begins to heal, the space is variably filled with hyperplastic and hyperkeratinized epidermis. The lamellae exhibit varying degrees of dysplasia, widening and shortening with a loss of primary or secondary lamellae. This condition results in decrease of surface area between the epidermal and dermal lamellae and therefore a decreased strength of the attachment. Concurrent with lamellar healing or repair is the continued hoof growth and the development of the characteristic distortion of the dorsal wall. The severity of the distortion of the hoof wall varies, and changes in the thickness of the hoof wall and divergence of the hoof wall from the parietal surface of the distal phalanx occur. The change in thickness of the hoof wall seems to be related to a change in the conformation of the coronary groove, so that it is wider and shallower. There are several potential causes for the redirection of the dorsal hoof wall away from the distal phalanx: the disparity of growth rate between the hoof at the heels and toes, the composition of the repair tissue between the hoof capsule and the distal phalanx, pressure on the distal surface of the hoof wall, causing continued distraction from the distal phalanx, and redirection of the dermal papillae of the coronary band.[3] In most horses, the new hoof wall growth from the coronary band is approximately parallel to the parietal surface of the distal phalanx, at least until it has reached the junction of the proximal and middle thirds of the hoof wall. At this juncture, the proximal and distal portions of the hoof wall form 2 distinct angles with the ground, separated by a margin between the hoof wall that is formed before the onset of laminitis and that is formed subsequently. This deviation is referred to as the lamellar wedge. In some horses, the newly formed hoof wall diverges from the parietal surface of the distal phalanx at the coronary band.

Displacement of the distal phalanx within the hoof capsule also causes the sole to drop, causing the concavity of the sole to disappear. As the new dorsal hoof wall grows out and reaches the ground surface, the white line becomes wider, reflecting the increased space between the stratum medium of the hoof wall and the parietal surface of the distal phalanx.

The exact causes of pain in chronically laminitic horses are undetermined, but pain is likely to be related to continued ischemia, inflammation, and trauma to the dorsal lamellae and ischemia or inflammation associated with bruising of the dermis of the sole immediately below the solar margin of the distal phalanx. Pain is also associated with the foci of infection causing increased subsolar or intramural pressure. In addition, contraction of the hoof may cause pain that is localized to the palmar/plantar aspect of the foot.[3]

CLINICAL EVALUATION

The diagnosis of chronic laminitis is seldom a challenge because the gait and appearance of the foot are characteristic of the disease, and radiographic examination usually removes all doubts. Occasionally, nerve blocks are necessary to localize the pain in the foot of mildly affected horses and are interpreted in conjunction with hoof tester application and radiographs.

Horses with chronic laminitis present in several ways: (1) as the continuation of acute laminitis, (2) as the recurrence of past chronic laminitis, or (3) with an unknown history, because the acute phase was never observed or the horse was purchased without knowledge of the disease.

Full evaluation of the history, the horse, and the digits is important in determining the prognosis and treatment.[6] The severity of the initial acute phase is the best indicator of the extent of the original damage and hence a major factor in prognosis. The duration of the disease since the acute phase gives some indication as to how much the lamellar repair process may have stabilized the distal phalanx within the hoof capsule. How lame the horse is, including how willing it is to walk, how stiffly it walks, how willing it is to lift up a foot, and how much it lies down, correlates neither with the prognosis as well as it does in acute laminitis nor necessarily with the clinical appearance of the foot or the changes observed by radiography. How the animal preferentially places its foot may indicate the distribution of lamellar injury; for example, a horse that preferentially bears its weight on its heels reduces the tension in the dorsal lamellae and the compression of the sole beneath the dorsal margin of the distal phalanx. Similarly, a horse that lands on one side of its foot may protect the contralateral wall or sole. In addition, the way a horse moves is an adjunct to determining the placement and type of shoe to use. Observation of the hoof wall, sole and white line along with palpation of the coronary band provides clinical indicators for the pathologic processes that have occurred within the digit, including capsular distortion, displacement of the distal phalanx, presence of infection, and secondary contraction of the hoof or flexor apparatus.[4,6,7] Of great importance is the necessity to evaluate the structures of the foot, especially the palmar/plantar area. As a rule, it is this section of the foot that is recruited to assume additional load in an attempt to unload the dorsal hoof wall. If the mass and integrity of these structures are inadequate to accept additional load, this creates another challenge to the clinician in redistributing the weight of the horse.

RADIOLOGY

The lateral radiograph has always been considered the gold standard for evaluating acute and chronic laminitis, but it limits the evaluation of the distal phalanx to 1 plane. It does not help in the identification of an asymmetric medial or a lateral distal displacement of the distal phalanx. Therefore, the author considers it crucial that a dorsopalmar (DP) (dorso 0° palmar) radiographic projection be included as part of the radiographic study for either acute or chronic laminitis.[2,4,8,9] An oblique DP view may also be included to evaluate the margin and integrity of the distal phalanx. Good-quality radiographs are required to visualize the osseous structures within the hoof capsule as well as the hoof capsule itself. Radiopaque markers can be used to determine the position of the distal phalanx in relation to surface landmarks.

The radiographic features of chronic laminitis are well documented.[10] The following observations from a lateral radiograph are important in guiding treatment: the thickness of the dorsal hoof wall, the degree of dorsal capsular rotation, the angle of the solar surface of the distal phalanx relative to the ground, the distance between the dorsal, distal margin of the distal phalanx and the ground, the position of the distal interphalangeal joint, and the thickness of the sole.

The DP radiograph is examined to determine the horizontal position of the distal phalanx in the frontal plane. Asymmetric distal displacement of the distal phalanx is present on either the lateral or medial side, if an imaginary line drawn across the articular surface of the distal interphalangeal joint or between the foramens of the semilunar canal of the distal phalanx is not parallel to the ground, the joint space is widened on the affected side and narrowed on the opposite side, and the width of the hoof wall appears thicker than normal on the affected side (**Fig. 2**). If the position of the coronary band is visible on the radiograph, then the distance between the coronary band and the palmar processes of the distal phalanx will be greater on the affected than the unaffected side.[3] The location of gas pockets is determined by correlating the findings of the lateral and DP radiographs. The margin of the distal

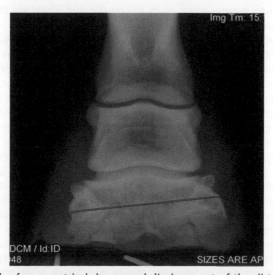

Fig. 2. Radiograph of asymmetrical downward displacement of the distal phalanx on the medial side. Note a line drawn through the foramens of the semi lunar canal are not parallel with the ground. Also note the disparity in the joint space from the lateral to the medial side and the thickness of the medial hoof wall.

phalanx is evaluated for the presence of pedal osteitis, sequestra, and marginal fractures on the oblique DP view.

With the advent of digital radiography, an image can be generated on site during the initial examination of chronic laminitis and also can be used immediately after treating the horse to access the accuracy of the farriery.

Venograms of the foot can be performed and may indicate the presence of filling defects in the digital vasculature, signifying a poor prognosis; namely, filling defects in the lamellar vessels, the circumflex area, and the terminal arch. The scope of venograms and the technique to perform a proper venogram are discussed in issues 1 and 2 of this series.

Hoof Care

It is not possible to directly reattach the mechanically separated lamellae; hence, the return of the mechanical function of the wall is a gradual process that may take up to 9 months barring complications. It is important to maintain an environment that enhances natural healing and/or the efficacy of other therapies. In case of chronic laminitis, this is rest and hoof care.[4] Absolute stall rest in the early stages of chronic laminitis is imperative, because movement of the horse is associated with increased stress placed on the damaged lamellae. Rest must be balanced against some form of exercise that is needed to restore normal function of the hoof capsule, which is achieved with repeated expansion and contraction of the hoof as the animal moves.

The mainstay of hoof care is therapeutic farriery.[2,4,7,11] In considering hoof care for horses with chronic laminitis, there are 3 goals of therapy: to stabilize the distal phalanx within the hoof capsule, to control pain, and to encourage new hoof growth to assume the most normal relationship to the distal phalanx possible.[2,4,7] It is necessary to stabilize the foot so that there is no further injury to the remaining or new lamellar attachments that are being formed. It is desirable to control the horse's pain for humane reasons as well as to restore limited function as the affected foot or feet heal to spare the other limbs from excessive weight bearing. Encouraging the foot to return to normal form, both physically and anatomically, is the surest way to optimize future function.

Attempting to stabilize the distal phalanx within the hoof capsule is important to prevent further rotation/displacement, promote healing, and decrease pain. Therefore, understanding how the stability of the distal phalanx within the hoof capsule affects the convalescence of a chronically laminitic horse is important. But there is no direct measure of stability except for pain, and the obvious progression of displacement determined by radiographs is associated with severe instability. The best indication available that the distal phalanx is more stable is that the horse is more comfortable because increased stability decreases tissue trauma.[2,4]

To achieve the goals outlined earlier, there are several farriery principles that should be followed.[2,4,5,7] Stabilizing the hoof capsule requires decreasing the stress on the most-damaged lamellae. Therefore, the principles are to reduce the load on the most severely affected wall by transfering it to a less severely affected wall, to recruit all available ground surface of the foot to bear weight, and to decrease the moment about the distal interphalangeal joint as necessary. To summarize these principles in simplistic farriery terms (1) recruit all available ground surface that is capable of bearing weight, (2) position breakover appropriately, and (3) provide heel elevation, if necessary. Pain caused by lamellar stress and injury is in part controlled by increasing stability within the foot. Pain associated with subsolar ischemia, trauma, and bruising is decreased by avoiding direct pressure on the ground surface of the foot immediately below the margin of the distal phalanx. The most important principle in limiting the residual capsular rotation as the hoof initially grows out is to eliminate load on the distal, dorsal hoof wall. There are a limited, although steadily increasing, number of methods and materials available to the veterinarian and farrier to apply these principles, but the variety of ways in which they can be applied is even greater. Above all, focus should be maintained on principles and not methods.

THERAPEUTIC FARRIERY
The Trim

The trim is the underlying basis for treatment of all horses with chronic dorsal capsular/ phalangeal rotation. The immediate objective of the trim is to realign the ground surface of the hoof capsule with the solar surface of the distal phalanx. To do this realignment accurately and consistently, it requires radiographic guidance. The long-term objective of trimming is to restore the best possible anatomic relationship between the distal phalanx and the hoof capsule. Before initiating the trim, the horse should be observed walking in a straight line and on turns. The degree of lameness and the landing pattern of the horse should be assessed and noted.

The angle between the solar margin of the distal phalanx and the ground surface of the hoof is approximately 2° to 5°, and the distance from the dorsal, solar margin of the distal phalanx to the ground surface of the hoof is approximately 15 to 20 mm (**Fig. 3**). These measurements vary slightly based on the conformation, size, and breed of the horse, but without prior radiographs, they serve as working reference points. Therefore, the plane of the trim can be estimated from the radiograph by drawing a line that is approximately parallel and 15 to 20 mm distal to the solar margin of the distal phalanx. Depending on the degree of rotation and the amount of sole growth after the injury, the distance from the dorsal margin of the distal phalanx to the ground surface is frequently less than normal. It is important to preserve the thickness of the sole up to 15 to 20 mm because thinner soles are associated with increased bruising and pain. However, in horses in which the thickness of the dorsal sole is less than 15 to 20 mm, the ground surface of the hoof cannot be realigned to the solar margin of the distal

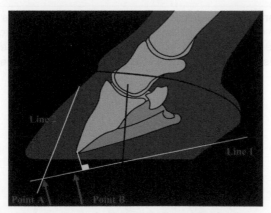

Fig. 3. A schematic representation of a lateral radiograph of a foot with dorsal capsular rotation. Black line shows the center of rotation. Line 1 is drawn approximately parallel and about 15 mm distal to the solar surface of the distal phalanx. Line 2 is drawn parallel and approximately 15–18 mm dorsal to the parietal surface of the distal phalanx. Point A at the intersection of line 1 and line 2 is the furthest dorsal point the toe of the shoe should be set. Point B is approximately 6 mm dorsal to the dorsal margin of the distal phalanx and is the approximate location of the point of breakover. (*Courtesy of* Dr Andrew Parks, University of Georgia.)

phalanx from the toe to the heels without decreasing the thickness of the sole. Therefore, in such horses, the walls and sole can only be trimmed palmar to the point where the distance from the solar margin to the ground surface of the hoof capsule is greater than 15 to 20 mm. Consequently, the dorsal and palmar aspects of the ground surface of the hoof capsule may form 2 different planes after being trimmed (**Figs. 4** and **5**). The junction between the 2 planes is seldom palmar to the widest point of the foot but can be located anywhere in front of this point to the toe. The other consequence of trimming the foot in this manner is that lowering the heels causes increased tension in the deep digital flexor tendon, which may increase the pain associated with weight bearing and movement. The uneven ground surface of the hoof and the increase in deep digital flexor tendon tension should be addressed at the time of shoeing.

To place the trim in a practical prospective, the frog is trimmed to the point where it is solid and pliable. A line is then drawn across the widest part of the foot with a felt-tipped marker. This line gives a referable guideline because it remains fairly constant and is the point where information from the radiograph can be transferred to the foot. From this line, the heels are lowered or moved palmarly or plantarly according to the depth of the sole noted on the radiograph. It is desirable to complete the trim with the heels of the hoof capsule and the frog on the same plane, if possible (**Fig. 6**).

Some horses such as those with metabolic disease may be satisfactorily treated with trimming alone. Such horses usually have adequate sole depth, can be trimmed with a single sole plane, have minimal phalangeal rotation, and are comfortable walking on soft surfaces with or without low doses of analgesics. Boots with foam pad inserts may be used to make barefooted horses more comfortable, but the author would rather rely on deep bedding and walking on deformable surfaces. If barefoot care is desired, but trimming to realign the distal phalanx with the ground is not possible without either reducing the thickness of the dorsal sole or creating 2 planes on the ground surface of the foot, it may be possible to realign the distal phalanx in gradual steps over time.

Shoes

It is readily apparent that no single prescription, shoe type, or device is effective in treating all horses with chronic capsular and/or phalangeal rotation due to several reasons such as the disease varies so much in its initial severity, the difference in individual foot conformation, horses present at various stages of the disease, and the progression and

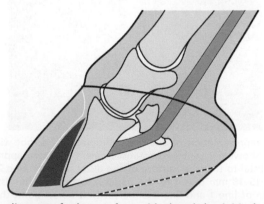

Fig. 4. A schematic diagram of a horse's foot with chronic laminitis that has severe dorsal capsular rotation. The dotted line represents line 1 in **Fig. 3**. Trimming along this line will result in the ground surface forming 2 different planes.

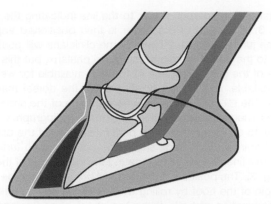

Fig. 5. After trimming along line 1 from radiograph in **Fig. 3**. Note that the dorsal and palmar aspects of the ground surface now form 2 different planes.

previous treatments are highly varied. However, there are guidelines that have been proved useful and can be adapted to the needs of an individual horse.[2,4,7]

GENERAL PRINCIPLES FOR FARRIERY

There are 3 main considerations involved in shoe selection and the shoeing technique: (1) where to position the point of breakover, (2) whether to provide support for the ground surface of the frog and sole and if so which type and how, and (3) whether to elevate the heels.[4] A brief discussion of these considerations, because they apply to the practical treatment of chronic laminitis, may be helpful.

The objective of moving the point of breakover palmarly, compared with normal shoeing practices, is to improve the ease of movement by decreasing the stresses within the dorsal lamellae. There is some debate as to where the optimal position for the point of breakover should really be in horses with dorsal capsular rotation. However, a good guideline is to draw a line on the radiograph from the distal, dorsal

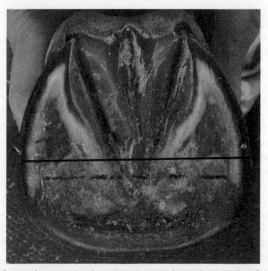

Fig. 6. Heels of hoof capsule moved palmarly/plantarly from the middle of the foot. This creates 2 planes on the ground surface of the foot. Black line denotes the widest part of the foot.

margin of the distal phalanx perpendicular to the line indicating the desired plane of the trim (see **Fig. 3**). The point of breakover is then positioned approximately 6 to 9 mm dorsal to the junction of the 2 lines. Some clinicians will position the point of breakover palmar to the dorsal margin of the distal phalanx, but this can significantly decrease the area of the ground surface of the foot available for weight bearing and render the foot unstable. In addition, positioning of the dorsal margin of the shoe warrants attention. The most dorsal point where the toe of the shoe should be positioned is best determined by drawing a third line on the radiograph, which is parallel to and approximately 15 to 18 mm from the parietal surface of the distal phalanx (see **Fig. 3**). The dorsal margin of the shoe should be positioned no further dorsally than the intersection of this line and the line indicating the ideal plane of the ground surface of the foot (see **Fig. 3**). The position of the point of breakover can be moved palmarly to the dorsal margin of the hoof by rolling the toe of the shoe, setting the shoe palmarly, or by a combination of both. If the toe of the shoe impinges on the dorsal margins of a thin sole immediately below the dorsal margin of the distal phalanx, the pressure causes bruising and ischemia and the horse experiences more pain.

The objective of supporting the sole and frog is to reduce weight bearing by the wall and thereby reduce the stress on the lamellae. It also increases the ground surface in the palmar/plantar section of the foot. The ground surface of the frog and sole can be supported, in part or fully, by a bar shoe, by pads, or by a synthetic composite. Bars only support part of the ground surface of the foot. Pads are usually placed between the shoe and ground surface of the foot. However, pads do not usually extend distally into the space between the branches of the shoe and may place pressure on the dorsal sole beneath the distal phalanx, and therefore, they do not provide maximal support. Synthetic polymers, such as impression material (Equilox Pink Impression Material, Eqilox International Inc, Pine Island, MN, USA) or polyurethane (Equi-Pak, Vettec Inc, Oxnard, CA, USA), mold to the ground surface of the foot and fill the space between the branches of the shoe and therefore provide the greatest degree of support to the ground surface of the foot under the sole and frog. The sole and frog support must be carefully tailored to the individual horse. Specifically, support provided immediately below the dorsal margin of the distal phalanx must be avoided or modified in horses with thin dorsal soles that are sensitive to pressure.

The objective of elevating the heels is to decrease the tension in the deep digital flexor tendon, which decreases the moment about the distal interphalangeal joint, with the intention of decreasing the stresses within the dorsal lamellae. This heel elevation is usually most appropriate in horses with phalangeal rotation that land toe first when walking in a straight line. The amount of heel elevation required varies between 2° and 6°. Heel elevation may be obtained with wedged shoes, pads, or rails (described later). The efficacy of heel elevation is best judged by the comfort of the horse, both at rest and during walking. How a horse lands is a good guideline that the amount of heel elevation is appropriate. Ideally, the heel elevation is such that the horse just lands heel first. If a horse lands markedly heel first, there is too much heel elevation, whereas if it lands toe first, there is not enough heel elevation. This concept assumes that other causes of pain have been precluded, particularly dorsal sole pressure. Prolonged heel elevation causes heel contracture, which potentially causes the heels themselves to become painful. Therefore, the least heel elevation necessary should be used and removed as rapidly as possible, compatible with the improvement in lameness.

An experienced clinician may well have a good idea of what measures are effective based on history, physical examination, and radiographs. For horses with dorsal capsular/phalangeal rotation, (1) moving the point of breakover palmarly is beneficial; (2) providing sole and frog support is based on the severity of the gait, the thickness of the sole, and the response of the horse to hoof tester application over the sole; and (3) elevating the heel, and the degree of elevation, is based on the severity of the lameness and whether the foot lands flat, heel first, or toe first. Knowing when to remove various aspects of the supportive care follows a similar process in reverse.

TYPES OF SHOES

Similar results may be obtained with several, if not many, different ways of shoeing. Success with any given technique increases with the experience of both the veterinarian and the farrier. Shoes such as egg-bar shoes, heart-bar shoes, reverse shoes, aluminum rail shoes, and the wooden shoe all have merit and have had their successes and failures. The author has been most successful using a wide web aluminum shoe or a wooden shoe.

Wide Web Aluminum Shoe

A wide web aluminum shoe forms an inexpensive, simple, and basic therapeutic shoe. Any one of the various brands that are manufactured can be used. The shoe is lightweight; yet the web is wide and sturdy, the shape can be easily altered, and it can be glued to the foot with a composite (Equilox International Inc), if desired. The toe of the shoe is made into a blunt shape, and the shoe is fitted to the trimmed foot again, using the radiograph as a template. The line drawn across the middle of the foot can act as a guideline for placing the shoe. The thickness of the web of the shoe is tapered using a grinder to move the point of breakover in a palmar/plantar direction. The branches of the shoe at the quarters can also be beveled with a grinder to provide an enhanced mediolateral breakover. The heels of the shoe should not extend excessively beyond the heels of the hoof capsule. Heel elevation can be achieved by the use of rails or by inserting a bar wedge of varying degrees between the shoe and the foot. Rails are narrow, wedge-shaped distal extensions that are applied to the axial side of the ground surface of the shoe. As such, they elevate the heels and ease mediolateral breakover. The rails can be made in different heights and can be attached to the shoe by welding or gluing the rails (**Fig. 7**). There is also a commercial system available

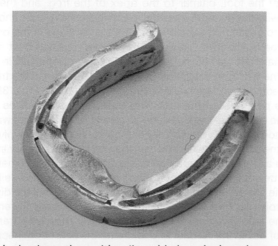

Fig. 7. A wide web aluminum shoe with rails welded on the branches.

that has rails of different heights that can be bolted to the shoe (Equine Digital Support System, EDSS Inc, Penrose, CO, USA). Sole and frog support is achieved by applying impression material between the branches of the shoe. The wide web aluminum shoe provides improved breakover, heel elevation, and sole and frog support.

Wooden Shoe

The wooden shoe may provide additional advantages over the traditional shoes that are commonly used to treat chronic laminitis.[2,8,9] One major advantage may be its ability to distribute weight evenly over a specified section of the foot due to its flat, solid construction. This ability is helpful when trying to recruit ground surface in the palmar/plantar section of the foot to shift the load from the dorsal lamellae, when the structures in this section of the foot are less than optimal.

Other advantages are
- Simplicity of construction; simple plywood
- Mechanics such as breakover and heel elevation can be fabricated into the shoe
- Beveled perimeter of the shoe concentrates the load under the distal phalanx
- Solid base of the shoe aids in maximum recruitment of surface area in the palmar/plantar section of the foot to accept load
- Solid base combined with an appropriate impression material places an even pressure and load across the palmar/plantar section of the foot.

The shape of the wooden shoe is derived by using the Natural Balance shoes (EDSS Inc, Penrose, CO, USA) shoe as a template; an 1.125-in plywood is cut out using an angle saw, with the perimeter being beveled at an angle of 45°. This bevel not only moves the breakover palmarly but also moves the medial and lateral weight-bearing surfaces axially, enhancing mediolateral breakover. After the foot has been trimmed as described earlier, the shoe of appropriate size is fitted to the trimmed foot, and placement of the shoe is determined by superimposing corresponding lines drawn across the widest part of the foot and by a line drawn across the middle of the block. The bevel on the front of the shoe is then increased with a rasp until the point of break-over is positioned to correspond to an imaginary vertical line drawn through the dorsal coronary band to the ground. A thin layer of impression material is applied between the ground surface of the foot, palmar to the apex of the frog, and the shoe and then allowed to cure with the horse in a weight-bearing position. Just enough impression material is used to fill the frog sulci and create a level plane in the palmar section of the foot. The shoe is attached with screws inserted through pilot holes previously drilled in the distal hoof wall (**Figs. 8** and **9**). Screws are placed in the area of the heel quarters of the foot to maintain the 2 planes created during the trim. The wooden shoe is further secured by placing 2-in casting tape (Vetcast Plus, 3M, St Paul, MN, USA) around the perimeter of the foot. The casting tape enhances the attachment as it will follow the contour of the diverging angles of the distal hoof wall and the bevel in the wooden shoe. Alternatively, screws can be screwed into the plywood, adjacent to the margin of the distal hoof wall, and the shoe can be secured by incorporating the screw heads into a 2-in casting tape that is placed around the perimeter of the foot. A wedge pad may be applied to the foot surface of the shoe to provide heel elevation, if needed. If the sole has prolapsed below the level of the wall or if the distal phalanx has penetrated the sole, the foot surface of the shoe is recessed to remove any direct pressure from the sole. The author uses the wooden shoe as a transient device to help produce hoof wall at the coronet and to create the sole depth necessary to realign the distal phalanx.

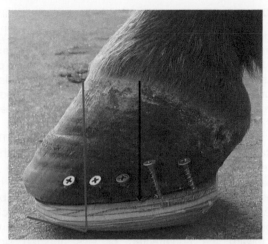

Fig. 8. A wooden shoe applied to the foot with impression material. Black arrow is the widest part of the foot. Red line denotes the point of breakover on the ground surface of the shoe.

FOLLOW-UP FARRIERY

Horses with chronic laminitis should have shoes applied with adjusted breakover, sole and frog support, and heel elevation. As the tissues heal, the horse becomes more comfortable and the foot conformation improves, and the farriery principles can then be slowly modified and eliminated in reverse order. There seems to be some intrinsic shortening of the musculotendinous deep digital flexor unit over time, when heel elevation is maintained continuously. When increased stability and comfort are achieved, heel elevation should be gradually removed.[2,4] With additional stability, the sole and frog support can be removed. Eventually, the horse may be shod normally or left barefoot. However, in some horses with permanent dorsal capsular rotation, the shoes may need to be repeatedly reset with the aid of radiographs, although heel elevation and sole and frog support are no longer needed.

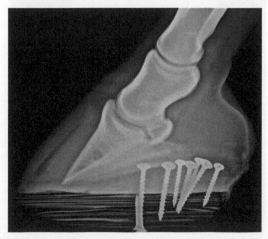

Fig. 9. Radiograph of a laminitic foot with a wooden shoe applied. Note the toe of the foot unloaded.

MEDIOLATERAL ROTATION OF THE DISTAL PHALANX

Mediolateral rotation is a less common condition than dorsal capsular rotation, and less is known about treating horses with this type of displacement.[2,4,9] The increased use of the DP radiograph reveals a higher incidence of this condition than was previously recognized. In the author's opinion, mediolateral rotation is driven by foot conformation because it has only been observed when the foot is offset to the lateral side placing disproportionate load on the medial side of the foot. One of the early signs of mediolateral displacement is a noticeable lack of hoof wall growth at the coronet on the affected side. The incidence of mediolateral displacement seems to increase when horses with the offset-foot conformation have had excessive heel elevation applied in the earlier stage of laminitis. This type of displacement is difficult to treat, and the response seems better if treated early. Theoretically, the hoof capsule can be stabilized in relation to the distal phalanx by reducing the weight bearing on the affected side and by increasing the weight bearing on the contralateral side. In other words, the GRF can be shifted toward the nonaffected or less affected side of the foot (**Fig. 10**). This shift is best accomplished by extending the shoe on the contralateral side to act as a lever and hence act as a mild wedge. The author has had success in controlling mediolateral rotation in a limited number of horses by applying either the rail shoe or the wooden shoe in combination with impression material and by setting the shoe tight on the affected side and wide on the unaffected side (**Fig. 11**). When the wooden shoe is used, a slight increase to the bevel on the lateral side of the shoe seems to increase the benefit. Before applying the shoe, any flare should be reduced on the affected side using a rasp on the adjacent outer hoof wall. This technique has visibly improved comfort, promoted hoof wall growth at the coronet on the affected side, and/or abolished the evidence of mediolateral rotation over time. This technique seems

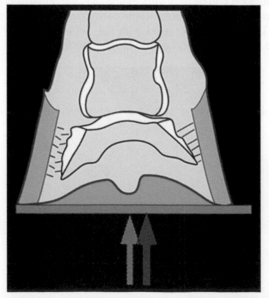

Fig. 10. Illustration shows the mechanics of moving the GRF away from the affected side of the foot by placement of the shoe. Grey color under hoof is impression material.

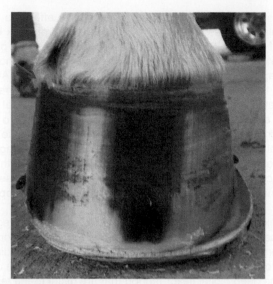

Fig. 11. Unilateral displacement with wooden shoe fitted with extension toward the lateral side. Note the lack of hoof wall growth at the coronet on the medial side coronet (*red arrow*).

promising, but because the complication rate with this condition seems to be high, the prognosis for treating this pattern of displacement is still less favorable than it is with dorsal capsular/phalangeal rotation. Unless the hoof wall on the medial side is completely detached, the author has been reluctant to resect the hoof wall because it may provide some stability and prevent collapse. If the margin of the hoof capsule is detached and impinges on the coronet, a thin strip of hoof wall can be removed, which immediately increases comfort. Identifying this type of rotation in the early stage may change the outcome in many cases.

CASTS

One useful technique that the veterinarian or farrier may use is application of a fiber-glass foot cast with compliant impression material against the sole and frog.[6] This technique is particularly beneficial in the horse with chronic laminitis that has poor quality and integrity of the hoof wall and is continually suffering from bruising of the feet. If applied properly, these casts may be worn for more than 1 to 2 months, before changing is necessary. After appropriate trimming, as previously described, impression material is applied to the palmar one-half of the foot, ie, from the apex of the frog palmarly. Cast padding is placed over the heel bulbs, and 1 roll of 3-in cast material (Vetcast Plus, 3M, St Paul, MN, USA) is applied to the foot. The material may be manipulated to alter the angle of the foot, point of contact, and point of breakover. The toe region should be protected from wear by the use of a composite. The cast seems to give circumferential support to the hoof wall preventing the stretching of the lamellae at the ground surface. Furthermore, the cast material helps the foot to expel moisture thus maintaining a healthier environment.

SURGICAL TREATMENT
Deep Digital Flexor Tenotomy

There are 3 instances in which deep digital flexor tenotomy is primarily indicated in horses with phalangeal rotation.[4] First, it is indicated for horses showing progressive rotation of the distal phalanx despite more conservative efforts to stabilize it. This technique particularly applies to horses in which the distal phalanx is already penetrating the sole of the foot. Second, it is indicated for horses with persistent severe discomfort, showing little to no growth of the sole or dorsal hoof wall despite apparent radiographic evidence of stability of the distal phalanx. After deep digital flexor tenotomy, there is frequently a dramatic increase in the rate of hoof wall and sole growth along with decreased pain. Although a deep digital flexor tenotomy is considered a salvage procedure, some horses may return to limited athletic performance. Third, deep digital flexor tenotomy is warranted to correct severe secondary flexural deformities that may develop during the later stages of treatment. The author believes that a tenotomy is contraindicated in horses with dorsal capsular rotation when accompanied by mediolateral displacement because this leaves the lamellae on the unaffected side of the foot as the only source of support for the distal phalanx.

Deep digital flexor tenotomy performed in the midmetacarpal region is relatively simple and can be performed under local anesthesia. When tenotomy is performed in the midmetacarpal region, rather than in the pastern region, the distal interphalangeal joint seems to be more stable when the animal moves because of the soft tissue attachments to the deep digital flexor tendon that are distal to the tenotomy site and proximal to the digital sheath. Furthermore, if a second tenotomy is necessary, the adhesions associated with the first tenotomy would preclude this area and the mid-pastern site could be used.

The author prefers to do the farriery before surgery. The foot is trimmed as described previously. After deep digital flexor tenotomy, the toe of the foot is prone to lift off the ground or flip as the animal rocks back on its heels or as it walks. This movement is because of the GRF moving palmarly as a result of transection of the tendon. This tendency can be countered by relatively short heel extensions that can be accomplished by placing the heels of the shoe at a short distance palmarly to the heels of the hoof capsule. Of greater concern to the author is the tendency of the distal interphalangeal joint to subluxate in a distopalmar direction, secondary to the lack of support of the navicular bone by the deep digital flexor tendon. In addition to heel extension, mild heel elevation ($2°–3°$) further aids in countering the tendency of the distal interphalangeal joint to subluxate.

Grooving and Hoof Wall Resection

Continued divergence of the dorsal hoof wall away from the parietal surface of the distal phalanx after the distal wall has been relieved of weight bearing may respond to coronary band grooving or dorsal hoof wall resection.[4] Coronary band grooving mechanically dissociates the new proximal wall from the older distal wall. In addition, it may enhance hoof growth by the coronary band proximal to the groove by some mechanism secondary to reducing pressure at the coronary band. The groove grows out as the new wall migrates distally.

Resection of the dorsal hoof wall may be partial or complete. It is indicated to improve the direction and rate of new hoof growth when other methods have failed or to debride draining tracts associated with necrotic tissue between the wall and distal phalanx. A complete hoof wall resection removes the entire wall from the weight-bearing surface of the wall to the coronary band. A partial resection extends a variable distance proximally from the weight-bearing surface. Therefore, rather than dissociating the proximal and distal hoof walls, the distal wall is simply removed. This approach allows debridement of the more superficial, hyperplastic epidermis. However, what is remaining of the lamellar attachments to the dorsal hoof wall is now functionless, potentially increasing the tendency of the dorsal margin of the distal phalanx to impinge on the soft tissues of the immediately adjacent sole. Also, stress is now concentrated on the hoof wall at the margins of the resection, increasing the tendency for separation within the hoof wall at these points. This stress is compounded by the lack of the tension band that the dorsal hoof wall provides between the medial and lateral quarters. Therefore, the dorsal hoof wall is resected far less frequently. Other than providing drainage when necessary, the author justifies resection only when the hoof wall is completely detached from the epidermal or dermal lamellae.

Treatment Failure

There are many reasons why the treatment of laminitic horses is not successful. The overwhelming severity of the initial disease is the most important reason, particularly when followed by persistent infection.[1,2,4,8,9,11,12] Also, financial constraints are important because the treatment can be very expensive, long, and exhausting. Therefore, many owners stop treatment as the full implications of the cost or the psychological or physical toll of the rehabilitation process become apparent.[12] Failure of owners to comply with recommendations from veterinarians and farriers is not uncommon. On the other hand, a successful outcome is invariably enhanced by merging the veterinary and farrier expertise along with owner compliance.

REFERENCES

1. Hunt RJ. Chronic laminitis. In: White NA, Moore JN, editors. Current techniques in equine surgery and lameness. 2nd edition. Philadelphia: WB Saunders; 1998. p. 548–52.
2. O'Grady SE, Parks AH. Farriery options for acute and chronic laminitis. Proceedings Am Assoc of Equine Pract 2008;54:355–63.
3. Hood DM. The mechanisms and consequences of structural failure of the foot. 2. In: Hood DW, editor. The veterinary clinics of North America, vol. 15. Philadelphia: WB Saunders; 1999. p. 437–61.
4. Parks AH, O'Grady SE. Chronic laminitis. In: Robinson NE, Sprayberry K, editors, Current therapy in equine medicine, vol. 6. St. Louis (MO): WB Saunders; 2008. p. 550–60.
5. O'Grady SE. Realignment of P3 – the basis for treating chronic laminitis. Equine Vet Edu 2006;8:272–6.
6. Hunt RJ. Equine laminitis: practical clinical considerations. Proceedings Am Assoc of Equine Pract 2008;54:347–53.
7. Parks AH, O'Grady SE. Chronic laminitis: current treatment strategies. In: O'Grady SE, editor. The veterinary clinics of North America, vol. 19:2. Philadelphia: WB Saunders; 2003. p. 393–416.
8. O'Grady SE, Steward ML. The wooden shoe as an option for treating chronic laminitis. Equine Vet Edu 2006;8:272–6.
9. O'Grady SE, Steward M, Parks AH. How to construct and apply the wooden shoe for treating three manifestations of chronic laminitis. Proceedings Am Assoc of Equine Pract 2007;53:423–9.
10. Redden RF, Hood DM. Clinical and radiographic examination of the equine foot. Proceedings Am Assoc of Equine Pract 2003;49:174–85.
11. Nickels FA. Hoofcare of the laminitic horse. In: Ross MW, editor. Diagnosis and management of equine lameness. WB Saunders Company Inc; in press.
12. Moyer W, Schumacher, James, et al. Chronic laminitis: considerations for the owner and prevention of misunderstandings. Proceedings Am Assoc of Equine Pract 2000;46:59–61.

Chronic Laminitis: Foot Management

Scott Morrison, DVM

KEYWORDS

• Founder • Foot management • Horseshoe • Sinker
• Derotation • Laminae • Tenotomy

THE ROLE OF LOADING AND PRESSURE ON DAMAGED LAMINAE

The distal phalanx (DP) is suspended within the hoof capsule via the laminar attachments that are located around the entire parietal surface of the DP and collateral cartilages. The normal foot is not completely dependent on these laminae for support. The arch of the sole and durable outer sole callus are also designed to support some portion of the load.[1,2] In most healthy, barefoot horses, the texture and conformation of the sole can be readily recognized as supporting structures. However, many domesticated shod horses lack a functional sole and probably depend more on the laminar interface for support. The sole is often suspended off the ground, disengaged from weight bearing, atrophied, or sometimes even intentionally and radically trimmed out to form a convex contour. When a foot with a thin sole is affected by laminitis, complete mechanical collapse of the foot may result. It has also been reported that weak feet with thin soles are more likely to develop a supporting limb laminitis than are strong robust feet with thick soles.[3]

Knowledge of the normal digital loading patterns can be helpful in formulating a foot support plan to aid recovery from laminitis. Most importantly, the normal foot tends to load the toe region during stance. Pressure mat studies show the center of pressure (COP) to be located dorsal to the center of articulation of the distal interphalangeal (DIP) joint, just behind and slightly medial to the apex of the frog.[4] However, variations in limb position and conformation are common in horses and can affect the location of COP in the normal, healthy foot. When the normal limb is loaded, the fetlock displaces downward, putting the deep digital flexor tendon (DDFT) under tension, which in turn pulls on the DDFT insertion site on the palmar (plantar) DP. This creates slight rotation around the DIP joint. For this reason, the COP is located dorsal to the center of the DIP joint.

Measurements made before and after surgery showed that transection of the DDFT in laminitis cases shifted the COP from just behind the frog apex to directly beneath the center of the DIP joint in all 3 cases studied. (Scott E. Morrison, unpublished

Rood and Riddle Equine Hospital, PO Box 12070, Lexington, KY 40580, USA
E-mail address: smorrison@roodandriddle.com

Vet Clin Equine 26 (2010) 425–446
doi:10.1016/j.cveq.2010.06.003
0749-0739/10/$ – see front matter © 2010 Published by Elsevier Inc.

vetequine.theclinics.com

data, 2008). This caudal shift repositioned the COP to a point that might create less stress on the toe region during stance.

EVALUATING DAMAGE TO THE LAMINITIC FOOT

Damage to the laminitic or foundered hoof capsule is evaluated by observing and sometimes measuring the relative displacement of structures from their normal architecture. Most cases of chronic laminitis have some degree of laminar separation and rotational displacement of the DP in the toe region; a smaller percentage has sinking (vertical displacement of the DP) in addition to rotation.

Rotation of the DP is the most common form of displacement. It may occur alone or be combined with medial, lateral, or vertical sinking (total circumference detachment). The prevalence of rotation in the toe region as a common finding probably relates to the tendency of horses at stance to load the dorsal regions of the foot. Laminae in the toe region are under more tensile strain than are the laminae in the quarters and heels (structures that expand and contract during locomotion and weight bearing).

In addition, the heel has other supporting structures, such as the frog, whereas the toe is primarily suspended by the laminae. It is possible that laminar damage may be uniform in the acute stages of the disease, with separation occurring first in regions of the foot under the most load. It is my experience, after observing many laminitic cases, that in horses with mismatched feet, the more upright or clubfoot experiences more rotation than the opposing foot. This could be a result of the already increased tension on the dorsal laminae from the preexisting mild tendon contracture. Conversely, the foot with excessively low heels generally develops rotation less readily than the more upright foot. The low-heel foot, however, seems more susceptible to sinking in the quarters. Research by Barrey[5] showed that when compared with feet with a normal hoof angle, feet with a lower hoof angle have an increased load in the heel region and feet with a higher hoof angle have an increased load in the toe region. Therefore, hoof conformation may influence loading patterns and the type of DP displacement that occurs when laminitis damages the foot.

THE STAGES OF LAMINITIS

The progression of laminitis can be broken down into several stages. The earliest stage is developmental laminitis, in which the trigger factors are activated and blood flow changes to the foot occur. This phase is usually set in motion by some other systemic ailment. The laminae are not compromised at this stage.

The second, or acute, phase is defined by 2 factors: the onset of foot pain and the presence of an easily detected digital pulse. Most horses exit the acute phase and subsequently enter the third, or subacute, phase. These cases recover with conservative treatment as long as the inciting cause is resolved.

The others enter the chronic phase, which is defined as more than 72 hours of foot pain and/or DP displacement[6] (rotation, sinking, or both). The chronic phase can be further broken down into the chronic compensated (stable) and the chronic uncompensated (unstable) cases.

A chronic compensated foot is one in which the DP has been displaced and then stabilized to some degree. "Stabilized" in chronic laminitis means that the bone is no longer moving and that the foot generates new sole and wall tissue, in all regions of the foot, although this growth is often slowed or distorted by the disease.

On the other hand, in the chronic uncompensated cases, the DP remains unstable and constantly shears and compresses the sensitive sole and coronary band, causing areas of repressed wall and/or sole growth. These cases usually suffer from chronic abscesses and severe pain.

TREATMENT OF THE ACUTE LAMINITIC FOOT

Treating the horse in the acute phase requires a thorough examination of the horse and the treatment of any systemic conditions. Like most other musculoskeletal injuries, the initial approach should include immobilization of the compromised tissue, rest, and systemic use of antiinflammatory medications. Because it is not possible to accurately determine the extent of laminar damage, all acute cases should be treated as unstable emergencies. Care should be taken to be as nontraumatic as possible to the hoof to protect the fragile laminar interface. The horse should be handled delicately and not be moved unnecessarily. However, the patient should be moved to a deeply bedded stall.

Lateral radiographs are necessary to serve as a baseline to compare future progress or deterioration. A quick, nontraumatic foot examination is required to rule out other causes of bilateral lameness.

Once the diagnosis of acute laminitis is made, mechanical strategies to limit or prevent DP displacement should be implemented. These include (1) recruitment of other structures into weight bearing (frog, sole, bars), (2) decreasing the moment arm around the DIP joint, and (3) redistributing the weight from the most stressed regions to least stressed areas. The feet should be placed in some type of temporary, easily removable, support.

Because most feet tend to rotate, there is a valid argument for wedging up the heels of horses, in the acute phase, to decrease the rotational force exerted by the DDFT. Wedging the heel has been shown to decrease strain on the DDFT.[7,8] Redden[3] recommends elevating the heels 10° and moving the break-over point back far enough so that the horse rocks forward, creating a 20° palmar angle. Redden reports that these mechanics significantly reduce the incidence of supporting limb laminitis (**Fig. 1**).

After the initial examination, with radiographs taken and foot support in place, the case should be confined to strict stall rest. It is recommended that grain or highly soluble carbohydrate feed sources be removed from the diet. Even if the inciting cause was not carbohydrate overload, any possible source of further laminar insult should be avoided. Medical therapy aimed at reducing inflammation (nonsteroidal antiinflammatory drugs, dimethyl sulfoxide, omega 3 fatty acid supplements), improving lamellar blood flow (acepromazine, isoxuprine, pentoxyphylline), preventing platelet aggregation (aspirin, heparin), and inhibiting matrix metalloproteinases (doxycycline) should be considered. Continuous cryotherapy for 72 hours during the developmental stage has been shown to be effective in preventing or decreasing the severity of acute laminitis[9] and may have some therapeutic merit for cases already in the acute phase. I prefer to use cryotherapy during the acute phase for the first 72 hours.

Strict stall rest and foot support are maintained until the patient can ambulate normally for 1 week without antiinflammatories and has no radiographic signs of displacement. If the feet were placed in 10° wedges, the wedge height should be reduced by half and then reevaluated in 1 week. If, at anytime, the horse appears less comfortable, then the removed wedge should be replaced. Another attempt to reduce the heel elevation should be tried after 1 week of walking soundly.

After the horse has been walking soundly for 1 week without antiinflammatories and with only a 5° wedge, the feet should have the first set of shoes nailed or glued on. Gluing the shoes on is less traumatic and is a more conservative approach at this stage; however, gluing is more expensive and may be cost-prohibitive in some cases.

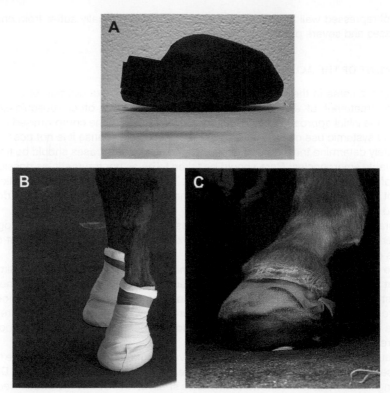

Fig. 1. (*A*) Nanric ultimate cuff (Nanric, Lawrenceburg, Kentucky, USA). The 10° wedge heel and rolled toe allow the foot to rock forward, decreasing tension on the DDFT. Sole support material is added and (*B*) the cuff bandaged or (*C*) adhered (shown) with acrylic or epoxy to the hoof wall.

The first set of shoes should have sole or frog support and a rolled or rockered toe to help decrease forces on the laminar interface (**Fig. 2**).

Because it is unknown how compromised the laminae are after the acute phase, a conservative and cautious approach is instituted when reintroducing the horse back to normal activity during the next 30 days. Frequent monitoring and examination of the feet during this period are required to detect signs of inflammation or structural damage. If any displacement occurs, the foot is considered to have entered the chronic phase of the disease and a revised treatment program begins.

HEEL ELEVATION IN THE ACUTE PHASE

Although most acute cases respond favorably to heel elevation, there is a subpopulation of cases that becomes more uncomfortable after a wedge is applied. A possible explanation for this is most likely the degree of lamellar damage in the quarters and heel regions. Heel elevation decreases tension on the DDFT, shifts the COP toward the heels, and increases strain on the quarters and heels.[10] This strain could cause pain if the laminae of the heel and quarter regions are compromised. Because tensile strain is potentially decreased in the dorsal regions with heel elevation, shear and compressive forces are increased. An analogy is to imagine that the unstable DP slides forward during heel elevation, causing compression and shear on the dorsal

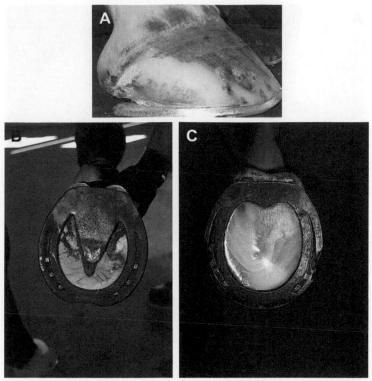

Fig. 2. (*A*) Aluminum shoe with a rockered toe to help decrease strain on the anterior laminar attachments. The shoe can be glued or nailed depending on the foot type and wall quality. (*B*) Steel heartbar shoe. (*C*) Sole support is added for axial support.

laminae and sole corium. Because the laminar suspensory apparatus is designed to mainly oppose tensile forces, the increased shear and compressive forces in the toe create tissue damage and pain.[11]

When horses react negatively to wedge therapy, the wedges should be removed and the foot left at its natural angle. In my experience, these cases do well in sole support and a system that eases break over in all directions or reduces the moment arm around the DIP joint. This support can be achieved with the use of several hoof appliances, including wooden clogs,[12] boots, wall or foot casts, Sigafoos Series II shoes (Sound Horse Technologies, Unionville, PA, USA), handmade shoes, dental impression putty, or the Equine Digital Support System (Penrose, CO, USA) (**Fig. 3**).

As long as the mechanics are present and the device can be applied quickly and nontraumatically, it does not matter which system is used.

RESTRUCTURING THE CHRONIC COMPENSATED (STABLE) FOOT

Feet in this category are out of alignment but do possess some stability. When observing a chronic, but stable foundered foot, one can appreciate the attempt of the foot to rebalance the forces acting upon it after structural failure has occurred in the dorsal laminae. The hoof produces excessive growth in the heels and less growth in the toe to balance the pull of the tendon against the compromised laminae (**Fig. 4**).

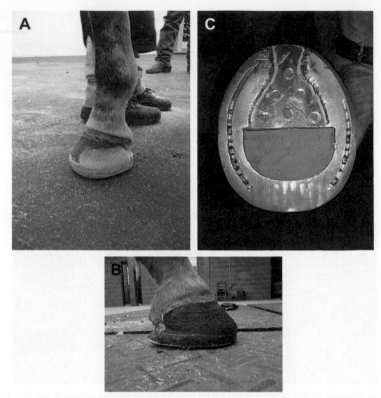

Fig. 3. (*A–C*) When horses react negatively to wedge therapy, the wedges should be removed and the foot left at its natural angle. In the author's experience, these cases do well in sole support and in a system that eases break over in all directions or reduces the moment arm around the DIP joint. This can be achieved with the use of several hoof appliances including (*A*) wooden clogs, boots, wall or foot casts, (*B*) Sigafoos Series II shoes, (*C*) handmade shoes, dental impression putty, or the Equine Digital Support System.

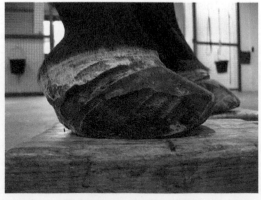

Fig. 4. Chronic laminitic foot with hoof capsule distortion.

In laminitic ponies with 6° to 13° of DP rotation, the COP was located palmar to the center of rotation of the DIP joint.[13] This is most likely the result of hoof capsule distortion and altered limb position or posture. The hoof capsule distorts, with increased heel growth, to rebalance the forces of the weight of the horse and the tension of the DDFT against the compromised laminae. In fact, in slowly progressing chronic laminitis cases, the mechanical failure may be self-limiting by hoof capsule distortion,[14] in which the heel is elevated by increased wall growth while the toe wall growth is slowed, thereby decreasing tension on the DDFT. This adapted hoof morphology should be observed and respected when devising a treatment plan.

Although most laminitic feet have laminar damage or failure isolated in the toe region, some cases present with laminar failure in the medial side or lateral side (medial/lateral sinkers, sometimes called horizontal plane laminitis) or around the entire foot, known as overt sinkers. As long as there are signs of continuous wall and sole growth in all regions, some sinkers can be classified as compensated.[6]

It is important to repeat that a hoof compromised by chronic laminitis is unable to respond appropriately to normal loading forces. Unlike a healthy hoof, the region under the highest load grows the most slowly. In overloaded regions, tissue is compressed thus compromising normal perfusion and tissue regeneration. However, because all the growth centers (coronary and sole corium) are intact in the chronic compensated case, these feet require only special trimming and shoeing to redistribute the load and correct the hoof capsule growth pattern. Eventually, once the foot is rebalanced with the aid of special shoeing, the hoof capsule distortion resolves. The long-term goals of managing the chronic, compensated laminitis case are (1) to increase dorsal sole depth, (2) to promote even toe and heel wall growth, (3) to eventually have a DP with a normal (0°–5°) palmar angle, and (4) to ensure that the horse is comfortable. The long-term goal is also to use the simplest mechanics possible to maintain a normal sole depth and palmar or plantar angle.

The trim and the shoe are the 2 components to the management of the foot. The goal of performing the trim is to establish DP alignment, balance, or even weight distribution. The shoe is designed to offer support, to ease break over in all directions, and to address the pull of the DDFT.

The foot is first prepared by trimming the heels back as much as possible without invading the live sole. A live sole is defined as a tightly compact sole with a greater moisture content than the dead exfoliating sole. With the limitation and restrictions of each foot type in mind, the heels should be trimmed back as far as possible. Care should be taken not create soreness by trimming the heels too short. The angle of the sole should routinely be palpated with thumb pressure to ensure that the heel trim is not too short. Because some cases have some degree of medial or lateral sinking, in addition to rotation, the medial-to-lateral balance of the DP is also corrected as much as possible with the trim.

Obviously, because the heel height is reduced, a more normal orientation of the DP to the ground is established and the base of support is moved palmarly. However, this shift puts more tension on the DDFT and dorsal laminar interface. This shift can, in fact, mechanically initiate further rotation. This issue is addressed by the shoe, which usually consists of a raised heel and a heavy rolled toe to facilitate break over. A combination of heel elevation and moving the break-over point to a more palmar position are effective ways to decrease the influence of the DDFT on the DP.

The amount of heel elevation or wedge should be at least equal to the amount of heel trimmed off the hoof. This may seem redundant to some: why trim the heel off the foot and then replace it with a wedge? The answer is simple: even weight distribution. The trim reestablishes the relationship of the DP to the ground, and the wedge takes tension off the DDFT.

An analogy would be a person standing on tiptoe with the bottom of the foot at a 45° angle to the ground. With this foot position, all the weight is concentrated on the toe as opposed to someone standing flat on a board that is raised 45° to the ground. In both situations, the bottom of the foot (palmar/plantar angle) is 45° to the ground, but the weight distribution on the bottom of the foot is different. The person standing on the board (the wedged shoe) has more even weight distribution along the bottom of the foot, whereas the person on tiptoe has the weight concentrated entirely on the toe (**Fig. 5**).

The second component of the shoe is to ease break over and reduce the moment arm around the DIP joint. Placing the break-over point at the natural COP of the foot greatly decreases resistance to movement when moving straight ahead. I usually place the dorsal break-over point directly beneath the dorsal coronary band (**Fig. 6A**). This point is also the approximate location of the COP for most feet.

Rolling the quarters of the shoe reduces resistance when turning. Because the lamellar interface is susceptible to shear forces, turning is particularly painful and potentially damaging; thus, easing medial and lateral break over is required. The quarters should be rolled to ease medial and lateral break over, at a point close to the plumb line dropped straight down from the coronary band in the quarters, at the widest part of the foot (see **Fig. 6B**).

The third component of the shoe is support. Axial support refers to the incorporation of other solar surface structures within the margins of the perimeter hoof wall into weight bearing. Weight can be distributed to the frog, sulci of frog, sole, and bars to help take load off the laminar interface.

The entire solar surface can be loaded with synthetic materials such as polyurethane, silicone, and elastomer. These products distribute the load over a larger surface area and are easy to use. There is a large variation in the hardness of the different materials available. The more firm materials offer more support but are less forgiving to thin, weak, painful areas, whereas the softer materials are more forgiving but offer less support.

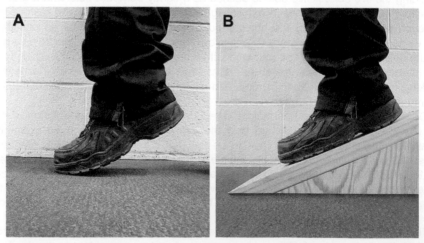

Fig. 5. Weight concentrated on the toe in the photo on the left compared with shared weight distribution along the entire plantar surface of the foot in the photo on the right.

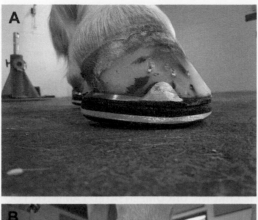

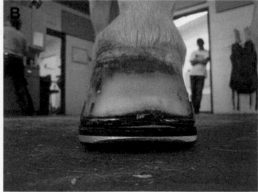

Fig. 6. (*A*) Placing the break-over point at the natural COP of the foot greatly decreases resistance to movement when moving straight ahead. (*B*) The quarters should be rolled to ease medial and lateral break over, at a point close to the plumb line dropped straight down from the coronary band in the quarters, at the widest part of the foot.

Most cases respond well to materials that are close to the hardness of a freshly trimmed frog. However, some cases have regions of the foot too painful to be used for weight bearing. These instances require more strategic axial loading such as the mechanics offered by heart bars, heel plates, or general solar loading with a combination of products of different hardness or by trimming material away from sore areas. A thorough examination of the foot is essential to determine which support method is the best.

A method that I find consistently reliable is to use a sole support material beneath a solid plate, such as a heel plate or treatment plate. This method provides even, constant loading in a controlled and protected manner. A firmer product with more support can be used when it does not have direct contact with the uneven ground surface. This combined mechanical plan alters the load distribution on digital structures, promotes even sole or wall growth and eventually rebalances the foot.

These customized shoeing systems are left in place until the sole depth in the toe matches the sole depth in the heel (indicating that the palmar surface of the DP is parallel to the shoe) and the new growth rings, parallel to the coronary band, have grown at least one-third the way down the hoof wall.

At this stage, the shoeing mechanics are slowly scaled down. Most cases are maintained in a small (1°–2°) wedged shoe that has the toe rolled from the plumb line below the dorsal coronary band forward. Some cases are weaned down to just a barefoot trim pattern, which consists of trimming the heels down modestly and rolling the toe, again from the dorsal coronary band forward, as explained for the chronic compensated foot. I recommend these cases have radiographs taken 3 to 4 times a year to make sure they are maintaining proper sole depth and DP alignment. Occasionally, some of these cases have to go back to wearing the shoe for a period of time to realign and rebuild sole depth (**Fig. 7**).

If cases do not respond to these shoeing mechanics, they are considered to be in the uncompensated (unstable) classification of chronic laminitis.

RESTRUCTURING THE CHRONIC UNCOMPENSATED LAMINITIC FOOT

Restructuring the chronic uncompensated (unstable) foot is often difficult. This foot type typically has massive vascular damage, secondary infections, and severe damage to tissue-generating structures such as coronary and sole coria (**Fig. 8**).

The initial approach to the unstable foot is often similar to the acute laminitic foot. I usually perform a venogram as part of the initial diagnostic workup to better assess the

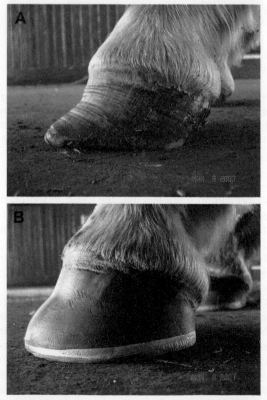

Fig. 7. (*A, B*) Chronic laminitic foot with heel trimmed down, wedged shoe, and rockered toe applied. The trim and shoe provide more even weight distribution along the solar surface of the DP, ease break over, and decrease tension on the DDFT.

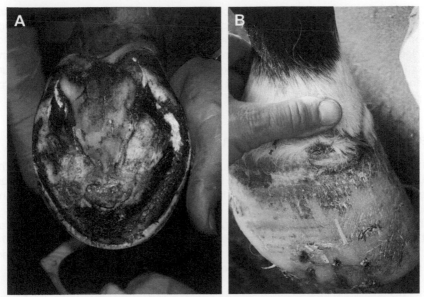

Fig. 8. Uncompensated cases have damage to the sole corium (*A*) or coronary band (*B*) and are unable to regenerate sole and/or wall in areas.

extent of instability and tissue compression.[15] The information gained from the external examination of the foot, venogram, and radiographs combines to dictate which treatment modalities need to be implemented.

Practically speaking, there is no systematic approach to dealing with every high-scale laminitic foot. Each case is different, and every foot is unique. Treating these feet requires experience, good judgment, and a well-coordinated effort by the farrier, veterinarian, and owner or manager, combined with adequate nursing care.

However, there are several techniques available that can be used to restore normal growth, stability, and DP alignment and, ultimately, to rehabilitate these feet. It is important to set goals and document landmarks that are useful in determining whether progress is being made and how much improvement to specific structures or parameters has been achieved. In addition, it is important to realize at which point the goal of reasonable long-term soundness is no longer obtainable and if the best option is euthanasia.

The most important short-term goal for the treatment of the chronic, uncompensated foot is to preserve or restore the integrity of the coronary band and sole corium and thus their vasculature. The ultimate goal is to maintain the health of the DP and eventually reestablish normal DP alignment and adequate sole depth.

Secondary complications such as bruising, abscesses, osteomyelitis, seromas, and coronary band shear lesions are consequences of digital instability and tissue compression. For this reason, these problems cannot be successfully resolved without formulating a plan to relieve the displacement forces and eventually realign the DP. Depending on the extent of damage and the modalities already tried, most cases can be treated by rebalancing the foundered foot with shoeing mechanics previously described for the compensated and acute conditions.

If the DP has penetrated the sole corium or if the foot fails to show continuous improvement with shoeing mechanics alone, a deep digital flexor tenotomy is often warranted. Trying to treat a DP that has penetrated the sole with shoeing alone takes far too long, and the bone suffers too much inflammation and demineralization, which becomes a source of pain throughout the life of the animal.

A deep digital flexor tenotomy is the fastest way to counteract rotational forces and restore perfusion and tissue mass to the dorsal regions of the foot. The horse's future soundness is not determined by the fact it has had a tenotomy; soundness is limited by the pathology in the foot. Preservation of DP health should be the priority.

DEEP DIGITAL FLEXOR TENOTOMY AND REALIGNMENT SHOEING TECHNIQUE

Transection of the DDFT allows for immediate realignment of the DP in relation to the ground surface. I prefer to shoe the horse before surgery because often the shoe must be glued on and the surgical preparation for the tenotomy may make the foot wet and unsuitable for gluing.

The goal of realignment shoeing is to glue a shoe onto the trimmed and prepared foot in a position that places the shoe parallel to the palmar (ground) surface of the DP.[16] In addition, the shoe should also provide enough heel extension to prevent the toe from hyperextending after transection of the DDFT.

HOOF PREPARATION FOR REALIGNMENT SHOEING

Each horse is sedated with detomidine IV and an abaxial sesamoid nerve block with local anesthetic is performed to facilitate the shoeing and radiography procedure. The heel is trimmed down as much as possible without invading the live sole (**Fig. 9**A, B). A lateral radiograph should be taken after the heels are trimmed (see **Fig. 9**C).

Using the lateral radiograph as a blueprint, several measurements should be made to assure proper shoe alignment (see **Fig. 9**D). A straight line should be drawn beginning from the most palmar aspect of the ground surface of the hoof, and parallel to the ground surface of the DP. This first line represents the shoe.

This line can be transferred from the radiograph to the hoof capsule using the following technique: drop a plumb line from the dorsal coronary band to the ground surface on the foot and notch this point on the hoof capsule. On the radiograph, drop the same plumb line and note where this line intersects the line that represents the shoe. This point is often below the ground surface of the hoof capsule; therefore, the next step is to measure the amount of space below the hoof where these 2 lines intersect (see **Fig. 9**D). This measurement is the distance the shoe has to be wedged up, off the foot, at the notch mark.[15]

The shoe should be forged from aluminum or is a manufactured shoe with a welded-in heel plate. The heel plate helps hold in the sole support and offers additional support to the palmar aspects of the foot. The sole support material is mixed and applied to the sole. The shoe is firmly placed onto the foot at the same angle as on the radiograph (see **Fig. 9**E). The impression material may be molded at this stage into a toe wedge to achieve proper shoe alignment.

The position of the shoe must also be checked at this stage; it should be sitting off the sole at the notched mark in the wall at the same distance that was measured previously on the radiograph. Once the proper angle is achieved, the shoe is glued in place using fiberglass cloth impregnated with acrylic adhesive (see **Fig. 9**E, F). The shoe is only glued in the heel and quarter regions, and the toe is left open. Gluing the toe is contraindicated in a laminitic foot.

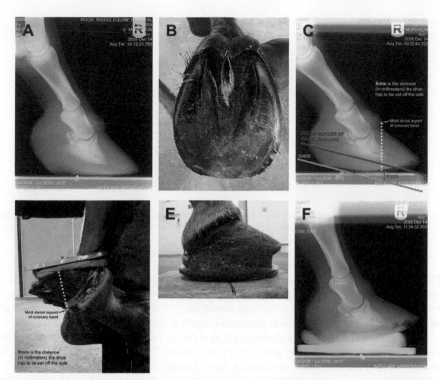

Fig. 9. (*A*) Radiograph of a foot nonresponsive to shoeing, with chronic abscessation, and continued bone remodeling. (*B*) Heels are trimmed down. (*C*) After heel trim, a lateral radiograph is taken as a blueprint for shoe alignment. A line is drawn beginning at the point of the heel, parallel to the solar surface of the DP, will be the shoe line. The distance between the shoe line and the sole is measured beneath the anterior coronary band. (*D*) The shoe is set flush to the heel and elevated off the sole beneath the anterior coronary band the same distance as determined from the radiograph. (*E*) The shoe is adhered to the foot with acrylic and fiberglass cloth. (*F*) Radiograph showing proper alignment of the shoe to the solar surface of the DP.

This shoeing method is adequate for most high-scale cases with severe mechanical failure limited to the toe region. These feet generally respond with significant dorsal sole growth during the next 4 to 6 weeks (**Fig. 10**).

However, if the foot shows damage in either the heel or quarter regions, such as medial or lateral sinking, the shoe may be set slightly lower on the side opposite the sinking side, that is, on the nonsinking side of the foot. For example, if the foot shows sinking to the medial side, the shoe may be set into the sole support slightly lower on the lateral side to shift the foot's weight distribution to the lateral heel. Regardless of the location of the damage to the foot, the DP should be parallel to the ground in the frontal and sagittal planes after shoeing.

DEEP DIGITAL FLEXOR TENOTOMY PROCEDURE

When shoeing is complete, the feet should be wrapped in plastic to keep the acrylic adhesive dry during the surgical preparation. All the laminitis-related tenotomies are performed at the midcannon region, unless there is scar tissue or evidence of an

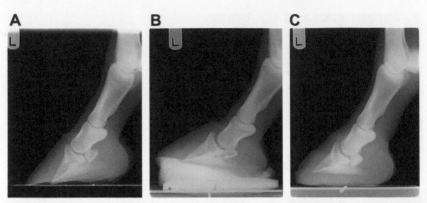

Fig. 10. (*A*) Foot at presentation with DP penetrating sole. (*B*) Same foot after tenotomy and realignment shoeing. (*C*) Same foot 3 months later; at this stage, the foot is left barefoot, with normal sole depth and alignment.

old tendon lesion; in that case, the procedure is performed at the pastern level. The limb is desensitized with a high 4-point nerve block and ring block in the proximal, metacarpal/metatarsal region with local anesthetic. (If the procedure is performed at the pastern level, only the abaxial sesamoid block is required.)

The surgical site is clipped and prepared. A 0.75- to 1-in skin incision is made on the lateral aspect over the DDFT in the midcannon region. The tissue is dissected around the DDFT using Metzenbaum scissors. A pair of small malleable retractors is used to isolate the tendon, and the DDFT is completely transected using a No. 15 blade. The skin is closed with 1-0 Supramid suture (Supramid Extra II S Jackson Inc, Alexandria, VA, USA), using vertical mattress pattern. The metacarpal/metatarsal region is bandaged with a nonadherent dressing and cotton bandage.

If the procedure is performed at the pastern level, the incision is made on the midline of the palmar pastern, just above the heel bulbs. The incision is continued through to the DDFT sheath and is about 1 to 1.5 in long. The DDFT is isolated with mosquito forceps, exteriorized, and completely transected. The tendon sheath is closed with 2-0 Vicryl suture (Vicryl Ethican Inc, Johnson & Johnson, NJ, USA) in a simple continuous pattern. The skin is closed with 1-0 Supramid vertical mattress pattern. The incision is covered with a nonadherent dressing and bandaged from the hoof to the metacarpus.

Postshoeing or tenotomy lateral radiographs should be taken to ensure perfect shoe alignment. Subluxation of the DIP joint is a normal finding. The subluxation is more pronounced in some cases, but does not seem to create any long-term problems and usually is corrected during the next 2 or 3 shoeings as the tenotomy site heals. Each case is re-shoed in the same manner at 5-to 6-week intervals, until there is even sole depth in the toe and heel regions and the palmar DP is parallel to the ground.

PROGNOSIS FOR CASES MANAGED WITH DEEP DIGITAL FLEXOR TENOTOMY AND DEROTATION SHOEING

Transection of the DDFT is a controversial treatment for chronic laminitis. This controversy is largely attributed to the variation in personal experience with the procedure and the differing success rates reported in literature.[17,18] The reported discrepancy in success rates is most likely the result of variations in foot pathology and the quality of foot management accompanying the procedure.

At Rood and Riddle Equine Hospital, we reviewed the records of 245 tenotomy cases, all of which received an identical realignment shoeing protocol, as previously described.[19] Success rates were determined for criteria such as degree of bone disease, solar penetration, sinking, number of limbs involved, and whether the affected feet were front or hind. Having success rates for different factors may help the clinician estimate a prognosis for similar cases requiring the procedure. Cases were considered a success if they were at least pasture-sound for 1 year after the procedure.

Bone disease was determined on the lateral radiographic view only and was classified as none, moderate, or severe. Moderate bone disease cases had one or more of the following: slight remodeling or lipping at the tip of the DP but no obvious bone loss, marginal rim fractures, or demineralization or divot on the distal, dorsal, and parietal surfaces. Significant bone disease had obvious bone loss approaching the terminal arch and shortening of the dorsal parietal surface (**Fig. 11**).

Cases with no bone disease and no signs of sinking or penetration had an 83% success rate after the procedure. Cases with moderate bone disease and no sinking or penetration had a 93% success rate. Cases with severe bone disease and no sinking or penetration had a 44% success rate. Cases with sinking had an 18% success rate. Cases with penetration into the sole (with no sinking or bone disease) had an 88% success rate.

The number of limbs involved or a differentiation between the front and hind limb had no effect on overall prognosis. Of all the successful cases, 13% returned to athletic use (4 of those were sinkers).

No cases with severe bone disease returned to athletic use. It is interesting that cases with moderate bone disease had a better success rate than the cases with no bone disease. A possible explanation for this success rate is that bone disease takes time to develop in the DP; at least 45 days are required, although osteomyelitis can cause bone loss much more quickly and therefore infers some degree of successful response to treatment to develop. Very unstable acute cases with a healthy DP (no bone disease) may have been euthanized before bone disease had a chance to develop.

The overall amount of rotation did not affect prognosis; even cases in which the DP had penetrated the sole did well as long as there was no severe bone disease or sinking.

The tenotomy procedure has the most success in cases that have a fairly healthy DP and in which mechanical failure is isolated to the toe regions. Although tenotomy may be helpful in rehabilitating acute sinker syndrome, those cases have an extremely poor prognosis regardless of the treatment. The 18% success rate for the tenotomy in sinker cases in our study does not reflect our entire sinker caseload. Many sinkers were euthanized without attempting treatment; however, 18% of the sinkers that were treated using a tenotomy as part of the treatment were a success.

For a tenotomy to be successful, several criteria must be met: proper case selection, timing of the procedure, realignment shoeing must be considered part of the tenotomy procedure, and finally, the limb needs to be used (handgrazing or small pen turnout if possible).

WHEN TO PERFORM A TENOTOMY

Timing of the procedure is critical. The procedure should be performed before the patient experiences advanced bone disease.

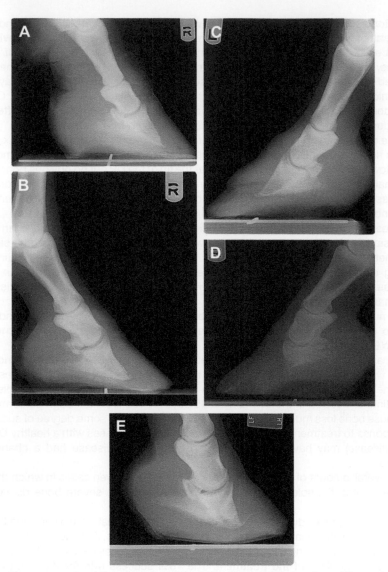

Fig. 11. Three examples. (*A*) A divot or notch at the distal parietal surface, (*B*) marginal rim fractures and remodeling, or (*C*) a change in the contour of the tip of the DP without any obvious bone loss are all signs of moderate bone disease. (*D, E*) Obvious bone loss with shortening of the dorsal surface of the DP is considered significant bone disease.

If the DP is severely compromised, it serves as a chronic source of pain. After surgery, these cases do not load and use the limb normally. They quickly heal with a contracted tenotomy site, and abundant scar tissue may form. These cases also tend to heal with a large amount of scar tissue and adhesions to the superficial digital flexor tendon and suspensory ligament. Over time, this tissue contracts, creating a combined superficial and DDFT contracture.

Another aspect of timing the tenotomy procedure is realizing that the goal is to return the limb to full weight bearing as soon after surgery as possible; therefore, it may be beneficial to treat infections or perform any necessary debridements sometime before the anticipated tenotomy. This may not be possible always, because most infections are secondary to tissue compression by the displaced DP and the tenotomy and realignment shoeing is often necessary to treat the infection.

After the tenotomy, I prefer to have the case hand walked or hand grazed or put into a small paddock to encourage loading of the limb. If the case remains on strict stall rest, with the horse resting the limb or lying down, the tenotomy site heals in a contracted position, and nothing is gained from the procedure. For this reason, I prefer to perform the tenotomy as soon as possible.

It is my opinion that many clinicians wait too long to perform the procedure, and as a result, the foot suffers irreparable damage. This is why the procedure receives a low rate of success in some studies. The chronic, uncompensated case should be regularly evaluated, and a judgment should be made before the secondary complications arise (osteomyelitis, coronary band shear lesions). If shoeing alone fails to rehabilitate the foot, surgery needs to be performed in a timely manner.

The most important aspect of the tenotomy procedure involves pre- and postsurgical management of the foot. Combining the surgery with the appropriate trim and shoeing is imperative for long-term success. Performing the transection without realignment shoeing offers only short-term clinical improvement and most likely does not affect the survival rate.

PRESERVATION OF THE CORONARY BAND

When the DP is severely displaced and the hoof capsule unstable, the coronary band is often internally compressed. The coronary cushion is compressed by the extensor process of the DP, and the coronary papillae become kinked or crimped; as a result, the coronary papillae produce hoof wall growth in an abnormal orientation. The hoof wall, which is normally produced in a proximal-to-distal orientation, is instead produced outward in ripples, creating abnormal wall growth; the wall later displays this abnormality as prominent growth rings or ridges.

In cases of coronary band compression, the coronary corium is still intact but hoof wall growth is just slowed in this region. If the displacement advances, the coronary band shears or separates because the soft tissue structures are further displaced beneath the fixed rigid hoof capsule. The area of separation is called a coronary band shear lesion.

Coronary band compression can occur anywhere in the toe in a rotational displacement or in the quarters if the foot is sinking medially, laterally, or vertically.

CORONARY BAND GROOVING

To preserve the coronary band and restore normal hoof wall growth, proper shoeing mechanics should first be implemented. In addition, the technique of coronary band grooving has proven to be a good adjunct treatment in this scenario.[20] This technique can preserve the coronary band from developing a shear lesion if addressed early and can speed up hoof wall growth in that region.

The hoof wall growth rings are a useful guide to determine which area to groove. Following the pattern of constricted growth rings, the hoof wall is grooved using a 0.25-in dremel, or the edge of a farrier rasp, at a point distal to the coronary groove; 0.75 in below the hairline is recommended (**Fig. 12**). The entire wall thickness is carefully grooved until small areas of hemorrhage are evident.

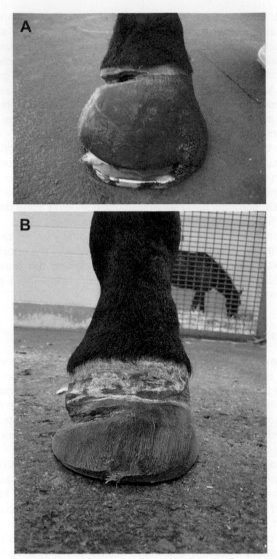

Fig. 12. (*A*) A hind foot with rotation and lateral sinking. The lateral coronary band has ceased growth and has a palpable ledge, but no shear lesion or separation. Subcoronary band grooving was used to restore normal growth and prevent separation. (*B*) Same foot 5 months later.

PROXIMAL HOOF WALL RESECTION

If the coronary band develops a shear lesion and significant compression, often the coronary band cannot regenerate because of severe pinching by the proximal hoof wall. When coronary band separation is followed by swelling and pain, a proximal hoof wall resection is required to regenerate the coronary band and ensure proper hoof wall growth.

The area resected should include all of hoof wall below the shear lesion and should taper off to a healthy coronary band at either end. The resected area should be about

0.5 to 1 in distal to the coronary band at its apex and taper off to a healthy coronary band at either end. A semielliptical shape is drawn on the hoof capsule to mark the area to be resected. A dremel, the edge of a farrier rasp, or cast cutters can be used to cut through the hoof wall. Then, using forceps, the transected piece of hoof is removed and the area firmly packed with antiseptic soaked gauze (**Fig. 13**).

The area should epithelialize within 10 to 14 days. True stratum medium hoof wall should be regenerated by the coronary band over the next few months. Failure of the tissue to epithelialize or continued impingement of the corium by the proximal aspect of the transected wall is an indication for further distal resection.

Topical products containing zinc may speed up epithelialization. Disinfected amniotic membrane as a wound dressing over the resection site has been shown to speed up epithelializaton.[21]

In many cases, the use of a foot cast is required if resections are needed in the quarter and heel regions. Immobilization of the hoof capsule and more uniform weight distribution by the cast may help stabilize the foot and encourage epithelialization.

MEDIAL OR LATERAL SINKING (DISPLACEMENT)

Depending on lower limb conformation, occasionally a laminitic foot sinks to either the medial or lateral side. Some of these cases are caused by the use of heel wedges to prevent rotation in the acute stage. Although wedging does decrease the rotational forces on the DP and thus the tension on the dorsal laminae, heel wedges shift the ground reaction force to the heels and put stress on the quarters. In this way, a strategy to decrease rotation may inadvertently cause sinking in the quarters.

Sinking is most accurately detected by palpation of the coronary band. A palpable cavitation or ledge is a sign of sinking. Radiographs typically show a soft tissue opacity or coronary halo in the region of the coronary band. Once medial or lateral sinking is

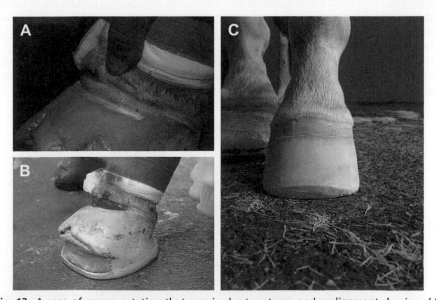

Fig. 13. A case of severe rotation that required a tenotomy and realignment shoeing. (*A*) The anterior coronary band was separated (shear lesion), creating swelling and pain on palpation. (*B*) A partial resection was performed to relieve the compression and restore normal growth. (*C*) Same foot 1 year later.

detected, the wedge should be removed and the horse placed flat into a soft rubber pad or boot. This technique allows the horse to mold the rubber pad into the most comfortable configuration and take stress off the compromised areas. Coronary grooving should also be implemented at this stage in the appropriate regions.

Sinking feet that do not respond to the aforementioned treatment are placed into a foot cast with a 0.5-in carpet felt or elastomer sole support placed on the sole surface. After the foot cast is set, I apply polymethyl methacrylate adhesive (Equilox) on the ground surface of the cast in a mild dome shape.[22] This method allows the foot to break over in all directions; it loads the axial regions of the foot and unloads the hoof wall perimeter (**Fig. 14**).

In cases in which the vertical displacement advances to shear lesions around the perimeter wall, the horse is usually euthanized. In some unilateral cases or special circumstances, complete hoof capsule ablation combined with a lower limb cast or transfixation pin cast has successfully rehabilitated some feet to reasonable pasture soundness.

After hoof capsule ablation or partial hoof wall resection, the hoof heals first through lamellar epithelialization. The duration of this process can vary from weeks to months depending on the amount of compression on the exposed area. The foot can take several months to begin generating hoof wall from the coronary band.

Dealing with infections while the foot is regenerating a hoof capsule can be challenging. The extent to which these feet can be rehabilitated is questionable. The laminar attachments are always compromised to some degree. For this reason, these cases must be intensely managed and monitored. Often, special footing, shoes, boots, and exercise restrictions are necessary for the remainder of the horse's life.

INFECTIONS IN THE FOUNDERED FOOT

Because of the chronic tissue damage and decreased perfusion to certain areas of the foot, tissue necrosis and infection are common sequelae in high-scale laminitis cases. Infections can vary from a gravel or seedy toe caused by the stretched white line to subsolar or submural abscesses or to osteomyelitis of the DP.

Formulating a mechanical plan using shoeing and/or surgery is a critical first step to alleviate compressed tissue and restore perfusion before any other treatment for infection can be effective. Most superficial infections are resolved with alleviation of

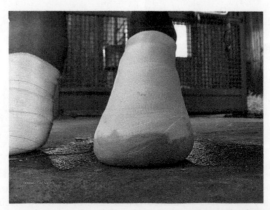

Fig. 14. A foot cast used to treat a sinker case. Sole support is placed on the sole. The bottom of the cast has a dome shape made from acrylic, to ease break over in all directions.

tissue compression and realignment of the DP. However, deeper infections are often more difficult to resolve. Methods to treat osteomyelitis of the DP include surgical debridement, regional limb perfusion, systemic antibiotic therapy, and larval therapy.[23,24]

I have had great success treating chronic infections with gentle surgical debridement followed by larval therapy and appropriate antibiotic therapy. Larval therapy uses disinfected maggots to debride necrotic tissue. This therapy has the advantage of removing only necrotic or infected tissue without structurally compromising the fragile foot. Larval therapy avoids removing adjacent healthy tissue as is sometimes done with surgical debridements (see the article by Morrison elsewhere in this issue for further exploration of this topic).

SUMMARY

Successful foot management of laminitis cases begins with understanding the differences in mechanics between the normal horse foot and the laminitic foot. Early and accurate diagnosis and evaluation of cases with pertinent images should place the case in a category, acute or chronic, so that a plan of action can begin immediately. Chronic cases need to be differentiated as compensated or uncompensated, and, as a result, a series of relevant and timely foot management practices, therapies, and minor surgeries can be used if the condition deteriorates. Monitoring the ways in which the DP might be displaced during the course of the treatment increases the chance for early intervention and a more successful outcome. It is always possible that a horse can recover from laminitis. It requires, above all, a dedicated and cooperative team, working together, throughout what is sure to be a challenging undertaking.

REFERENCES

1. Bowker R, Page B, Ovnicek G. Morphology of the hoof wall and foot of feral (wild) horses versus that of domestic horses. 12th Annual Bluegrass Laminitis Symposium. Louisville (KY), January 29–31, 1998. p. 65–72.
2. Hood D, Taylor D, Wagner I. Effects of ground surface deformability, trimming, and shoeing on quasistatic hoof loading patterns in horses. Am J Vet Res 2001;62(6):895–900.
3. Redden RF. Preventing laminitis in the contralateral limb of horses with non-weightbearing lameness. Clin Tech Equine Pract 2004;3:57–63.
4. Hood DM. Center of digital load during quasi-static loading. 12th Annual Bluegrass Laminitis Symposium. Louisville (KY), January 29–31, 1998. p. 47–62.
5. Barrey E. Investigation of the vertical hoof force distribution in the equine forelimb with an instrumented hoof boot. Equine Vet J 1990;9:35–8.
6. Hood DM. The mechanisms and consequences of structural failure of the foot. Vet Clin North Am Equine Pract 1999;15:437–61.
7. Willemen MA, Savelberg HH, Barneveld A. The effect of orthopaedic shoeing on the force exerted by the deep digital flexor tendon on the navicular bone in horses. Equine Vet J 1999;31:25–30.
8. Eliashar E, McGuigan MP, Wilson AM. Relationship of foot conformation and force applied to the navicular bone of sound horses at the trot. Equine Vet J 2004;36:431–5.
9. Pollitt CC, Van Eps AW. Prolonged, continuous distal limb cryotherapy in the horse. Equine Vet J 2004;36:216–20.

10. Thompson KN, Cheung TK, Silverman M. The effect of toe angle on tendon, ligament and hoof wall strains in vitro. J Equine Vet Sci 1993;13:651–3.
11. Collins S. Hoof loading and biomechanics. The 5th International Equine Conference On Laminitis and Diseases of the Foot. West Palm Beach (Fl), November 5–8, 2009. p. 72–9.
12. Steward ML. How to construct and apply atraumatic therapeutic shoes to treat acute or chronic laminitis in the horse. AAEP Proceedings, vol. 49. Lexington (KY); 2003. p. 337–46.
13. McGuigan MP, Walsh TC, Pardoe CH, et al. Deep digital flexor tendon force and digital mechanics in normal ponies and ponies with rotation of the distal phalanx as a sequel to laminitis. Equine Vet J 2005;37:161–5.
14. Wilson A, McGuigan P, Pardoe C. The biomechanical effect of wedged, eggbar, and extension shoes in sound and lame horses. AAEP Proceedings, vol. 47. Lexington (KY); 2001. p. 339–43.
15. Redden RF. A technique for performing digital venography in the standing horse. Equine Vet Educ 2001;3:172–8.
16. Redden RF. Shoeing the laminitic horse. In: Ric Redden, editor. Understanding laminitis. Lexington (KY): The Blood Horse Inc.; 1998. p. 60–79.
17. Allen D Jr, White NA 2nd, Foerner JF, et al. Surgical management of chronic laminitis in horses: 13 cases (1983–1985). J Am Vet Med Assoc 1986;189:1604–6.
18. Hunt RJ, Allen D, Baxter GM, et al. Mid-metacarpal deep digital flexor tenotomy in the management of refractory laminitis in horses. Vet Surg 1991;20:15–20.
19. Morrison SE. Deep digital flexor tenotomy and realignment shoeing for chronic laminitis. The Fifth International Equine Conference On Laminitis and Diseases of the Foot. West Palm Beach (Fl), November 5–8, 2009. p. 50–1.
20. Ritmeester AM, Ferguson DW. Coronary grooving promotes dorsal hoof wall growth in horses with chronic laminitis. AAEP Proceedings, vol. 47. Lexington (KY); 1996. p. 212.
21. Long CG, Schultz LA. How to use hoof-wall resection and amniotic membrane as a treatment for coronary-band prolapse. Proceedings of the 52nd Annual Convention of the American Association of Equine Practitioners; 2006. p. 501–4.
22. Morrison S. Foot management. Clin Tech Equine Pract 2004;3:71–82.
23. Morrison SE. How to utilize sterile maggot debridement therapy for infections in the horse. AAEP Proceedings. Lexington (KY); 2005. p. 51.
24. Sherman SA, Morrison SE, Ng D. Maggot debridement therapy for serious horse wounds - a survey of practitioners. Vet J 2007;174:86–91.

Maggot Debridement Therapy for Laminitis

Scott Morrison, DVM

KEYWORDS

• Maggot • Debridement • Chronic laminitis • Abscess
• MDT • Larval therapy

In the treatment of chronic foot infections, certain species of blowfly larvae have proved beneficial because they debride necrotic tissue, disinfect surrounding areas, and stimulate healing. Unlike surgical debridement, maggot debridement therapy (MDT) is a nontraumatic, minimally invasive method to treat infections in a foot compromised by laminitis.

Feet affected by chronic laminitis often develop tissue damage and infections secondary to distal phalanx displacement. This leads to compression and shearing of sensitive tissues. Additionally, compromised blood supply and damage to the protective hoof capsule barrier may contribute to the development of infections. Therefore, to adequately treat an infection of the horse's foot, a mechanical strategy must first be in place to address the instability of the distal phalanx and hoof capsule. Because tissues and their blood supply are compromised by the disease process, normal debridement and repair processes are hindered.

Larval therapy aids in the debridement and repair phase of wound healing. It is significantly more effective in débriding chronic pressure ulcers in humans when compared with more conservative and conventional treatments.[1] The salivary secretions of blowfly larvae contain proteolytic enzymes and disinfecting compounds that kill bacteria and break down necrotic tissue. Ultimately, these breakdown products are ingested by the larvae. Other compounds in salivary secretions have been shown to stimulate fibroblasts and promote granulation tissue.[2] It has been theorized that the physical movement of the larvae may also aid in the stimulation of granulation tissue.

Medical grade maggots are currently available for clinical use by human physicians and veterinarians. The green bottle fly (*Lucilia sericata*) is recognized as the blowfly species of choice for medicinal use. The eggs are disinfected, transferred to sterile vials, and shipped overnight for clinical use.[3] Newly hatched larvae should be used within 2 to 3 days and should be kept at room temperature if going to be used in this time frame. If the intended time of use is beyond 2 days, the larva should be refrigerated until the time of application. The recommended dose is 10 larvae per square centimeter of necrotic tissue.[4]

Rood & Riddle Equine Hospital, PO Box 12070, Lexington, KY 40580, USA
E-mail address: smorrison@roodandriddle.com

Vet Clin Equine 26 (2010) 447–450
doi:10.1016/j.cveq.2010.06.002
0749-0739/10/$ – see front matter © 2010 Published by Elsevier Inc.

vetequine.theclinics.com

The wound should be prepared by gently swabbing loose necrotic tissue and exudates from the wound and then lavaging with saline. If surgical debridement is required to remove a bone sequestrum, or a large area of necrotic tissue, then application of the larvae should be delayed until all bleeding has stopped. Removal of any grossly necrotic tissue from the treatment area, before application of the larvae, facilitates the debridement process. The larvae are removed from the vial with sterile gauze and gently applied to the wound site. An absorbent layer of gauze should be placed over the site, with gentle pressure, and then bandaged to the foot. To facilitate protection and ease of management, the larvae are often applied beneath a hospital/treatment plate or placed into a window cut into a foot cast (**Fig. 1**).[5] If a shoeing application requires a gluing process with an acrylic or urethane, it is recommended to wait at least 24 hours before applying the larvae to the wound. Often the vapors from the adhesives kill the newly hatched larvae.

The absorbent layer of gauze should be changed daily in extensive infections with copious exudates or at a minimum of every-other-day in less severe infections. As the larvae digest the necrotic tissue, they secrete an ammonia/urea compound that may aid in the disinfection of surrounding tissue. Excessive accumulation of this compound can be slightly irritating to sensitive tissue, however. An application of sterile maggots usually lasts 5 to 7 days in a wound before the larvae become satiated and fully grown. At this time, the mature maggots are lavaged from the wound and replaced with fresh batches as needed.

Infections associated with certain bacteria are difficult to manage with larval therapy. In these instances, the maggots have not prospered. The bacteria most commonly associated with this occurrence are *Proteus* and *Escherichia coli* infections. *Proteus* is a bacterium normally found in the gut of maggot larvae and may be resistant to the larval secretions. In these instances I have found that soaking the foot in a chlorine dioxide or oxychlorosene solution before application of the larvae promotes a more livable environment for the maggots and increases their chances of thriving. Maggots, however, also fail to thrive in wounds with copious amounts of drainage and may require several days of lavaging/soaking before the successful application of larvae.

Adverse reactions to MDT are uncommon[6] and the only side effect observed has been irritation or hypersensitivity at the site. These infrequent cases show discomfort

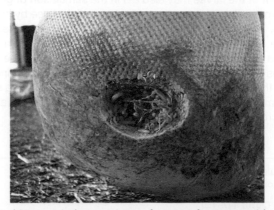

Fig. 1. Larvae placed into a window cut into a foot cast for a case with sinking and infections in the medial quarter.

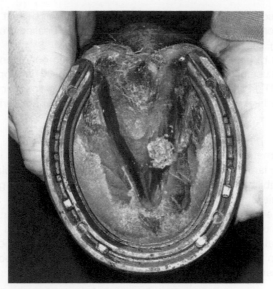

Fig. 2. Larval therapy in a chronic draining tract at apex of frog.

by stomping the limb or rubbing the bandage. To prevent contamination and secondary infection it is important to use sterile medical grade larvae. Spread of infection is possible if the larvae are handled inappropriately or nondisinfected larvae are used. The larvae used for debridement therapy are selected because they are noninvasive. Myiasis or tissue invasion is a potential complication if invasive fly species are used.

There seems to be no effect on the viability of the larvae if MDT is combined with other treatments, such as systemic antibiotic injections, regional limb perfusion with antibiotics, or soaking the feet in disinfectants before application (eg, dilute betadine or chorine dioxide).

MDT has been shown a safe and effective method to help treat various foot infections in the horse (**Fig. 2**).[5,6]

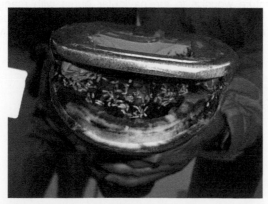

Fig. 3. MDT in the toe region of a horse with exposed sole corium. This case showed a deep digital flexor tenotomy and realignment shoeing.

Chronic laminitic cases of sepsis/necrosis within the hoof benefit from this procedure due to the noninvasive, continuous debridement and healing properties provided by the larvae (**Fig. 3**).

In those cases of high risk of developing severe septic conditions, application of maggots may be useful before massive necrosis develops. The prophylactic or early application of MDT, in cases of severe distal phalanx displacement or even solar penetration, is an effective way to prevent the establishment of more serious infections.

SUMMARY

MDT is a nontraumatic, minimally invasive method to treat infections in a foot compromised by chronic laminitis. A mechanical strategy must first be in place, however, to address the instability of the distal phalanx and hoof capsule. The green bottle fly is the blowfly species of choice for veterinary use. Larvae may be applied beneath a hospital/treatment plate or placed into a window cut into a foot cast. Adverse reactions to MDT are uncommon and the only side effect observed has been irritation or hypersensitivity at the site. Chronic laminitic cases of sepsis/necrosis within the hoof benefit from this procedure due to the noninvasive, continuous debridement and healing properties provided by the larvae.

REFERENCES

1. Sherman RA. Maggot versus conservative debridement therapy for the treatment of pressure ulcers. Wound Repair Regen 2002;10:208–14.
2. Horobin AJ, Shakesheff KM, Pritchard DI. Maggots and wound healing: an investigation of the effects of secretions from *Lucilia sericata* larvae upon the migration of human dermal fibroblasts over a fibronectin-coated surface. Wound Repair Regen 2005;13:422–33.
3. Sherman RA, Wyle FA. Low-cost, low-maintenance rearing of maggots in hospitals, clinics, and schools. Am J Trop Med Hyg 1996;54:38–41.
4. Sherman RA, Morrison S, Ng D. Maggot debridement therapy for serious horse wounds—a survey of practitioners. Vet J 2007;174:86–91.
5. Morrison SE. How to use sterile maggot debridement therapy for foot infections of the horse. Proceedings of the Annual Convention of the American Association Equine Practitioners. Seattle (WA): AAEP; 2005. p. 461–7.
6. Bras RJ, Morrison SE. Retrospective case series of 20 horses (2002–2009) sustaining puncture wounds to the navicular bursa with maggot debridement therapy as an adjunctive treatment. Proceedings of the Annual Convention of the American Association Equine Practitioners. Las Vegas (NV): AAEP; 2009. p. 241–50.

First Aid for the Laminitic Foot: Therapeutic and Mechanical Support

Patrick T. Reilly[a],*, Emily K. Dean, DVM[b], James A. Orsini, DVM[a]

KEYWORDS

- Laminitis • Orthotics • Impression material • Glue-on shoes

The treatment of Laminitis is probably more varied than of any other disease, and yet a large number of cases recover for even the poorest practitioner
  A.A. Holcombe, D.V.S. (US Department of Agriculture Special Report on Diseases of the Horse 1916 Pearson, Mitchner and colleagues, Washington, DC)

The first opportunity to mechanically treat the feet of a laminitic horse is generally in the acute phase. In the time frame of laminitis development, the acute phase is identified as the onset of clinical signs such as the onset of pain, elevated digital pulses, and adoption of the characteristic laminitic stance and gait. The acute phase continues until lamellar inflammation resolves and enters a subacute phase, the best outcome, or until the distal phalanx displaces downwards, relative to the hoof capsule. This displacement marks the beginning of the chronic phase of the disease.[1] The goals of mechanical treatment during the acute phase are to preserve the lamellar interface by reducing the forces that are compromising its integrity and to make the horse more comfortable.

At the turn of the twentieth century, many veterinarians were educated in horseshoeing, and this training exposed them to various methods of supporting the hoof. However, veterinary teaching hospitals, including the University of Pennsylvania, discontinued this hands-on approach to equine foot care in favor of a theoretic approach to education. Thus, the hands-on method of dealing with supportive hoof problems was removed from the veterinary curriculum. Addressing the immediate emergency needs of the horse with acute laminitis is one of the few instances during which a veterinarian of today is expected to apply a protective orthotic device to its foot. This instance, along with the sometimes-idiopathic presentation of laminitis, makes the decision-making process difficult.

[a] University of Pennsylvania, School of Veterinary Medicine, New Bolton Center, 382 West Street Road, Kennett Square, PA 19348, USA
[b] C.B. Miller and Associates, 39 Fields Lane, North Salem, NY 10560, USA
* Corresponding author.
E-mail address: reillypa@vet.upenn.edu

Vet Clin Equine 26 (2010) 451–458
doi:10.1016/j.cveq.2010.06.004
0749-0739/10/$ – see front matter © 2010 Elsevier Inc. All rights reserved.

vetequine.theclinics.com

There are an extraordinary number of variables to consider when confronted with an acute laminitic patient: (1) the cause and severity of the disease, (2) the breed and use of the horse, and (3) the environment and the financial limitations of the owners. Complicating this is a lack of evidence-based research on supportive orthotics for the horse. Considering that laminitis is the second leading cause of death in horses and the frequency of facing the management decisions (laminitis affects 2.1% of the horse population annually[2]), the importance of early decision making in managing these cases becomes apparent. Decisions are frequently based on anecdotal experience and information.

The following sections help the practitioner identify some of the commonly used and accepted methods of protecting the laminitic foot. The available materials and the theories behind their use are also presented.

SUPPORTING THE HOOF

A review of the scientific literature on the topic of supporting the laminitic digit reveals part of the problem. The practitioner has to decide on a course of treatment for the horse in the acute phase of laminitis, relying on literature that is either anecdotal or experiential in nature. Although practitioner experience is not to be discounted, the certainty of the comments made should be placed in context. The following passage recounts the cure for laminitis:

> "....if we only pull out the Sole and do not cut part of the hoof off also. This is not my bare opinion, but the experience of those who have had good success in curing foundered horses, who by rasping the hoof from the coronet to the very bottom in five or six places until they have made the blood come; and then applied their remedies to those places have made the horses sound, whom the drawing out the sole would not cure." The remedies are described as "mixing pitch and tar together with a sufficient quantity of hog's lard pouring the mixture boiling hot upon the sole and stuffing it up very carefully with Hurds and above them a piece of leather with splints."
> —The New Farrier's Guide 1721 W.Gibson p. 291–292.

The treatment methods used by the practitioners of the 1700s are obviously very different in nature from those methods used by "those having good success in curing foundered horses" today. However, anecdotal evidence is still relied on, and it is possible that today's methods will seem equally archaic to future clinicians.

Further complicating the discussions of studies critically assessing support for the equine digit during laminitis is that many of the evaluations are conducted on normal horses or cadaver specimens. The hypothesis that both laminitic and nonlaminitic feet respond to external forces in a similar manner is misleading. For example, some in vitro studies have recorded compressive radial strain forces in the region of the stratum internum in the diseased foot, whereas tensile forces were observed in the normal foot. This difference underscores the need to understand the laminitic foot before determining the methods for its support.

THE PHYSICAL EXAMINATION

Most of the treatment options available to the clinician involve shifting the weight-bearing forces from compromised areas of the foot (ie, the lamellar interface) to areas more capable of supporting the patient's weight, remembering that the sum of the forces should remain the same. These areas should be identified for each foot by physical examination of the horse, observation of the gait, and hoof tester or digital pressure sensitivity.

GOALS OF MECHANICAL SUPPORT

- Provide axial support to unload the diseased laminae.
- Reduce the lever forces on the laminar interface.
- Change the mechanical forces on the foot in the dorsal/palmar plane to reduce the pull of the deep digital flexor tendon (DDFT) on the distal phalanx.

There are several good options available to the equine practitioner to assist in meeting these basic mechanical goals. Advances in new materials make this a minimally invasive, cost-effective, and practical approach, in an ambulatory setting. Each of the treatment options has advantages and disadvantages, with little scientific evidence to support one method over the other.

TO SHOE, OR NOT TO SHOE?

One of the first decisions to be made in managing an acute laminitis case is the decision whether to remove or leave the shoes on the horse. There are many variables to consider in the latter decision, particularly the appropriateness of the shoes. Shoes with toe grabs or traction devices intuitively would seem to mechanically compromise the foot, as might a similar shoe at the end of its shoeing cycle. Alternatively, many normal horses accustomed to wearing shoes might become foot sore without their shoes, and this might further compromise an acute laminitic patient.

Every change or adjustment made to the foot has the potential to produce both positive and negative mechanical results. Therefore, the clinical approach has to be individualized to the patient with the treatment objectives clear in mind.

FOAM PADS

The use of foam pads, taped to the feet, gained attention in the 1980s as a quick and easy method to support the diseased hoof. This protocol was originally described by Mathew Frederick and marketed by a farrier, Gene Ovnicek as part of the Equine Digital Support System. Alternatively, many practitioners use a 1.5-in foam insulation purchased from a hardware or building materials store. This foam is easily cut with a narrow blade and fits most hoof shapes. The process of applying the foam pads is simple, with one caveat being the thicker the pad the greater the chance for slippage between the foot and pad, especially as the foam compresses. The literature recommends removal of horseshoes before foam pad application; however, many clinicians find that by leaving the shoes on, there is reduced slippage of the foam pad.

Theoretically, expanded polystyrene pads (styrofoam material), being easily compressible, should result in a reduction in laminar forces on the digits. This is because the collapsing foam reduces the abaxial levers that occur during movement and thus preserve the dermal-epidermal bond. Furthermore, as the pad conforms to the entire foot, the sole, frog, and bars become part of the weight-bearing surface of the foot resulting in distribution of the horse's bodyweight over a larger surface area.

The inexpensive cost and ease of application are advantages of expanded polystyrene pads. However, the ease of mechanical deformation is also a limiting factor. When used in larger breed horses, the pads can collapse in less than 24 hours, requiring regular replacement. When using the foam pads for laminitis, some protocols recommend removing the dorsal portion of the compressed pad, adding the remainder to a new pad, and reapplying the combination to the horse's foot.

Although open-cell foams, such as expanded polystyrene, are effective for short periods, closed-cell foams provide similar effects but last much longer. Many common items, such as wrestling and horse trailer mats and gardening knee pads, can be easily cut into hoof-shaped pads and applied to the foot.

LILY PADS

Named by its developer Ric Redden because "every frog needs a lily pad," they were designed for emergency support. Made from urethane and trimmed so as to not extend beyond the apex of the frog, they are taped to the hoof. The Lily Pad can also serve as a palmar/plantar extension and as a mild heel wedge (Lily Pad, Nanric Inc, Lawrenceburg, KY, USA; www.nanric.com). Although easy to apply, the specific effect of the Lily Pad on the mechanics of the foot varies depending on the shape of the foot and the presence or absence of shoes.

MODIFIED ULTIMATE CUFF

This cufflike orthotic is available in 5 different sizes and fits most nondraft breeds. It can be taped or glued to the hoof. Silicone impression material is generally applied to the palmar/plantar sole. Attached to the cuff is a 20° heel elevation. This helps unload the DDFT and transfers weight to the palmar/plantar half of the foot. The directions suggest that the ideal angle of the coffin bone is 20° relative to the ground surface (Nanric Ultimate, Nanric Inc, Lawrenceburg, KY, USA; www.nanric.com). By using adjustable wedges, the degree of heel elevation can be modified. In normal feet, heel elevation is believed to benefit dorsal laminar blood circulation. However, the effect on circulation in the laminitic foot remains to be critically evaluated.

IMPRESSION MATERIAL

The use of silicone-based polymeric putty is one of the most popular methods for sole support in the laminitic horse. First introduced by a farrier, Rob Sigafoos, these materials are commonly used in the dental industry to create molds and are referred to as dental impression materials. There are several varieties commercially available in the equine industry, and they range in base metal composition (platinum or tin) and in their physical properties. Impression materials are generally mixed in a 1:1 ratio by volume but differ in time from mixing to polymerization (range 2–10 minutes). The firmness of the final product is usually measured on the A-Shore scale, varying from 25 (the approximate hardness of a rubber band) to 75 (the hardness of a tire tread). Under loads, these silicone polymers tend to absorb force in a linear fashion.

The general principle is to custom fit axial support to the foot. The surface area for weight bearing is increased by using the frog, sole, and the lamellar attachments of the bars. Impression material can be applied with or without shoes and can be taped in place.

In the authors' experience, impression material affords a flexible, simple, and consistent support for the foot. The following mechanical support protocol is routinely used in horses at the George D. Widener Hospital at New Bolton Center (**Fig. 1**).

If the horse presents with acceptable shoes, the foot is cleaned off loose debris. The silicone impression material components are mixed until uniform in color and applied to the solar surface of the hoof, extending beyond the surface of the horseshoe.

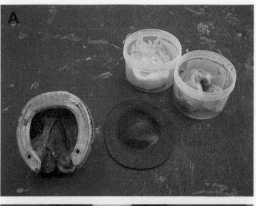

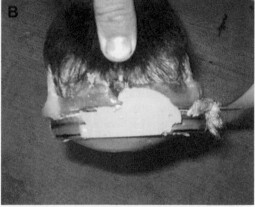

Fig. 1. (*A*) A 2-part silicone impression material and a rigid convex plate that are fabricated to size. An alternative is 1/8 in acrylonitrile butadiene styrene plastic that is heat molded with a butane torch. (*B*) The foot with impression material in place between the sole and the convex domed sole plate.

1. The impression material, in the prepolymerized state, is taped in place over the shoe. In a deep concave shoe, tape is not always needed because the polymerized pad interlocks with the shoe and is held in place.
2. The convex plate is positioned over the silicone and lightly taped or stretch wrapped in position.
3. The foot is allowed to weight bear until the silicone has polymerized approximating 5 minutes, depending on the individual properties of the material used.
4. Once the silicone is fully set, the outer tape and convex plate are removed, and the patient is evaluated for comfort.

HEART BAR SHOES

Heart bar shoes are commonly used in the treatment of the horse with laminitis. Amongst users, the concept is similar but methodologies vary. Basically, a plate covers the frog to support the distal phalanx. In addition, the solar corium is only minimally impacted, and therefore the circulation of the digit is preserved. The bar, being entirely located within the dimensions of the frog, allows varying amounts of pressure to be applied, depending on the clinicians preference.

The effectiveness of the heart bar shoe, in preventing displacement of the distal phalanx, is continually debated. In one trial, low pressures (<1300 N) on the frog created palmar displacement of the distal phalanx. However, higher loads did not affect the position of the bone within the hoof wall.[3] In another study, using an open toe shoe with a caudal plate reduced the compressive strain on the dorsal hoof wall by 23% when compared with a similar foot without a shoe.[4]

GLUE-ON SHOES

The use of polymer adhered horseshoes represents a major advance in the application of horseshoes. Glue-on shoes offer distinct advantages over mechanically attached shoes. The need to pound on feet that are inflamed and painful seems intuitively counterproductive. Thus, in laminitic patients, the atraumatic application of glue-on shoes is being used with increasing frequency. There are 2 categories of glue-on shoes:

1. Direct, the shoe is bonded directly to the hoof wall with adhesives.
2. Indirect, an intermediary attachment system (fabric or urethane cuffs) bonds the shoe to the hoof.

The most commonly used adhesives such as polymethyl/cyclohexyl methacrylate and urethanes react exothermically; the total energy released depends on the quantity and thickness of the repair. The choice of adhesive varies depending on the product and application required.

The variety of advanced glue-on shoes now equals nail-on horseshoes. The materials used for glue-on shoes, in general, require a greater financial investment than other options.

CLOGS

The clog was first introduced by Michael Steward, a veterinarian in Oklahoma.[5] Originally fabricated from plywood, the thick clog reduced the mechanical forces associated with hoof wall breakover while maintaining the integrity of the hoof; modifications are easily made to the clog itself. To reduce sole pressure under the distal margin of a displaced distal phalanx, the clinician removes material and creates a concavity corresponding to the margin of the distal phalanx in the surface of the shoe. Silicone impression material is commonly incorporated to support the palmar/plantar hoof.

The original design was attached using screws placed through the hoof wall at the heels. The clog can also be attached to the hoof using adhesives and fiberglass casts.

FOOT CASTS

Foot casts, using materials commonly found in a veterinarian's ambulatory vehicle, are used to stabilize the hoof. One procedure, described by Huskamp,[6] uses 2 rolls of plaster cast material and a heel elevation. The first roll is positioned approximately 2 cm palmar to the apex of the frog and is molded to fit the frog, lateral sulci, and bars, creating a 15° to 20° wedge. The second roll is applied circumferentially and secures the wedge to the sole of the hoof. The wedge moves the quarter and frog compression forces in a palmar/plantar direction, relative to the center of rotation of the distal interphalangeal joint. The technique aims to reduce the pull of DDFT on the distal phalanx and ultimately the dorsal hoof wall. Strain gauges on the surface of the hoof showed that the longitudinal compressive strain on the dorsal hoof wall was reduced by 60%. Strain on the DDFT was also reduced, and loading was transferred to the quarters.[7] Commercially available casting materials (plaster of Paris and fiberglass) can be used, and impression material and clogs can be incorporated into the cast.

REDUCING THE WEIGHT OF THE HORSE

In the treatment options previously discussed, the total body weight of the horse remains unchanged, and therefore the effect on the feet is similar. One of the real goals in managing the acutely laminitic patient is to reduce the tension on the lamellar interface. Several methods have been described to achieve this goal: a horse can be (1) suspended in a sling, (2) floated in water, or (3) fitted with weight-reducing orthotics. Each case has to be assessed individually with consideration given to the severity of the clinical signs and temperament of the patient. All the methods have potential drawbacks that must be individualized to the specific patient to minimize complications. Furthermore, these modalities are time consuming, labor intensive, and expensive. Length of treatment and financial constraints cannot be ignored, especially as the case moves into the chronic phase of laminitis.

BEDDING/CONFINEMENT

The application of an orthotic device is important to the mechanics of the laminitic foot, but equally important is the quality of the surface on which the horse has to stand. Stabling the acute laminitic horse on deep sand is advocated for many of the mechanical reasons already discussed. Providing a variable surface that can contour to the horse's foot and provide comfort is the goal. Deep bedding, using shavings at least 6-in deep, is advocated and is also used as an enticement for the horse to lie down. In one case, using an instrumented horseshoe on a laminitic horse, the peak forces on the hoof were recorded to be reduced by 25% in deep shavings as compared with a firm, unyielding surface. Reducing activity levels is beneficial because it lessens the forces on the compromised interface between the laminae of the hoof capsule and the distal phalanx.

SUMMARY

The acute laminitic patient must be closely monitored for increasing discomfort, metabolic derangement, and ongoing displacement of the distal phalanx, which are signs that indicate a progression of the disease. Mechanical support, medical treatments, and environmental management affect the outcome. Serial digital radiographs combined with clinical monitoring are important to better transform the treatment course of these acute care patients.

The many options presented in this article allow for flexibility and effective management of the acute laminitic patient and permit each modality to be combined in infinite ways for hoof support. For instance, impression materials alone can be used to support the foot, foam pads combined with impression material can support the palmar/plantar hoof, and impression material can be combined with a foot cast. These are just a few examples that are available to the attending clinician. There is no right or wrong answer to the question "how do I manage the acute laminitis patient?" If one modality is ineffective, it can be changed, combined with another, or removed altogether. The goal remains the same—support the foot and stop the progression of the disease to the chronic phase.

REFERENCES

1. Hood DM. Laminitis in the horse. Vet Clin North Am Equine Pract 1999;15:287–94.
2. USDA. Lameness and laminitis in U.S. horses. Fort Collins (CO): USDA: APHIS: VS, CEAH, National Animal Health Monitoring System; 2000.
3. Olivier A, Wannenburg J, Gottschalk RD, et al. The effect of frog pressure and downward vertical load on hoof wall weight-bearing and third phalanx displacement in the horse—an in vitro study. J S Afr Vet Assoc 2001;72(4):217–27.
4. Hobbs SJ, Mather J, Rolph C, et al. In vitro measurement of internal hoof strain. Equine Vet J 2004;36(8):683–8.
5. Steward ML. How to construct and apply atraumatic therapeutic shoes to treat acute or chronic laminitis in the horse. In: American Association of Equine Practitioners 49th Annual Convention, 2003. p. 337–46.
6. Huskamp B. Anmerkungen zur orthopä dischen Behandlung der Hufrehe. Pferdeheilkunde 1990;6:3–9 [in German].
7. Hansen N, Buchner HH, Haller J, et al. Evaluation using hoof wall strain gauges of a therapeutic shoe and a hoof cast with a heel wedge as potential supportive therapy for horses with laminitis. Vet Surg 2005;34(6):630–6.

Index

Note: Page numbers of article titles are in **boldface** type.

A

Acute founder
  defined, 392
  prognosis of, factors influencing, 401
Acute inflammatory laminitis, chronology and severity score in, 353–354
Adrenocorticotropic hormone, for endocrinopathic laminitis in horses and ponies, 380
Analgesia/analgesics
  conventional, for chronic laminitis, 322–327
  nonconventional, for chronic laminitis, 327
Anesthesia/anesthetics, for chronic laminitis, 328–329
Anti-inflammatory drugs, nonsteroidal, for chronic laminitis, 323–324
Apoptotic effects, in glucocorticoid-associated laminitis, 280
Artifact(s), digital venography and, 345–346

B

Bedding/confinement, in chronic laminitis management, 457

C

Calcium channel $\alpha_2\delta$-ligands, for chronic laminitis, 327–328
Carbohydrate(s), nonstructural, factors affecting content in grass, 361–365. See also
  Nonstructural carbohydrates (NSCs), factors affecting content in grass.
Cast(s), foot
  farriery for, 421
  in chronic laminitis management, 456–457
Catabolic effects, in glucocorticoid-associated laminitis, 280–281
Chromium, in reducing risk for endocrinopathic laminitis, 374
Chronic laminitis
  clinical evaluation of, 410
  described, 407–408
  evaluation of, 426
  farriery for, **407–423**
    follow-up, 419
    for casts, 421
    for mediolateral rotation of distal phalanx, 420–421
    general principles for, 415–417
    in surgical treatment, 421–423
    in treatment failure, 423
    shoes, 414–415
      types of, 417–418
    trim, 413–414

Vet Clin Equine 26 (2010) 459–466
doi:10.1016/S0749-0739(10)00061-1
0749-0739/10/$ – see front matter © 2010 Elsevier Inc. All rights reserved.

Moving?

Make sure your subscription moves with you!

To notify us of your new address, find your **Clinics Account Number** (located on your mailing label above your name), and contact customer service at:

Email: journalscustomerservice-usa@elsevier.com

800-654-2452 (subscribers in the U.S. & Canada)
314-447-8871 (subscribers outside of the U.S. & Canada)

Fax number: 314-447-8029

Elsevier Health Sciences Division
Subscription Customer Service
3251 Riverport Lane
Maryland Heights, MO 63043

*To ensure uninterrupted delivery of your subscription, please notify us at least 4 weeks in advance of move.

Printed and bound by CPI Group (UK) Ltd, Croydon, CR0 4YY

03/10/2024

01040454-0006